Gerontological Nursing

Current Practice and Research

Gerontological Nursing

Current Practice and Research

Virginia Burggraf, RN, C, MSN
Washington, DC

Richard Barry, MDiv, MLS
Washington, DC

SLACK Incorporated, 6900 Grove Road, Thorofare, NJ 08086-9447

Publisher: John H. Bond
Acquisitions Editor: Amy E. Drummond
Associate Editor: Jennifer J. Cahill
Art Director: Linda Baker

Gerontological nursing: current practice and research/[edited] by Virginia Burggraf, Richard Barry.
p. cm.
Includes bibliographical references and index.
ISBN 1-55642-284-9 (alk. paper)
1. Geriatric nursing. 2. Aged—Diseases—Prevention. I. Burggraf, Virginia. II. Barry, Richard.
[DNLM: 1. Geriatric Nursing—methods. 2. Health Promotion—United States. 3. Nursing Research. WY 152 G37715 1996]
RC954.G475 1996
610.73'65—dc20
DNLM/DLC
for Library of Congress 96-16712

Some material contained in this book has been revised from articles published in the *Journal of Gerontological Nursing*. The chapters have been adapted, revised, and expanded for the purpose of this book.

Printed in the United States of America

Published by: SLACK Incorporated
6900 Grove Road
Thorofare, NJ 08086-9447 USA
Telephone: 609-848-1000
Fax: 609-853-5991

Contact SLACK Incorporated for more information about other books in this field or about the availability of our books from distributors outside the United States.

Last digit is print number: 10 9 8 7 6 5 4 3 2 1

DEDICATION

This book is dedicated to our parents,
Phyllis and Angelo Bottone and Agnes and Jack Barry.
They were our first teachers and caregivers, inspiring us to
succeed and always to care about others.

CONTENTS

ACKNOWLEDGMENTS

A wonderful sense of humor and an ease about working together sustained us during these many months. Many individuals assisted with graphics, converting disks, and our initial mailing and solicitation of authors. Thanks to Ken Kauffman, Frank Pretlow, and Robbi Kimball, respectfully. Conference calls with John Bond and Jennifer Cahill assured us that this book was indeed a team effort. Special thank you to all our expert authors who provided us with high quality manuscripts within a few months. Numerous gerontological nurses were surveyed to develop a future perspective, to them we are very grateful. Lastly, to you the reader and caregiver of older persons, thank you for believing in us. We have a personal interest in the provision of high quality care to older persons; when our time arrives, we will know that we had a stake in the provision of that care. Our focus from the inception of this text has been the clinician and patient to assist your practice and the research spawned by the ideas presented.

CONTRIBUTING AUTHORS

Dolores M. Alford, PhD, RN, FAAN
Dallas, Texas

Nagia S. Ali, PhD, RN
Muncie, Indiana

Loretta J. Aller, RN, MSN
Kent, Ohio

Richard Barry, MDiv, MLS
Washington, DC

Lisa Begg, DrPH, FAAN
Pittsburgh, Pennsylvania

Brenda Bergman-Evans, PhD, RN, CS
Omaha, Nebraska

Nancy Bergstrom PhD, RN, FAAN
Omaha, Nebraska

Ann Blaylock, RN, CS, MNSc
North Little Rock, Arkansas

Mary Bliesmer, DNSc, RN, GNP-C
Mankato, Minnesota

Rebecca Brady, BSN, RNC, CNA
Cleveland, Ohio

Virginia Burggraf, RN, C, MSN
Washington, DC

Frances Kathleen Bushnell, RNC, EdD, MPH
Nashville, Tennessee

Carolyn L. Cason, RN, PhD
Little Rock, Arkansas

Francis R. Chester, MPA, RN, CPQA
Cleveland, Ohio

Darlene Clark, RN, MS
University Park, Pennsylvania

Vicki S. Conn, PhD, RN
Columbia, Missouri

Janet Cuddigan, PhC, RN
Omaha, Nebraska

Cheryl Dellasega, GNP, PhD
University Park, Pennsylvania

Margaret Dimond, PhD, RN, FAAN
Seattle, Washington

Maggie Donius, RN, MN
Mt. Angel, Oregon

Marge Drugay, ND, RN, C
Glenview, Illinois

Pat Earle, MS, RN
Mankato, Minnesota

Diane Feeney Mahoney, PhD, RN, CS, GNP
Boston, Massachusetts

Marlene Frost, PhD, RN
Rochester, Minnesota

Carla Groh, PhD, RN, CS
Detroit, Michigan

Jennifer Hayden Merritt, MSN, RN, CDE
Ann Arbor, Michigan

Amy Helmuth, RN, MS
Harrisburg, Pennsylvania

Diane M. Holt, RN, MS, CS, GNP
Madison, Wisconsin

Donald J. Joyce, OMI, MLS, MDiv
Washington, DC

Janet Kwaiser Kuhn, EdD, RN
Villanova, Pennsylvania

Evelyn Lancaster, RN, BSN, PHN
San Diego, California

Deborah Lekan-Rutledge, MSN, RNC, CCCN
Chapel Hill, North Carolina

Susan K. Madson, RNC, MSN
Raleigh, North Carolina

Delores McCreary, RN, MS
Altoona, Pennsylvania

Marycarol McGovern, PhD, RN
Villanova, Pennsylvania

Rebecca Miller, MS, RN
Springfield, Missouri

Martha Mitchell Funnell, MS, RN, CDE
Ann Arbor, Michigan

Joye A. Norris, EdD
Raleigh, North Carolina

Linda L. Pierce, MSN, RNC, CRRN
Cleveland, Ohio

Henry M. Plawecki, RN, PhD
Hammond, Indiana

Judith A. Plawecki, RN, PhD
Hammond, Indiana

Joanne Rader, RN, MN, FAAN
Portland, Oregon

Rosanne Radziewicz, MSN, RN, CS
Cleveland, Ohio

Judith P. Salter, MSN, RN, CRRN
Cleveland, Ohio

Judith S. Schainen, RN, CS, PhD
Seattle, Washington

Patricia Schan, RN, MS
Hershey, Pennsylvania

Sharon Schreck, RN
Cleveland, Ohio

Sue G. Taylor, PhD, RN, FAAN
Columbia, Missouri

Johannah Topps Uriri, MNSc, RNP, CS
Little Rock, Arkansas

Harriet Van Ess Coeling, PhD, RN
Kent, Ohio

Ann L. Whall, PhD, RN, FAAN
Ann Arbor, Michigan

Joyce White, DrPH, CRNP
Pittsburgh, Pennsylvania

Nancy Wieler Fishman, RN, MPH
Pittsburgh, Pennsylvania

Karen Willette, MS, RN
Mankato, Minnesota

Winifred WindRiver, RN, MSN
Pelham, Massachusetts

Rozanne Winger, PhD, RNP, C
Little Rock, Arkansas

PREFACE

The genesis for this text commences with a unique partnership between research and practice. Professionally working together, a gerontological nurse grant writer and a medical librarian collaborated frequently on gerontological issues needing in-depth research into clinical topics. The meshing of these professional skills has ensured the successful application and awarding of many grants to support the clinical practice of nurses. Our collective vision is to apply our talents to write a text that would provide gerontological nurses with current information in the areas of research and practice.

Analysis and reflection upon resources, medical and technological advances, the information explosion, as well as demographic realities of the aging population, hasten the necessity for up-to-date data/information and research findings. The current status of this text is reflected in the fact that this effort has taken approximately 18 months from inception to publication. This was our original vision which could only become a reality with the support of SLACK Incorporated, as well as the gifted authors who all consented to share their expertise.

The Healthy People 2000: National Health Promotion and Disease Prevention Objectives, specific to the elderly, provided the selection criteria for inclusion in this compendium. The Objectives list three goals to be achieved by the year 2000:

1. Increase the span of healthy life for Americans.
2. Reduce health disparitics among Americans.
3. Achieve access to preventive services for all Americans.

We concentrated solely on the objectives specific to the elderly.

HEALTH STATUS

Reduce:

- Suicide among white males
- Death by motor vehicle accidents (age 70+)
- Death from falls and fall-related injury particularly in ages 85+
- Death from residential fire
- Number of persons who have difficulty performing two or more personal care activities so as to enhance independence
- Significant visual impairment
- Epidemic related pneumonia and influenza deaths
- Pneumonia-related days of restricted activity

Increase:

- Years of healthy life to at least 65 among Blacks and Hispanics

RISK REDUCTION

Increase:

- Percentage of individuals who regularly participate in light to moderate activity for at least 30 minutes a day
- Immunization levels for pneumococcal influenza among the chronically ill older population
- The percentage of older persons who receive, within appropriate intervals, screening and immunization services at least one counseling service.

SERVICES AND PROTECTION

INCREASE:

- Percentage of recipients of home food service
- Percentage of older adults who have the opportunity to participate yearly in at least one organized health promotion program through senior centers, life care facility, or community-based setting serving the older adult
- Percentage of states in the United States that have design standards for signs, signals, marking, lighting, and other roadway environmental improvements to enhance visual stimuli and protect the safety of older drivers and pedestrians
- The proportion of primary care providers who routinely review with their patient prescribed and over-the-counter medications each time a new medication is prescribed
- The usage of the oral care system
- The proportion who receive clinical breast examinations and mammograms
- The number of women age 70+ with uterine cervix who receive Pap tests

EXTEND:

- Long-term institutional facilities, the requirement of oral examinations, and service provided to new admissions no later than 90 days after entering a facility

As comprehensive as one attempts to be, there are always some gaps. Page constraints and our intention to be timely with this initial presentation led us to limit the number of Objectives to be covered. As nurses become more familiar with the health promotion/disease prevention goals of *Healthy People 2000*, they will develop clinical implications and research protocols based on this document.

As editors, we took the liberty to commission original articles when it was difficult to find current manuscripts that fully met the criteria. The chapters on pressure ulcers, quality of life, alcohol, patient education, and spirituality were not intrinsic to the stated objectives, however, were felt to be of major importance to the emotional and physical well-being of older adults. The body-mind-spirit, holistic approach to patient care is intrinsic to nursing and vital in the care of the older adult.

Although only a portion of *Healthy People 2000* Objectives are included, each chapter offers specific implications for gerontological nurses and a recent reference list to enhance your future activities. Providing this text to the vast gerontological nursing audience made us aware of the differing needs of all clinicians, as well as the diverse areas that nurses care for and about older persons. It is our hope that our readers will develop the suggested areas for research, contact individual authors for additional assistance and implement the clinical directives that accompany each chapter/topic. The elderly persons we encounter in our practice will demand from us not only knowledge and skill but also a caring attitude conveying trust and acceptance. Would we want anything less than this?

Editing, not an easy chore, focused on providing key concepts, underlying principles, and quality scientific methodology. We hoped to blend these concepts into a book that was timely and worthy of use by professional nurses working with elderly patients. Quality patient care will continue to be the driving force behind our work so that nurses can have access to current information that addresses their clinical practice and research initiatives.

This book is published at a time when health care is in turmoil, and professional nursing care is being compromised. For all patients and for those older persons we serve, the lack of professional nurses to care for them can prevent the goals listed in the *Healthy People 2000* Objectives from becoming a reality. Gerontological nurses must address the challenges ahead with expert clinical and research skills. We hope this information helps you in meeting those challenges.

—Virginia Burggraf, RN, C, MSN, and Richard Barry, MDiv, MLS

FOREWORD

We are almost there. The year 2000 is fast approaching. Will we, as citizens and nurses, be able to reach our health goals? Maybe. Maybe not. The historic document *Healthy People 2000: National Health Promotion and Disease Prevention Objectives*[1] has provided the American people only one decade to meet the goals/objectives suggested by a "national strategy for significantly improving the health of the Nation."

We know, in America, what it takes to be healthy and to improve our quality of life. However, knowing what to do and doing it are two different things. If the American people really want to start anew in the next millennium, there must be national efforts to improve health throughout the lifespan. No longer can we afford to be a "sick" society where our monies and our energies are spent treating preventable diseases. We can no longer believe that physicians and other health providers will accept the burdens of our "errors of living" and expend valuable and limited resources on our follies.

Diseases and traumas will be with us into the next century and beyond. We do not have to experience them in the amount and severity that they are health problems today. By taking care of ourselves, by promoting and protecting our health, we will be able to use our resources for enhancing our quality of a healthy life.

These goals are being met in various stages, and total success cannot be achieved until all Americans accept, to the best of their ability, the responsibility for their own health and well-being. Complicating this self-responsibility—even when it can be achieved—are the social and environmental barriers that arise from lack of total commitment to health and wellness by communities and governments. For example, even if individuals do not smoke, their lungs may become diseased from environmental pollutants, if communities, businesses, and governments do not address these issues.

Nurses, at all levels, have been working very hard to achieve these goals. What does all of this mean to the profession of nursing? The American Academy of Nursing (AAN) at their Wingspread Conference in 1987[2] on Wellness and Health Promotion throughout the lifespan published recommendations for nurses to follow in promoting health and wellness.

In October 1992, Alford and Futrell[3] published the AAN's Long-Term Care Expert Panel's working paper on Wellness and Health Promotion for Older Adults. This paper also made recommendations for nursing to use in caring for the elderly. There are exciting indications that visionary nurses are using the recommendations by opening wellness centers for older adults, where optimal functional abilities and healthy lifestyles are promoted. Gerontological Institutes, such as Case Western Reserve University, are being developed with the aim of engaging in research, education, and practice in gerontological nursing which encompass the health promotion goals for older adults.

Nursing texts (eg, Ebersole and Hess[4] and Stanley and Beare[5]) are major efforts to provide curriculum materials for teaching nursing students and others that older people can be and should be healthier.

The collection of papers in this volume are on themes reflecting gerontological nurses' current practices and research that address the goals for older people in *Healthy People 2000*. As a review of these papers and the general gerontological nursing literature show, nursing is making a valiant effort to reduce disease and disability in the elderly and to encourage them to improve the quality of their lives through health promoting and health protecting behaviors. Gerontological nurses are already arranging periodic health screenings for real or potential health problems. They are providing immunizations, they are teaching the elderly healthy lifestyle habits, and they are providing counseling and support to help the elderly cope with the developmental tasks arising from social, economic, and environmental changes in their lives.

These papers not only give readers evidence of what nurses have accomplished and are accomplishing to help meet the *Healthy People 2000* goals for older adults, but provide incentives to nurses to evaluate these accomplishments for quality, generalizability, and ideas to expand further health promotion efforts. One major research effort must be made to reduce the barriers to wellness and health promotion/protection, such as poverty, language, attitudes, and lack of access to health care, especially for the elderly. This compilation of well-chosen papers should give impetus to nurses to promote and help set policies to improve the health of the nation. Most of all, this volume should motivate nurses to set the example of healthy lifestyles (especially in weight control and avoidance of smoking), and should encourage nurses to be relentless in helping others, particularly the elderly, to be healthier.

Virginia Burggraf and Richard Barry are to be commended for this volume about nursing's contribution to making the *Healthy People 2000* Objectives a reality for older adults. We are well on our way to making the next millennium for those who will experience it, a much healthier life than that of our 20th century cohorts. As you, of the next millennium, enjoy the benefits of our efforts, think of us with affection, but continue our efforts to keep producing the means for future generations to be healthy.

—Dolores M. Alford, PhD, RN, FAAN
Gerontic Nursing Consultant
Dallas, Texas

References

1. Department of Health and Human Services. *Healthy People 2000: National Health Promotion and Disease Prevention Objectives.* (DHHS publication no (PHS) 91-50212). Washington, DC: U.S. Government Printing Office; 1991.
2. Duffy M, Pender N, eds. *Conceptual Issues in Health Promotion.* Report of Proceedings of a Wingspread Conference. Sigma Theta Tau International; Indianapolis, Ind; 1987.
3. Alford D, Futrell M. Wellness and health promotion of the elderly. *Nursing Outlook.* 1992;40(5):221-226.
4. Ebersole P, Hess P. *Toward Healthy Aging.* St. Louis, Mo: Mosby; 1994.
5. Stanley M, Beare P. *Gerontological Nursing.* Philadelphia, Pa: F.A. Davis Company; 1995.

Chapter 1

Health and Long-Term Care: A Perspective on the Older Adult

Virginia Burggraf, RN, C, MSN, and Richard Barry, MDiv, MLS

OVERVIEW

Long-term care has expanded from concentrating exclusively on the older adult to an inclusive perspective of all age and population groups needing health care over a prolonged period of time. For the older adult beset with disability and chronic illness, long-term care takes on an added challenge to maximize potential and prevent further disability. For the provider, the challenge is to protect and preserve a fragile system of health care that is threatening to collapse, to provide a system of integrated care, to maintain the elderly in the community, and to prevent additional chronicity and disability.

This chapter will briefly discuss the present state of health care in later life, develop priority considerations for long-term care of older people, and develop a role for the gerontological nurse care manager.

INTRODUCTION

The redefined perspective of long-term care now includes children with disabilities, the frail elderly, those with chronic illness, and the mentally challenged.[1] There is a strong possibility that the care needs of each of these diverse groups will become diluted. A recent Government Accounting Office (GAO) report discussed whether long-term care should consist of many different services aimed at helping people with chronic conditions compensate for limitations in their ability to function independently.[2] Although each group needing long-term care services fits categorically into a long-term care agenda, each has its own identity that demands individual attention and policy considerations. Each of these groups has one thing in common: a need for an ongoing commitment to an integrated system of primary and secondary prevention, as well as acute and rehabilitative services.

Future providers of care to older adults will require commitment not only to a knowledge of the patient population to be served but also commitment to new paradigm-defined practice protocols based on prevention of additional chronicity, community-based services, and consistency of care that preserves quality.

THE OLDER ADULT: NEEDS AND PRIORITIES

Today, people who are 65 years of age can be expected to live approximately 17 years longer and have an active life in the community well into their seventh decade. Women can expect to live until about 84 years of age.[3] In 1990, there were 31 million people older than age 65; this will increase to more than 70 million in the year 2030. The 1990 census figures indicated a 67.4 million population in the year 2050 (Figure 1-1),[4] and the 1980 census predicted 52 million people older than 65 for the same year.

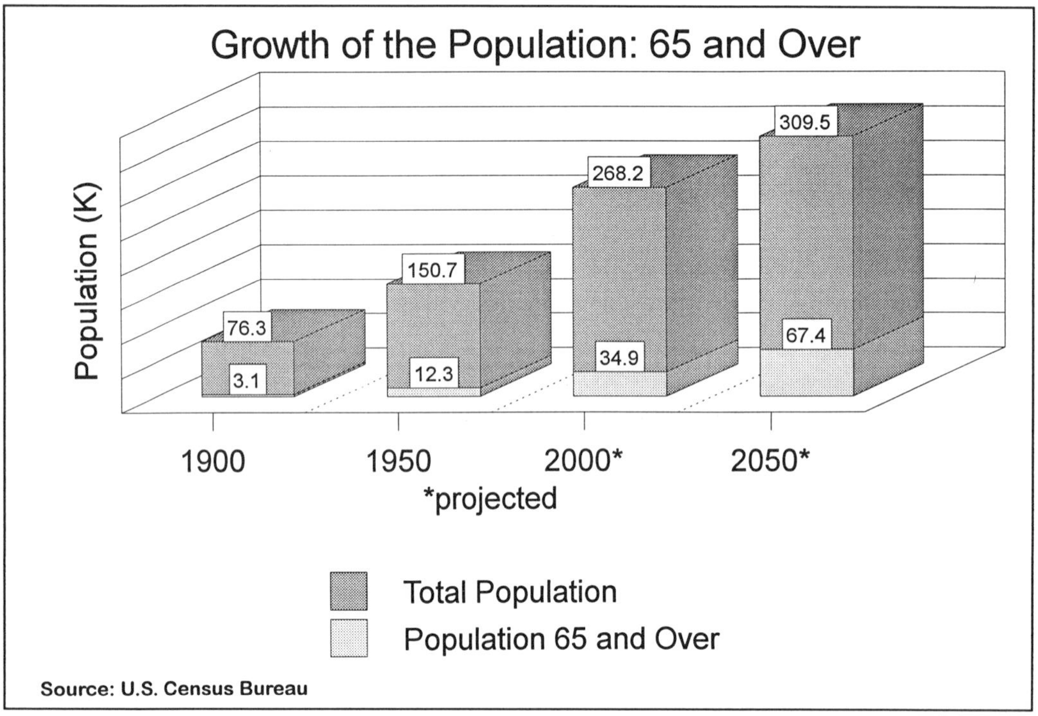

Figure 1-1. Growth of United States population.

A tremendous diversity exists in this older population regarding income, minority status, environment, and age. The 1990 data indicated that those older than 75 were more likely to be poor, with elderly women nearly twice as likely as elderly men to be poor or near poor.

Alarmingly, elderly Hispanics were twice as likely and elderly blacks were three times as likely to be poor. In the next 30 years, it is projected that the combined proportion of minority people older than 65 is expected to be 17%, which is nearly double today's proportion among older Americans.[5]

These population projections have implications not only for the preservation of life and the quality of that state but also for the providers needed in the future to care for these millions of older people. These statistics have implications for planners of facilities, corporations and their workers, and consumers themselves to play an active role in their health care,

Women comprise 69% of the over-65 age population, and it is anticipated that there will be five women for every two men older than 75 in the year 2000. At present, there are 1.6 million elderly in institutions and 5.7 million at home or in community settings.[2] Poverty is also projected to be a greater problem for older women when the baby boom generation reaches retirement.[5] The inability of women to afford basic services will need to be considered since they will comprise the largest segment of the older population.

TABLE 1-1

Chronic Conditions of the Older Adult: Ages 65-74 Years of Age*

Condition	Number
Arthritis	475
Hypertension	352
Hearing Impairments	343
Cataracts	172
Sinusitis	154
Diabetes	109
Bronchitis	63
Ulcer	33

*Conditions per 1000 people.
Source: U.S. National Center for Health Statistics, Vital and Health Statistics.

Considering the formidable trends toward longer life, it is essential to coordinate knowledge with the realization that our growing population of 30+ million people have increasing health demands. Table 1-1 illustrates the chronic conditions of people 65 years of age and older.[6] The crippling effects of arthritis, the disability associated with cardiopulmonary disease and diabetes, coupled with visual and communication disorders, are all major causes for concern. As severe as these statistics appear, they mask the growing trend that each additional decade past 65 brings with it increasing disability and chronicity.[3] The octogenarians are the fastest growing population group. It becomes apparent that acute and chronic illness accompanied by increased disability will be the future for older adults. It appears to be common sense that these disorders provide the future health care agenda for older adults; however, as these words are written, common sense does not seem to be the agenda dictating our present health care system. Nurses caring for older adults must advocate for the care provided to older patients and take on the additional challenge to preserve their identity as providers of that care.

PRIORITY CONSIDERATIONS IN LONG-TERM CARE

The political rhetoric of the early 1990s surrounding health care reform provided a glimmer of hope to policy makers and professionals involved in long-term care. The failure of the health care reform agenda creates a very tentative agenda for the older chronically ill person. Medicaid has largely subsidized the institutional care of older adults and Medicare the community-based care. As of this writing, these two federally subsidized programs are under considerable scrutiny, and decisions will be made that require careful consideration of a new paradigm to address the issues of cost and quality for an increasing population. A future perspective on health promotion and disease prevention is necessary in order to avoid this discussion in the next millennium. The baby boomers will demand a comprehensive health care package and will need incentives to stay well. It is clear that there are many tough choices required to address the needs of older adults in America. Nursing accepts the fact that delays in addressing long-term care issues will spell out hardship for many population groups.

Many of the concepts incorporated into *Nursing's Agenda for Health Care Reform*[7] provided the authors the opportunity to develop some guiding principles for a long-term care agenda. These are

- Access to all population groups experiencing chronic and disabling conditions
- A continuum of care design to reduce fragmentation as older adults move through the varied segments of the health care system
- A system with a full range of service, in which families are allowed to choose services best suited to their needs and that will delay hospitalization or institutionalization
- Care coordination (professional registered nurses) managing and transferring individuals into appropriate facilities (ie, day care, hospitals, institutions, nursing homes, and other facilities when needed)
- Community-based networks with multiple entry points into the system, using the least restrictive environment
- Emphasis on consumer responsibility for decisions made, an educational effort made to encourage people to make health care decisions in terms of quality of life rather than on the prolongation of life
- Provision of a continuum of care, beginning with acute care and integrating innovative "step up" approaches, until the individual is independent or prepared for an alternative lifestyle if more dependent.

The Policy Committee of the White House Conference on Aging (WHCoA) selected America Now and into the 21st Century: Generations Aging Together with Independence, Opportunity, and Dignity as the theme for the recent 1995 conference. WHCoA adopted many resolutions that can be the building blocks to direct the focus of care for older people.[8] In addition to the change in definition of long-term care, as previously discussed, this conference provided direction for all future discussion surrounding long-term care and older people. Post-conference activities will deal with these issues in the new millennium:

- Preserving a method of payment for health care, retirement, and future programs
- Promoting the quality of life as one ages
- Enhancing access to comprehensive care as well as promotion of a continuum of integrated care services
- Promoting economic security.

The task at hand is to look at these approaches and how they can be maximized. An initial look at the crisis in long-term care expenditures for the older adult may shed some light on how the present system can be altered.

Total expenditures for long-term care are projected to more than double by 2018, with more than twice as much spent on institutional care as was expended for home- and community-based care.[9] Nursing home care is projected to increase from $75.5 billion in 1993 to $168.2 billion in 2018.[10] Based on the chronic illness considerations (see Table 1-1) and the increased need for institutionalization, there will be a need for more nurses not only educated about care of older people but also nurses who will specialize in gerontological nursing.

Nursing homes will change their names to something akin to care centers and ally themselves with a community-based care service. The term nursing home has generated, here in America, a very negative place where older people receive inadequate care. These centers will provide the clinical laboratories for basic and graduate nursing students and will be a hub for continuity of care to the community and for hospice or respite care services. These care environments could be centered around academic institutions of learning, which would allow for maximum collaboration among professionals and provide clients with professional teams that could best meet their needs.

Home care services are much more desirable than institutional care, and the bulk of funding will be toward promoting community-based services. There will be a need to educate nurses not only in the aspects of community/family centered care but also in the administration of these centers. Nursing administration is presently moving away from acute care to home care. There will be a return to house calls by nurse practitioners whose offices will be in a car circuit riding in a nursing care district. In order to prevent disease and maintain ability in older people, this type of care will be necessary. Mobile van clinics will appear on certain days in areas to care for entire populations by locale. New experimental types of primary care environments will be attempted, and only those that are effective will remain. Adult day care centers will increase and be managed by nurses. Rehabilitation services will be offered here, and caregivers of the elderly will have an easier time with access to more resources. Adult day care services will be provided by corporations as an elder care option for families caring for older relatives.

GERONTOLOGICAL NURSING IMPLICATIONS

The next century will be a time of change for nursing and the way in which health care is administered. Nurses will be a model for the delivery of primary care to older persons and be visionary in their approach to their long-term care needs. Reflection of the specific implications that impact practice can provide well-developed, achievable goals for our generation and those who follow.

In order to reduce the fragmentation surrounding the present health care environment, older people must have a one-person nurse care/case manager to orchestrate their care. This framework begins with the patient's entry into the primary care setting and extends through all aspects of care and coordination.[11] To maximize ability, decrease existing chronicity and disability, and promote health, the nurse manager must assure adequate placement from one health care area to another. For older people, a full range of services needs to be available with follow-up to assess the adequacy and quality of the services offered. A person experiencing a stroke must have a team assembled that will address all aspects of rehabilitation, as well as nutritional, emotional, and physical health. The team must act quickly to assure that additional deterioration does not occur. Caregivers/family members are intrinsic to the coordination of care and must be considered in every decision made.

Designing inservice programs to educate professionals will be a necessity. The health care team must have specialized knowledge in order to work with older people and their families, other professionals, as well as multiple facilities. The number and range of informal caregivers will continue to increase, and many resources will be needed for them to continue to provide this vital care at home. Corporate programs will address the needs of caregivers as well as possible provision for the care of older adults. Many corporations have begun to address elder care as an option. The need for gerontological nursing education in occupational health will expand to address prevention initiatives as well as care of the older worker.[10]

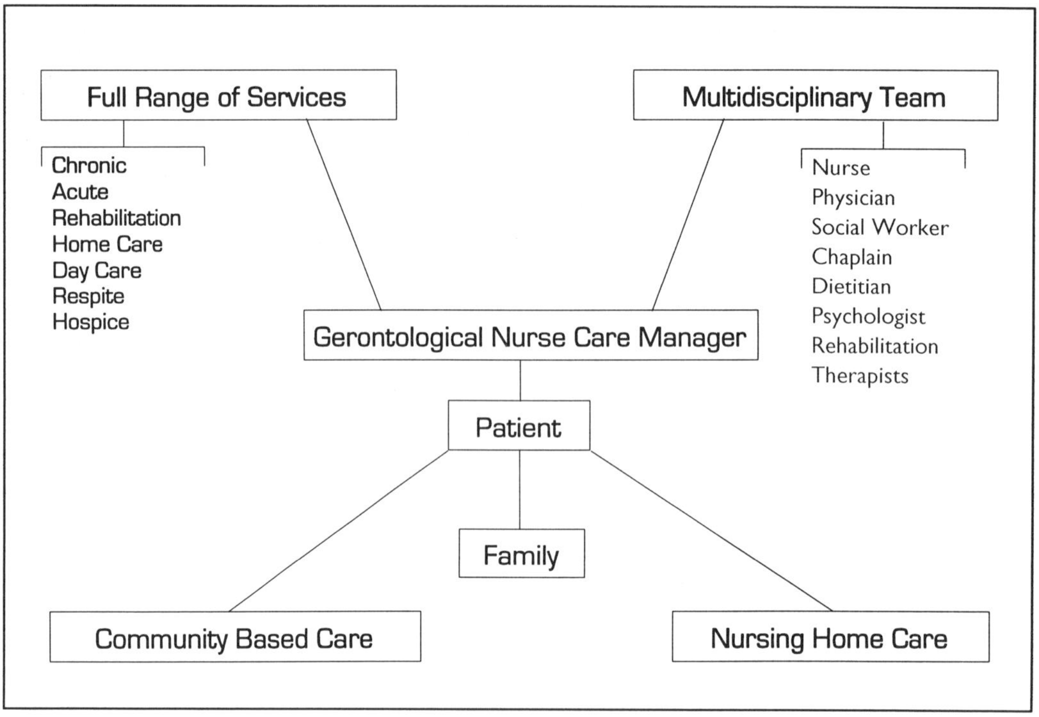

Figure 1-2. Coordination of the continuum of care for older people.

Figure 1-2 provides a diagram of the coordinated effort of the gerontological nurse care manager. The manager is the key to accessing the environments necessary to maximize the potential of the older person. Older people enter the health care environment frequently at any point of acute, episodic, or community-based care, and many move along a continuum to other centers of care. A multidisciplinary team must be assembled, based on the criteria (care maps) decided upon by the managed care or group insurance plans providing the coverage for the individual. The nurse manager is the patient advocate and works to assure that high quality care is the primary consideration. This model of care has the potential to provide quality in a cost-effective environment. Research is needed to validate patient outcomes.

Nurses working in these environments have the responsibility to

- Advocate for their older patients and maximize their potential
- Provide for a smooth transition from one patient care area to another
- Evaluate the quality and effectiveness of care provided
- Provide patient education materials for the client and family

- Work with the team to develop research methodologies that address health promotion and disease prevention modalities.

Academicians also have a responsibility to older patients and to share in the quality of care provided. They should:

- Educate students in the concepts of gerontological nursing
- Provide for a continuum of education for faculty to be educated about care of the older person
- Develop a curriculum base that is culturally sensitive to meet the needs of all groups
- Research and publish developments, trends, and outcome measures that impact on older people and the care provided them by registered nurses.[11]

In the next millennium, it will be more common for people to live productive lives past the age of 100. The challenge for nurses is to advocate for their patients in an age when economic issues often preempt the human and where less than professional is fast becoming a standard. No one can substitute for the unique care a nurse provides, delegates, or supervises. Anything less is unacceptable. Our collective voices must be heard in the board rooms of professional associations as well as in the offices of politicians who create the laws and establish the appropriations. Our future as gerontological nurses and the quality of care provided to our patients depend on this.

REFERENCES

1. American Nurses Association. *Position Statement on Long-Term Care*. Washington, D.C.: American Nurses Association; 1995.
2. U.S. Government Accounting Office GAO-HEHS-95-109. *Long-Term Care: Current Issues and Future Directions*. GAO. Washington, D.C.: Government Printing Office; 1995.
3. Young R, Olson E. *Health Illness and Disability in Later Life*. Newbury Park: Sage Publications; 1991.
4. U.S. Bureau of the Census. *1990 Census of the Population: Characteristics of the Population: General Social and Economic Characteristics*. PC80-1-CI. Washington, D.C.: Government Printing Office; 1993.
5. Public Policy Agenda. Older Americans of today and tomorrow. *Perspectives on Aging*. 1995;24(1):6-7.
6. U.S. Bureau of Health Statistics. *Statistical Abstract of the United States*. Washington, D.C.: U.S. Department of Commerce; 1995.
7. American Nurses Association. *Nursing's Agenda for Health Care Reform*. Washington, D.C.: American Nurses Publishing; 1993.
8. Conference on Aging. *Official 1995 White House Conference on Aging: Adopted Resolutions*. Washington, D.C.: U.S. Government Printing Office; 1995.
9. Vladek BC, Miller NA, Clauser SB. The changing face of long-term care. *Health Care Financing Review*. 1993;14(4):5-24.
10. Weiner JM, Illston LH. Health care reform in the 1990's. Where does long-term care fit in? *Gerontologist*. 1994;34(3):402-408.
11. Burggraf V, Barry R. Long-term care: providing for those with disability and chronic illness. *J Gerontol Nurs*. 1995;21(10):31-35.

Chapter 2

Older Women: Social Policies and Health Care

Margaret Dimond, PhD, RN, FAAN

OVERVIEW

The population of older adults in America is composed mostly of women. Many of these women are poor and have chronic illnesses. Current social, political, and economic structures that govern health care discriminate against all women, but particularly women who are poor and black. Income is a major predictor of quality health care. Many factors contribute to the poverty rates among older women, including discriminatory Social Security benefits, life histories of gender bias and inequitable compensation for work, and no compensation for years of caregiving to both young and old. Medicare, as the largest single source of payment for health care, also discriminates against women, since its emphasis is primarily on acute and hospital care. Older women have many chronic conditions that require community-based services that are not reimbursed by Medicare. The quality of health care provided to older women is diminished by health professionals' lack of knowledge about older women's health and by their failure to provide culturally sensitive care. Older women are beginning to take charge of their own health both at the individual level and through political action. Gerontological nurses can encourage and facilitate older women's more proactive approach to health care through political action, aimed at the elimination of the social, political, and economic causes of discrimination against older women, and thus ensure quality health care for all older women.

INTRODUCTION

The current and future demographic trends are unequivocal in their prediction of the gender distribution into the 21st century. Women will continue to outnumber men by increasing margins with increasing age, such that by 2020 the ratio of men to women older than 85 years is projected to be one man for every three women.[1] Given that the population of older adults in America is composed mostly of women, many of whom are poor and have chronic illnesses, it is clear that most of the issues of aging are women's issues.[2] How do the current political, social, and economic systems influence the experience of being old and female in America? Being old, female, and poor is sometimes characterized as "triple jeopardy," but the consequences of age, gender, and socioeconomic status are further heightened by ethnicity. Black women are at particular high risk of experiencing the final stage of life in poverty and poor health.[3] Any analysis of current social policy would be incomplete without the inclusion of all four concerns, since singly and in combinations these four factors jeopardize the health of all older women.

The greater risk to women, particularly black women, when compared to older men, is largely due to the fact that although women have lower mortality rates than men, women have greater morbidity due to chronic illnesses and more limitations in self-care.[4] The health care issues facing older women are not due solely to old age, but to "lifelong patterns of socioeconomic and gender stratification in the larger society."[5] In order to achieve solutions to health care issues of older women, root causes must be addressed. That is, "gender, race, and age discrimination in the labor market; unequal pay for comparable work; quality of income security programs for women; and a lifetime of devalued caregiving work"[5] are all factors that are operative for young and middle-aged women. These culminate in restrictive health care options and poor life quality for many older women. An analysis of health and health care for older women is complex, including as it does, issues that are not mutually exclusive, but highly interconnected. Thus, while the ideas presented in this chapter are organized by seemingly discrete headings, it should be understood that this strategy is mainly for heuristic reasons. The issues of poverty, ethnicity, and health care are highly interactive and reciprocal. This is particularly the case in the late life experiences of older women.

POVERTY AND OLDER WOMEN

Income is a major predictor of quality health care for older women. Although the economic trends show an improving outlook for older adults generally, it is inappropriate to generalize these trends to all old people, given the heterogeneity of the aging population. Among all older women, poverty rates for non-Hispanic (white), Hispanic, and black older women are widely divergent (13%, 25%, and 39%, respectively).[6] Living alone dramatically increases the rate of poverty among older women, particularly black older women. Fifty percent of older Hispanic women and nearly 60% of older black women who live alone are poor.[7] Marital status is also a factor in poverty levels of older women. Widowed older women are disproportionately poor. Living with family members is a strong predictor for the transition out of poverty for widowed older women. For those widowed older women who live alone, dependence on food stamps and Supplemental Security Income is a strong predictor of continuing impoverishment.[8]

The largest source of financial income for older adults is Social Security (nearly 40%).[1] Current Social Security policy provides some explanation for the disproportionate risk of poverty and lower income of older women.[9] Social Security benefits are based on the average monthly earnings (wages) of individuals over a lifetime. The current cohort of women older than 65 had shorter work histories and lower wages than men in the same age group. Single women in this age group were much less likely to have worked in jobs that offered employer pensions.[9] Most women currently older than 65 years of age have experienced work interruptions for childbearing and childrearing. For married women, these factors become more salient after the death of a spouse.[10] Briefly, with the death of a spouse, the older woman may receive either the survivor benefits from the husband's work or her own worker's benefits. She must choose between these options, but cannot receive both. The survivor benefit in the United States ranges between one half and two thirds the combined Social Security benefit of husband and wife while both are alive.[9,11] Given the 5- to 7-year shorter life expectancy for men, the impact of these policies is felt disproportionately by older women than older men. Sole dependence on Social Security, which is the case for many older women, is a sign of economic dependence and insecurity.[11] This economic insecurity is a major issue when older women try to negotiate the health care system. A major barrier to quality health care for older women is cost. Who pays for health care for older women?

PAYING FOR HEALTH CARE

Medicare and Medicaid are the largest sources of funding for the health care of older adults. These sources of health care financing have been of enormous value for all older adults. But, helpful as the Medicare legislation has been since its passage in 1965, it has also created significant problems. This is primarily due to its emphasis on acute and institutional care rather than community-based care. Here, as in the Social Security system, women are at greater risk than men. Most of the morbidity of older women is due to chronic conditions (eg, arthritis, osteoporosis and its sequelae, urinary incontinence, and depression). While these conditions may at times require hospitalization (covered by Medicare), most of the time they are managed in community-based settings (not covered by Medicare). Sofaer[12] has shown that the out-of-pocket costs for health care for older women (after taking Medicare reimbursement into consideration) far exceed those for older men.

As amended in the Medicare Catastrophic Coverage Act of 1988, Medicare covers almost all hospitalization costs (with the exception of inpatient psychiatric care) and sets limits on the fees that can be charged by physicians, but only if physicians agree to accept Medicare's fee schedule. Outpatient mental health services are covered in a very limited manner by Medicare.[13] Since 1988, Medicare covers between 50% and 80% of the cost of outpatient drugs after a deductible and the cost of mammograms, a significant benefit for older women.

Medicaid, health coverage for the poor, provides financial assistance for drugs, nursing home care, and custodial care in the home.[13] Among older men and women, women represent 62% of those eligible for Medicaid. Apart from the discrimination visited on older women by the public policies that govern payment of health care, what is the experience of older women once they get into the system? Do they receive the same quality of care as older men?

QUALITY HEALTH CARE FOR OLDER WOMEN

In a recent representative national survey by Louis Harris and Associates, Inc., 2500 women and 1000 men, ages 18 to older than 65, were interviewed about a wide variety of health issues. Women reported problems of communication and condescending behavior on the part of their physicians. Thirty-two percent of women reported changing their physicians because of communication problems, 25% reported that physicians "talked down to them," and 17% reported they were told their conditions were "all in their head."[14] All of these situations were reported significantly more often by women than men. Although these data were reported by a wide age range of women, there is no compelling reason why older women would experience these problems any less frequently than younger women. In fact, this report may underestimate the communication problems of older women and their physicians. Quality of care is clearly jeopardized by interactions such as these between physicians and female patients. On a positive note, the Task Force on Older Women's Health pointed out the need for better physician education about older women's health and recognition of gender differences in manifestation of disease and response to treatment in order to overcome biases in diagnosis and treatment.[4] The task force report notes specifically the need for greater knowledge of breast and lung cancer, menopause, osteoporosis, depression, urinary incontinence, and cardiovascular disease. Two recent publications referring to cardiovascular illness provide evidence of differential treatment of women and men, and the recognition by medical professionals of the need for intensive research and improved practice in this area. Young[15] found noticeable differences in the medical management of myocardial infarction of men and women. Men received significantly more information than women and were more likely than women to be referred to rehabilitation programs and diagnostic angiograms. The 1-year post myocardial infarction health of women in the study was poorer than men (eg, women reported more sick days, more shortness of breath, and overall greater limitations in functional ability). A special article in the *New England Journal of Medicine*[16] reports that in spite of the fact that 500,000 women die each year of cardiovascular disease, there exists very little information about preventive strategies, diagnostic testing, or responses to medical or surgical therapies in women. The reasons why women frequently receive less aggressive evaluation and treatment than men, particularly in the case of chest pain, is due to differences in pathology between men and women and possibly from suboptimal or delayed care.[16] These unknowns are due in part to the failure to enroll women in significant clinical trials in the past. It appears that the medical profession is becoming increasingly aware of its responsibilities in medical education and research to improve the quality of health care for older women. Improving the quality of the technical care of older women is important, but it will not address another important component of quality health care: culturally sensitive care.

CULTURAL SENSITIVITY

Older black women seeking health care are particularly concerned about access, lack of appreciation among health providers for heterogeneity among and within ethnic groups, and culturally insensitive care. Poor access to care may be due to several factors including lack of knowledge about available services and how to "work" the system, lack of health insurance and knowledge of how to acquire the health insurance to which they are entitled, unavailable or poor transportation, and perceived (and often real) discrimination by health care providers and ancillary workers in health care settings.[17-19] The belief that all black people, including those belonging to the same ethnic group, hold the same values and beliefs and practice the same health behaviors is incorrect. The following is often not recognized by health care providers:

> Ethnicity is not merely a set of artifacts and labels, language or dress, but rather a fluid concept that changes and adapts over time, changes among generations, and often re-emerges in later life as an integrating force in the transition to age, providing a sense of continuity of self and community.[20]

Failure to understand ethnic heterogeneity on the part of health care providers was responsible for the concept of "colorblind" care (ie, care provided without regard for race or ethnic diversity). And while intended to convey equality of care for all people, colorblind care has in fact, been responsible for the development of formidable barriers to care. So-called colorblind care can result in inappropriate or poor care because it does not take into account individual beliefs, customs, and language diversity. There is growing recognition among health care providers that curricula in health professional schools must include content in ethnogeriatrics if future cohorts of older adults are to receive culturally sensitive health care.[21] The factors in the current health care system that lead to discrimination against older women on the basis of age, gender, income, or ethnicity are beginning to motivate large numbers of these women to take control of their own health.

OLDER WOMEN TAKING CHARGE OF THEIR OWN HEALTH

Successful achievement of healthy aging is a combination of information and action. Older women need accurate information about the normal aging processes. If women are educated about normal aging and given time to assimilate and plan for aging changes, the outcome of successful aging will be enhanced. Women need to learn ways to take charge of and protect their own health, and they need accurate and current information about sources of paying for health care and eligibility criteria for health insurance. Knowledge resources to assist women in this endeavor include primary health care providers, both nurses and physicians. Older women need to ask nurses and physicians questions about their own health status, the meaning of symptoms, reasons for and results of diagnostic procedures, and the rationale for prescribed medications. Women should become familiar with the details of coverage included in Medicare, "More-than-Medicare" supplements, and private insurance policies. Although most older adults are reluctant to take what is perceived as a "handout," it is important for older women to be knowledgeable about the eligibility criteria for financial assistance such as Medicaid and Supplemental Security Insurance to ensure that if the need for this assistance arises, they can be confident about their right to this type of assistance. In addition to nurses and physicians, the factual information published by the American Association of Retired Persons (AARP) is an excellent resource for the acquisition of information about health care for older women. The topics covered in these publications are timely and accurate. Examples of information provided by AARP include topics such as exercise, nutrition, stress reduction, breast cancer, incontinence, depression, self-care, and menopause. Some older women will be motivated to take an active role not only in their own care, but to influence the health care system for the benefit of all older adults. For these women, there are opportunities to participate in political action, either through membership in political action groups or through direct communication with state and federal legislators. However, it is not enough simply to outline the ways that older women can take charge of their own health or influence health policy. Gerontological nurses have a responsibility to provide support and assistance, and to facilitate the active participation of older women in their own health behaviors.

GERONTOLOGICAL NURSING IMPLICATIONS

The implications for gerontological nurses of the changing social and political environment of health care for older women can focus on either care of individuals or care of populations. At the individual level, gerontological nurses are students with the major responsibility to stay abreast of the latest information on health promotion and the rapidly changing approaches to the management of myriad mostly chronic conditions that affect older women. They are educators whose knowledge of health promotion and chronic illness is shared with clients and families. They are counselors and coaches who guide and encourage older women in their pursuit of health. As advocates, gerontological nurses lead the efforts to increase access to culturally sensitive, quality care for all older women, regardless of their ability to pay or their ethnic group membership.

At the broader level of populations, some gerontological nurses will take responsibility for involvement in sociopolitical action to secure changes in social structures that will benefit older women and ensure quality health care now and in the future. To paraphrase Arendell and Estes,[5] such changes would eliminate discrimination in the labor market based on age, gender, or race, ensure equal pay for comparable work, quality income security programs for women, and recognition and remuneration for the invaluable work of all women caregivers (for the young and the old). Through political action, gerontological nurses can work to eliminate the root causes of discrimination against older women and ensure quality health care for all older women.

REFERENCES

1. Gilford D, ed. *The Aging Population in the Twenty-First Century.* Washington, D.C.: National Academy Press; 1988.
2. Dimond M. Older women's health. In: Fogel C, Woods N. *Women's Health Care.* Thousand Oaks, CA: Sage Publications; 1995:101-110.
3. Dimond M. Older women: social policies and health care. *J Gerontol Nurs.* October 1993;19:5-6.
4. Task Force on Older Women's Health. *J Am Geriatr Soc.* 1993;41:680-683.
5. Arendell T, Estes C. Older women in the post-Reagan era. *Int J Health Serv.* 1991;21:59-73.
6. *Poverty in the United States: 1991.* Washington, D.C.: U.S. Department of Commerce; 1992. Current Population Reports, Series P-60, No. 18.
7. *Poverty in the United States: 1992.* Washington, D.C.: U.S. Department of Commerce; 1993. Current Population Reports, Series P-60, No. 185.
8. Dodge H. Movements out of poverty among elderly widows. *J Gerontol.* 1995;50B:S240-S249.
9. Burkhauser R. Sharing prosperity across the age distribution: a comparison of the United States and Germany in the 1980's. *Gerontologist.* 1994;34:150-160.

10. *Social Security Bulletin Annual Statistical Supplement: 1993.* Washington, D.C.: Social Security Administration, U.S. Department of Health and Human Services; 1993:Tables 5.A14.
11. Smeeding T. Economic status of the elderly. In: Binstock R, George L. *Handbook of Aging and the Social Sciences, 3.* San Diego, CA: Academic Press; 1990:362-382.
12. Sofaer S, Abel E. Older women's health and financial vulnerability: implications of the Medicare benefit structure. *Women Health.* 1990;16:47-66.
13. Kane RL, Kane RA. Health care for older people: organization and policy issues. In: Binstock R, George, L. *Handbook of Aging and the Social Sciences, 3.* San Diego, CA: Academic Press; 1990:415-437.
14. *Commonwealth Fund Survey.* New York: The Commonwealth Fund; 1993.
15. Young R, Kahana E. Gender, recovery from late life heart attack, and medical care. *Women Health.* 1993;20:11-31.
16. Wenger N, Speroff L, Packard B. Cardiovascular disease and health in women. *N Engl J Med.* 1993;329:247-256.
17. Yeatts D, Crow T, Folts E. Service use among low income minority elderly: strategies for overcoming barriers. *Gerontologist.* 1992;32:24-32.
18. Hopper S. The influence of ethnicity on the health of older women. *Clin Geriatr Med.* 1993;9:231-259.
19. Johnson C. Differential expectations and realities: race, socioeconomic status and health of the oldest-old. *Int J Aging Hum Dev.* 1994;38:13-27.
20. Gelfand D, Baressi C. Current perspectives in ethnicity and aging. In: Gelfand D, Baressi C. *Ethnic Dimensions of Aging.* New York: Springer; 1987:5-17.
21. Brangman S. African-American elders: implications for health care providers. *Clin Geriatr Med.* 1995;11:15-23.

Chapter 3

Quality of Life From the Long-Term Care Resident's Perspective

Loretta J. Aller, RN, MSN, and Harriet Van Ess Coeling, PhD, RN

OVERVIEW

Historically, quality of life in long-term care has received only limited investigation. A review of current quality of life literature is presented with supporting research, investigating quality of life of residents in a long-term care facility. Physical environment, recreational activities, and social environment have previously been identified as being important, while the findings of this study support social environment and a desire to help oneself and others as the strongest elements affecting quality of life. Recommendations for further research are presented. Gerontological nursing implications resulting from the research provide specific suggestions for developing both individual and group programs to enhance the quality of life of those residents living in long-term care settings.

INTRODUCTION

Although the concept of quality of life is assuming increasing importance in health care literature, relatively few research studies describe factors that enhance quality of life in nursing homes.[1-3] Current literature has identified physical environment, recreational activities, and the social environment as three major factors that affect a resident's quality of life.[1,4-12] The general environment has been examined by looking at both physical and organizational structure. Physical aspects include such areas as architectural features, color, lighting, space, and privacy. The organizational structure includes facility policies, staffing, financing, and the presence or absence of residents' grievance council meetings.

LITERATURE REVIEW

Moos[10] has developed a conceptual framework for assessing the environment and suggests examining the physical and architectural features of a facility, in addition to the policy and programmatic resources available. Moos reported that the environmental system has a direct impact on the residents' stability, morale, health, and well-being.

Clark[4] also examined both the physical properties and organizational structure as components of quality of life for elderly residents in long-term care facilities. This study compared the physical settings of two nursing homes—a long-stay geriatric hospital ward and a hospital patients' club—in order to determine whether the size and physical structure had a direct impact on quality of life. Regarding organizational structure, Clark and Bowling predicted that a smaller environment might lead to flexibility in care practices and, subsequently, a better quality of life. While their initial quantitative survey results did not support this prediction, further qualitative analysis of additional observational data showed that staff mood and interaction in the club did make a difference in determining quality of life.

Oleson[13] found important differences when comparing nurses' and residents' perceptions of the relative importance of the environment in determining quality of life. Residents described their own internal environment, particularly their coping strategies and ability to adapt to their increased dependence and placement within the long-term care setting, as being important. In contrast, nurses thought that ensuring that residents had private space, personal possessions, and direct involvement in the decisions made regarding their care would improve residents' quality of life. Additionally, the physical structure and design of the institution were seen as being important whereas the residents did not comment on these factors.[13]

Individualized recreational activities, such as music, reading, and engaging in personal hobbies, have also been identified as factors influencing quality of life, as have group activities such as sing-a-longs, exercise sessions, and current-events readings.[4,12] Ross[12] explored the types of activities chosen and use of time in later life and related them to health and well-being. This study emphasized the need to individualize recreation for the elderly since the frequency, duration, location, and social context of activities are important determinants of perceived satisfaction.

While the physical and recreational environments have been shown to be important, the human relationships and social contact with others have been described as being far more crucial in determining quality of life.[1,8,12] The interaction between resident and nurse, and the subsequent bond that develops, rather than the color of the room or the administrative philosophy of the facility is the variable of greatest importance to the resident.[8]

Huss[6] conducted a study designed to explore the relationships between residents of long-term care facilities and the nursing staff, and the effect of these relationships on the residents' life satisfaction. Thirty subjects were interviewed from two intermediate care facilities. Researchers found that, although the nurse/resident relationship did not correlate significantly with life satisfaction, nurses did have an effect on residents' perceived life satisfaction when they assumed the role of a confidant. Those residents who reported having a confidant exhibited higher levels of life satisfaction.

A review of research suggests three factors that affect quality of life: physical environment, recreational activities, and social environment. Further study was conducted to confirm that these three factors did influence quality of life. Further research is needed to determine whether other factors, not identified, may also contribute to a person's quality of life. Much of the research that has been done in this area has been quantitative in design. Some researchers have identified the disadvantages of using quantitative methods to study quality of life. Najman[14] warns that studies employing only objective indicators may have little to contribute to our understanding the quality of life experience. Those who use these objective measures alone may simply be projecting their own values and priorities on others.[14] Sutcliffe[15] notes that because quality of life is a subjective concept, objective methodologies may limit the value of the outcome. Self-reports allow the individual, who may be a more reliable source than the health professional, to describe and determine such subjective content.[16]

A qualitative method was chosen by these researchers in order to confirm accepted factors and identify new factors that might more effectively reveal residents' personal goals and ideals.[17,18] The purpose of this study, therefore, was to allow the residents living in a long-term care facility to explain what quality of life meant to them by describing those activities and events that contributed to the quality of their lives.

METHOD

To identify what contributed to the quality of life of long-term care residents, a semistructured, open-ended format was used. This openness encouraged the expression of residents' true thoughts and feelings as they were encouraged to describe what, for them, constituted quality of life, rather than asking them concrete, structured questions that would have limited free expression and potentially masked emergent themes.

A convenience sample of eight subjects who were permanently residing in a 150-bed, long-term care facility in northeastern Ohio was utilized. West[19] noted the difficulty of finding good informants among institutionalized elderly. The social worker and the director of nursing compiled a list of subjects who met the criteria as described by Dobbert[20] of sources who are likely to provide valid data. The criteria indicated that participating individuals in the study were

- Comfortable and unstrained in interactions
- Generally open and truthful
- Able to provide solid answers with good detail
- Able to converse on a topic or related important issue
- Thoughtful and willing to reflect on what they said.[20]

Potential subjects who were legally incompetent or seen by the social worker and director of nursing as being unable to participate in a 20- to 30-minute interview were not considered as candidates. Out of 142 residents, only 12 met the criteria. The range in length of stay for these residents was 8 months to 7 years, with primary diagnoses including paraplegia, cerebrovascular accident, brain injury, and lower-extremity amputation. The actual sample included six women and two men between the ages of 44 and 90.

DATA COLLECTION

After obtaining consent from both the facility and the residents, 20- to 30-minute taped interviews were conducted with each subject. The sessions were conducted in the subjects' rooms with no one else in the rooms and the doors closed. Staff were given a brief description of the research study and were asked not to interrupt. The researcher began with open-ended questions such as "What does quality of life mean to you?" and "What gives your life quality or meaning?" If the researcher found that the subjects did not appear to understand the meaning of the original term, the terms life satisfaction and meaning were substituted for quality of life. Although the researcher had some semistructured questions on topics previous researchers had found to be components of the concept of quality of life (namely environment, recreation, and social interaction), those questions were only asked if prompts were necessary to continue the conversation. Because saturation was reached quickly (seven of the eight residents alluded to the importance of helping others, either through direct descriptions or as evidenced by the enthusiasm with which they spoke), the researcher decided to halt data collection upon completion of eight interviews to allow an analysis, which would direct the next stage of the research program.

DATA ANALYSIS

Each interview was reviewed, and direct quotations were transcribed. These transcripts were analyzed using traditional content-analysis procedures in an attempt to identify common themes.[21] Initially, nine content areas were identified: care given/caretakers; activities/hobbies; perception of health; visitors/friends/family; roommate/communication with other residents; environment/setting; comments regarding quality of life; food; and life before admission. Patient responses were then placed categorically into nine columns to allow the data to be analyzed comparatively between subjects. While looking for commonalities among content areas, three themes emerged that identified abilities important to the residents. Minor areas of disagreement were discussed and resolved, and both researchers collaboratively identified the three common themes after the nine content areas were developed and analyzed separately.

The importance of being able to interact with other residents was identified through responses such as "I've made a lot of friends since I've been here." Other typical comments: "I like to meet people" and "People are the most important thing." One theme identified was the subjects' ability to communicate with other residents and staff within the facility. The second emergent theme was that of the subjects' ability to care for themselves. Although they did not identify complaints concerning the care provided by the staff, the majority of the respondents felt that the ability to perform self-care activities provided them with a feeling of satisfaction and gave their lives a sense of quality. This was expressed in comments like "I want to do what I can for myself;" an amputee states "I get around and do a lot of little things—only with my hands now;" and "...the way I've been feeling, I haven't been able to get out and visit, and I don't like that."

A third theme, the strongest one, identifies the subjects' ability to care for or help others who were in more need than themselves. The number of times the theme was repeated, the verbal emphasis given to that particular comment, and facial expressions exhibited during the discussion were the determining factors of its strength. This analysis is supported by Goodinson,[22] who identified the need for results to be weighted by the individual, depending on the importance of a particular factor to that individual. As residents described the importance of their ability to care for others, they elaborated openly and spoke with more conviction than they had in any other area of the interview. Their care is reflected in statements such as "Quality of life, to me, is not only self-betterment, but the betterment of others" and "Helping the other people here...now that enhances my quality of life."

DISCUSSION

Of the three components previously identified in the literature (physical environment, recreational activities, and social environment), participants in this study discussed only the importance of social interaction with others as giving their lives quality when asked to describe quality of life in an open-ended manner. This finding supports the need for therapeutic relationships.[6]

Residents suggested that, although the environment (primarily physical) was "nice," it was not a determining factor in their quality of life. Likewise, residents noted the importance of recreational activities and hobbies, but described them as being more "to pass the time" than a meaningful part of their lives. Perhaps physical facilities and recreation would have been more readily noted if these needs were not being met; if they are, other concerns are discussed. Social interaction was identified by previous researchers as a factor affecting quality of life, and the respondents in this study reinforced this belief.

This study did identify two new findings as contributing to quality of life—the importance of caring for oneself and the importance of helping others. These components were not previously identified in the literature at the time this study was done. This study found that the subjects' ability to help others who were in more need than themselves emerged as the strongest theme. This finding has been reported in a recent study.[13]

This recent research compared the long-term care residents' and nurses' perceptions of quality of life and reported that the concept of resident usefulness was considered more important to residents than nurses. The loss of usefulness was considered to be more of a problem from the residents' perspective. This may be due to the tendency for nurses to focus on what they can do for residents, thereby fostering dependence, rather than building on the strengths and assets that residents already have to support independence.[13]

Previous gerontological studies have not found the concept of resident usefulness as a factor affecting quality of life. Ferrans did suggest that usefulness to others is a variable within the health and functioning domain of the concept of quality of life.[23] This research has been done with patient populations other than long-term care residents, specifically hemodialysis and breast cancer patients. Ferrans suggests her concepts might be applicable in the nursing home setting.[23,24]

GERONTOLOGICAL NURSING IMPLICATIONS

This study is best viewed as the first stage of a research program to investigate the impact of a new factor, namely the importance of caring for others, on quality of life. This research, limited by sample size, did elicit the importance of caring for self and others. A larger sample is recommended as well as a more highly controlled method to clarify the relative importance of this factor. Extended qualitative research could be performed using a variety of methods, such as listening to stories, videotaping, and observing behaviors that subjects confirm or refute, as well as the use of structured questionnaires. Further research is needed in this area.

Incorporating the results of this study can prove beneficial. Encouraging self-care and promoting independent decision-making can be beneficial in enhancing the well-being of nursing home residents.[13,25] This study found that quality of life is also enhanced when residents are able to assist others. Suggestions for enhancing each of these factors will be discussed.

Failure to accurately assess a resident's ability to provide self-care may lead to a phenomenon known as excess disability. In this situation, a resident may become more functionally disabled, due in part to staff's performing more care for the resident than is needed.[26,27] Such an error in assessment and subsequent plans of care may actually promote dependence. Only through changes in attitude and the elimination of the dependency-producing nature of nursing homes can individual autonomy and independence be promoted.[28]

Creative strategies to meet residents' needs for self-care must be identified. The potential for excess disability can be prevented by encouraging independent activities of daily living (ADLs) including bathing, dressing, eating, and self-medication as well as instrumental activities of daily living (IADLs). Additionally, other programs such as restorative ambulation and dining/feeding have proven helpful. Other suggestions include having residents assume more responsibility for their own environment such as making their beds, folding clothes, dusting, and washing windows.

As has been identified earlier, residents have indicated that, in addition to caring for themselves, caring for and helping others is important in enhancing their quality of life. Therefore, they should be permitted, if they desire, to participate in such activities that would allow them to assist others. Possible activities that could be integrated into their plan of care may be those that help others on an individual basis or those that benefit a larger group. Suggestions for one-on-one involvement include assistance with ADLs as described above, writing and/or reading letters and current events to those who may not be able, and praying with/for others. Activities that help others on a broader scale may include assisting staff by answering phones and with non-confidential paperwork such as stamping blank documentation records, preparing pre-admission charts, recording visitors and those in attendance at facility events, and becoming involved in or coordinating a birthday club in which they sing and/or give balloons to other residents, or lead or assist with religious programs. Outside the facility, residents can become involved in community events such as soup kitchens and clothing drives.

Caution on the part of the staff must be taken, however, to avoid resident misinterpretation of such creative suggestions. Personal experience shows that residents may perceive staff's efforts to promote resident independence to be a way for employees to get out of work. The interdisciplinary team must work collaboratively with residents and their families to explain that their intention is to enhance quality of life through increasing independence, self-care, and the care of others.

Each initiative to promote self-care and care of others must be presented as a positive endeavor and one that is an integral part of the facility routine so that it is not perceived as contrived or punishing.[29] In addition, risk management professionals should be consulted to ensure that interdisciplinary documentation supports specifically how such contracted activities are beneficial to the resident.

One means of helping residents understand that such activities are intended to be beneficial to them rather than the facility is through the use of contracting. Contracts are designed to collaboratively identify behaviors, either positive behaviors that can be reinforced or negative behaviors that can be discouraged and eventually changed.[29] To increase self-care and/or care of others, a written agreement may be developed by the residents and the interdisciplinary team that identifies specific behaviors such as making their beds a certain number of days per week with contingent reinforcement such as coupons to the snack or gift shop.

The finding from this study, that clients perceive that other factors in addition to those generally presented in the literature have as much, if not more, of an impact on their quality of life, also has implications for nursing care. This finding suggests that nurses, rather than assuming they know what will lend quality to a patient's life, ask patients what is important to them. Ferrans has begun to do this on a formal basis in developing a quality of life instrument that addresses not only content areas but also the relative importance of each area to a given patient.[23]

Nurses can assess on an individual basis what is especially important to patients by asking them what could be done to make their lives in the nursing home more rewarding. Very often these changes will relate to the patients' ideas of what is important in life or the goal of their life. Traditionally, quality of life scholars have assumed that personal happiness and comfort is the goal of all people. However, Holmes questions this single-minded-goal thinking. He suggests increasing one's understanding and helping others as additional and/or alternative goals. Holmes encourages patient participation in achieving whatever goals are important to a particular patient. This participation is a natural corollary to the holistic approach in which health care is viewed as a nurse-patient partnership.[18]

Furthermore, federal regulations require that facilities "must care for their residents in a manner and in an environment that promotes maintenance or enhancement of each resident's quality of life."[30] This responsibility and challenge to all long-term care providers for improving quality of life for residents is not only mandated by government regulations; as our study shows it has been demanded by residents that such a challenge be accepted. Maintaining an individual philosophy of promoting the highest level of independence in residents by promoting self-care and care of others may not be an easy task. However, the gain is significant, and the quality of life far greater because of the effort.

REFERENCES

1. Walker S, Rosser R. *Quality of life: Assessment and application.* Lancaster: MTP Press Limited, 1988:9-49.
2. Mukherjee R. *The quality of life: Valuation in social research.* New Delhi, India: Sage Publications, 1989:15-21.
3. Szalai A, Andrews F. *The quality of life: Comparative studies.* London: Sage Publications, 1980:7-17.
4. Clark P, Bowling A. Quality of everyday life in long-stay institutions for the elderly: An observational study of long-stay hospital and nursing home care. *Soc Sci Med.* 1990;30(11):1201-1210.
5. Cox C, Kaeser L, Montgomery A, Marion L. Quality of life nursing care: An experimental trial in long-term care. *J Gerontol Nurs.* 1991;17(4):6-11.
6. Huss M, Buckwalter K, Stolley J. Nursing's impact on life satisfaction. *J Gerontol Nurs.* 1988;14(5):31-36.
7. Kahana E. A congruence model of person-environment interaction. In: Lawton M, Windely P, Byerts T, eds. *Aging and the environment: Theoretical approaches.* New York: Springer, 1982:97-121.
8. Kayser-Jones J. The environment and quality of life in long-term care institutions. *Nurs Health Care.* 1989;10(3):121-130.
9. Koncelik J. *Designing the open nursing home.* Stroudsburg: Dowden, Hutchison, Ross, 1976.
10. Moos R. Specialized living environments for older people: A conceptual framework for evaluation. *J Social Issues.* 1980;36:75-96.
11. Paunonen M, Haggman-Laitila A. Life situation of aged home-nursing clients. *J Community Health Nurs.* 1990;7(3):167-178.
12. Ross M. Time-use in later life. *J Advanced Nurs.* 1990;15(4):394-399.
13. Oleson M, Heading C, Shadick K, Bistodeau J. Quality of life in long-stay institutions in England: Nurse and resident perceptions. *J Adv Nurs.* 1994;20(1):23-32.
14. Najman J, Levine S. Evaluating the impact of medical care and technologies on the quality of life: A review and critique. *Soc Sci Med.* 1981;15:107-115.
15. Sutcliffe J, Holmes S. Quality of life: Verification and use of a self-assessment scale in two patient populations. *J Adv Nurs.* 1991;16(4):490-498.
16. Zlotnick C, Decker R. Home visiting outcomes and quality of life measures. *J Community Health Nurs.* 1991;8(4):207-214.
17. Weick K. Organizational communication: Toward a research agenda. In: Putnam L, Pacanowsky M, eds. *Communication and organizations— an interpretive approach.* Beverly Hills, CA: Sage Publications, 1983:13-29.
18. Holmes CA. Health care and the quality of life: A review. *J Adv Nurs.* 1989;14(10):833-839.
19. West M, Bondy E, Hutchinson S. Interviewing institutionalized elders: Threats to validity. *Image J Nurs Sch.* 1991;23(3):171-176.
20. Dobbert M. *Ethnographic Research.* New York: Praeger, 1982.
21. Krippendorf K. *Content analysis: An introduction to its methodology.* Beverly Hills, CA: Sage Publications, 1980.
22. Goodinson S, Singleton J. Quality of life: A critical review of current concepts, measures, and their clinical implications. *Int J Nurs Stud.* 1989;26(4):327-341.
23. Ferrans CE. Development of a quality of life index for patients with cancer. *Oncol Nurs Forum.* 1990;17(3):15-19.
24. Ferrans C, Powers M. Quality of life index: Development and psychometric properties. *ANS.* 1985;8(1):15-24.
25. Faucett J, Ellis V, Underwood P, Naqvi A, Wilson D. The effects of Orem's self-care model on nursing care in a nursing home setting. *J Adv Nurs.* 1990;15(6):659-666.
26. Dawson P, Kline K, Wiancko D, Wells D. Preventing excess disability in patients with Alzheimer's disease. *Geriatr Nurs.* 1986;7(6):298-301.
27. Salisbury S. Preventing excess disability. In *Clinical Gerontological Nursing.* Philadelphia: W.B. Saunders Company, 1991.
28. Pearson A, Hocking S, Mott S, Riggs A. Quality of care in nursing homes: From the resident's perspective. *J Adv Nurs.* 1993;18(1):20-24.
29. Boehm S. Patient contracting. In: Bulechek G, McCloskey J, eds. *Nursing Interventions: Essential Nursing Treatments.* Philadelphia: W.B. Saunders Company, 1992.
30. Health Care Financing Administration. *The Long Term Care Survey.* Washington, D.C., Federal Register, Health Care Financing Administration, 1991.

Chapter 4

Nursing Home Quality Perceptions

Mary Bliesmer, DNSc, RN, GNP-C, and Pat Earle, MS, RN

OVERVIEW

The residents and nursing staff of two private nursing homes in a midwestern metropolitan community were sampled to measure the perceived importance and frequency of 17 specific Quality Care Indicators (QCIs) previously identified by the National Citizens' Coalition for Nursing Home Reform. Minimal to moderate congruence was found between resident and staff perceptions of the importance and occurrence of QCIs. Use of these validated QCIs for evaluating and improving nursing home care would demonstrate a commitment to quality that goes beyond responding to the requirements of external regulators. QCI will enhance the practice of gerontological nurses and, more importantly, provide residents with the motivation to accept responsibility for their care.

INTRODUCTION

One of our nation's most challenging health care problems is providing quality care for culturally diverse nursing home residents. Those of us who desire to evaluate and improve the quality of care provided in nursing homes must attempt to define this quality in specific terms even though it is a product of many factors.

Tellis-Nayak offers a simple statement about the subjective meaning of quality in a nursing home. "You have high quality when the nursing home resident is satisfied—with oneself, with the nursing home, and with the care one receives."[1] However, a consensus has not yet been reached concerning objective standards for quality of care measurement. Donabedian describes three categories from which inferences can be drawn about the quality of care:

- Structure—the attributes of the settings in which care occurs
- Process—what is actually done in giving and receiving care
- Outcome—the effects of care on the health status of patients and populations.[2]

Historically, structure and process approaches to quality measurement have been used extensively. Recently, the outcome approach has been emphasized. The Health Care Financing Administration has shifted its focus from merely looking to see if a facility has the capacity to provide care to looking at the quality of care that is actually being delivered.[3]

LeSage bases her concern about the quality of nursing home care delivery in the future on several factors: demographics, a possible decrease in functional level of future nursing home residents, governmental fiscal constraints, an inadequate regulatory environment, and possible conflicts between quality of care and life.[4]

A 1995 study that investigated the quality of life of community nursing home residents reported that the ability to perform activities of daily living was most closely associated with a positive perception of quality of life.[5] In this study, 120 residents answered a series of questions with more than 40% rating their quality of life as average and 45% rating it as outstanding or better than average.

QUALITY CARE INDICATORS

Consumer knowledge related to quality of care, especially in nursing homes, has not been appreciated until recently. However, Merry emphasizes that consumers are a force to be reckoned with,[6] and Davies asserts that information collected from consumers is valuable.[7] At this time, government regulation of long-term care may not receive the same high priority it had in the past. Kane suggests that the regulatory system collect information that is reliable, accurate, and derived from the residents themselves as much as possible. Also, the system should look at quality indicators that are meaningful to the residents, reflecting structures and processes they value and outcomes they desire.[8]

Roberts reports that residents' viewpoints about their care are increasingly being recognized as important because the institution is their "home." However, they caution that some nursing home residents may give prejudiced responses, choosing not to make negative comments about their care for fear of retaliation.[9] Nevertheless, consumers are the reason for the service, and health care providers should elicit their views in order to make an honest attempt to meet their needs.

The Joint Commission on Accreditation of Healthcare Organizations defines an indicator as an identified component or outcome that is indicative of either high- or low-quality care. "Indicators are measurable components of resident care that can be monitored so that long-term care professionals can determine the quality of services being provided."[10]

What residents view as important indicators of quality of care may differ from what caregivers view as important. Kolata reported specific results of a study that discovered the differing views of residents and nursing assistants about residents' concerns of daily life. What residents wanted most was to leave the home for short periods of time. Secondly, they wanted to use a telephone to contact family and friends. In contrast, assistants thought that residents would be most concerned with choosing their activities at the home, a choice that residents ranked fifth of 10. The aides ranked leaving the home third, and using the phone 10th.[11]

Indicators of quality of care judged as important to nursing home residents were identified in a study completed by the National Citizens' Coalition for Nursing Home Reform (NCCNHR) in 1985.[12] More than 450 residents from 105 nursing homes throughout the United States volunteered to participate in open-ended discussion sessions and provided a collective answer to the question "What is quality care?" Specific quality indicators were identified and ranked according to the number of times discussed: staff, environmental factors, food, activities, medical care, cleanliness, administration, religion, resident council/resident rights, and transportation.

RESEARCH QUESTIONS

Do other nursing home residents view these indicators as important? Do nursing staffs have similar views about these indicators? What is the perceived frequency of occurrence of these indicators of quality in nursing homes? Is there a positive relationship between reports of importance and frequency?

METHOD

Seventeen specific Quality Care Indicators (QCIs), identified in the NCCNHR study, were the basis of two slightly different instruments used to measure the perceived importance and frequency of quality indicators in two private nursing homes (NH-A and NH-B) in a midwestern metropolitan community during the summer of 1989. The specific quality indicators were the following: good staff attitude, prompt attention, home-like atmosphere, privacy in room, variety of food, broad range of activities, daily activity choices, physician availability, privacy with physician, room cleanliness, bathroom cleanliness, strong administration, practice of religion, rights respected, opportunity for community activities, vehicle transportation, and problem resolution.

Responses related to each QCI were elicited for both importance of the indicator and frequency of occurrence. Following are two examples of instrument items: "How important is it that a broad range of activities are available?" and "What percentage of time are a broad range of activities available?" The importance items were based on a 5-point scale: very important (5) to not important (1). The frequency items were answered on a percentage scale ranging from 100% to 0%.

Since not all residents in Nursing Home A (NH-A) were able to quantify their responses, the instrument was modified prior to use at Nursing Home B (NH-B). The importance items were changed; for example, "Is it important that a broad range of activities are available?" Items were answered no (1) or yes. If the answer was yes, the resident was then asked "How important: somewhat (3) or very (5)?" The frequency items were based on a 4-point scale: always (4) to never (1).

The instruments were completed by the author during interviews with 15 residents who were able and willing to participate in each setting. The interviewees were randomly selected from lists of residents provided by nurse managers. Five registered nurses (RNs), five licensed practical nurses (LPNs), and five certified nurses' aides (CNAs) were randomly selected from the staff lists at each home, and they completed the instrument on their own. All 15 members of the nursing staff at NH-A completed the instrument; 11 of the 15 selected at NH-B (four RNs, three LPNs, and four CNAs) completed the instrument.

All levels of nursing staff were included because each level had definite responsibilities for resident care. As much as 90% of resident care may be delivered by nurses' aides.[13] The same instrument was used with both residents and nursing staff in each setting to determine if there was quality perception agreement.

RESULTS

NURSING HOME A

NH-A has 76 beds and is the health care facility of a non-profit retirement community affiliated with the United Church of Christ. The ages of the 15 white female resident cases in NH-A ranged from 84 to 96 years. Twelve were widows, two single, and one married. The educational level of these residents was higher than the majority of the NCCNHR study subjects. Five had some college education and six had graduated from college. Length of time in NH-A ranged from 2 months to 11 years. It is not known whether these residents' characteristics were representative of the other residents in the home.

Not all residents rated either the importance or percentage of occurrence of the QCIs. They did not seem to understand some of the indicators (eg, strong administration) and could not personally relate to others (eg, problem resolution). Several said they didn't need a doctor often and didn't have any problems. The majority of those who chose to respond rated all of the QCIs as either very important or somewhat important. Notably, a small number of residents rated certain indicators as unimportant or somewhat unimportant: broad range of activities, community activities, and vehicle transportation. The resident's physical abilities and/or lack of desire were the reasons for these ratings.

The age range of the 15 nursing staff (five of each level) was 25 to 60 years. The length of time these staff members had worked at NH-A ranged from 3 months to 9.5 years; two CNAs did not provide this information. The great majority of the staff also rated the QCIs as important. The QCIs ranked by NH-A residents and staff as most important and most frequently occurring are listed in Table 4-1.

NURSING HOME B

NH-B has 172 beds in the health care center portion of a nonprofit retirement community affiliated with the Presbyterian church. The ages of the 15 white residents in NH-B ranged from 83 to 100 years. Nine women were widows, four were single. One man was married and the other was a widower. The residents were well educated; five had some college education, four completed college, and one completed graduate work. Length of time in NH-B ranged from 2 months to 4 years. As in NH-A, it is not known whether these residents' characteristics were representative of the remainder of residents.

More responses were obtained using the modified format and the majority of the residents rated the QCIs as important. However, certain indicators were again perceived as not important by some residents: broad range of activities, physician availability, privacy with physician, opportunity to practice religion, community activities, and vehicle transportation. As in NH-A, physical abilities and/or lack of desire were the reasons for these ratings.

Twice as many responses to frequency of occurrence were obtained than in NH-A. However, in both settings only six or less even rated three of the quality indicators: community activities, vehicle transportation, and problem resolution. It was often the case that they personally did not participate in community activities, "did not want to" or "were not able to" use vehicle transportation, and didn't have any problems.

TABLE 4-1

Quality Care Indicators: Most Important and Highest Occurrence

RESIDENTS	STAFF
Nursing Home A	
Most Important	
• Bathroom cleanliness	• Home-like atmosphere
• Good staff attitude	• Good staff attitude
• Opportunity to practice religion	• Opportunity to practice religion
• Rights respected	• Rights respected
• Room cleanliness	• Broad range of activities
• Prompt attention	• Prompt attention
• Variety of food	• Vehicle transportation
Highest Occurrence	
• Physician availability	• Home-like atmosphere
• Bathroom cleanliness	• Bathroom cleanliness
• Room cleanliness	• Room cleanliness
• Opportunity to practice religion	• Opportunity to practice religion
• Community activities	• Rights respected
• Good staff attitude	• Prompt attention
Nursing Home B	
Most Important	
• Good staff attitude	• Good staff attitude
• Prompt attention	• Prompt attention
• Privacy in room	• Privacy in room
• Problem resolution	• Physician availability
• Bathroom cleanliness	• Bathroom cleanliness
• Room cleanliness	• Room cleanliness
• Daily activity choices	• Privacy with physician
Highest Occurrence	
• Privacy with physician	• Prompt attention
• Opportunity to practice religion	• Opportunity to practice religion
• Bathroom cleanliness	• Bathroom cleanliness
• Room cleanliness	• Room cleanliness
• Daily activity choices	• Rights respected
• Rights respected	• Strong administration
	• Privacy in room
	• Problem resolution

The age range of the 11 nursing staff (four RNs, three LPNs, and four CNAs) in NH-B was 27 to 57 years. Length of time at NH-B ranged from 4 months to 14 years. All the staff rated the QCIs as important. See Table 4-1 for the most important and most frequent QCIs in NH-B.

DATA ANALYSIS AND INTERPRETATION

Ideally, there should be congruence between residents' and staffs' perceptions of the importance and occurrence of indicators of quality in a nursing home setting. However, minimal to moderate congruence of perceptions was found in this study. The importance of three QCIs was ranked highly by residents in both NH-A and NH-B: good staff attitudes, room cleanliness, and bathroom cleanliness. The importance of prompt staff attention and respecting residents' rights was ranked highly by nursing staff in both settings. Residents in both settings ranked three QCIs highly for frequency of occurrence: room cleanliness, bathroom cleanliness, and the opportunity to practice religion. Five QCIs were ranked highly by staff for frequency of occurrence in both settings: prompt attention, room cleanliness, bathroom cleanliness, opportunity to practice religion, and rights respected (see Table 4-1).

Range of nursing home activities, opportunity for community activities, and vehicle transportation were ranked very low in importance by residents in both settings, while daily activity choices and community activities were ranked very low by staff. Physician availability was given a middle to low importance ranking by the residents in both settings and the staff in NH-A; it was ranked at the top by staff in NH-B. Also, residents in both settings felt that physicians were available when needed, but staff did not agree.

The frequency of privacy when seeing their physician was given the top ranking by residents in NH-B but staff ranked this QCI frequency very low. Perhaps the physicians see these residents privately in their rooms when the staff is not aware of it. These comparisons demonstrate that residents and staff in these two nursing homes had differing perceptions of the importance and occurrence of several quality indicators. This showed the need for communication. The staff need to listen and talk with the residents about a variety of personal topics and issues.

The *t* test[13,15] was used to identify significant differences between perceptions of importance and frequency of the QCIs. A significant difference was found between resident and staff perceptions of the importance and/or frequency of several specific quality indicators (significance level of $<.05$). The residents in NH-A perceived the frequency of occurrence of all indicators higher than staff. Perhaps they didn't want to be critical of staff or they were receiving "higher quality care" than the staff thought was being provided. The residents in NH-B perceived the frequency of 11 of 17 indicators higher than staff.

Comparisons of perception of the importance of quality indicators also were made between nursing homes. No significant difference was found between the two staffs' perceptions of QCI importance. The only significant difference between resident groups was for problem resolution (t=-2.39, p=.041). However, the case numbers were small (NH-A=4 and NH-B=7). No comparison was made between perceptions of frequency of occurrence of the indicators because different scales were used for measurement in the two nursing homes.

Pearson's correlation[14] was used to discover the extent of the relationships between importance and frequency perceptions of the QCIs within each group (residents and staff) in each home. Significant moderate to strong positive relationships were found for 15 of the 17 QCIs in NH-A (Table 4-2).

The staff correlation results were not surprising since nursing personnel are in positions to influence these QCIs. If staff see the indicators as important, one would expect that they would attempt to implement them as well. The resident results that showed a strong relationship between the importance and frequency of only three indicators were not encouraging. One goal for measuring the improvement of the quality of care in a nursing home might be to demonstrate significant strong positive relationships between the importance and frequency for all indicators.

No significant relationships were found between the QCI importance and frequency perceptions of the residents in NH-B. The small number of subjects responding may be an influencing factor. Only two of the QCIs were found to have significant relationships between importance and frequency of occurrence as perceived by staff: good attitude (r=-.6500, p=.015) and vehicle transportation (r=.8729, p=.000). The negative relationship between staff attitude importance and frequency is both surprising and discouraging since good staff attitudes are extremely important to residents.

TABLE 4-2

Pearson's Correlation (NH-A)
Relationships Between Importance and Frequency of Occurrence

INDICATOR	GROUP	NUMBER OF CASES	*r*	*p*
Good staff attitude	Staff	15	.5766	.012
Prompt attention	Staff	15	.7519	.001
Home-like atmosphere	Staff	15	.7498	.001
Home-like atmosphere	Residents	5	.9855	.001
Privacy in room	Staff	15	.5384	.019
Variety of food	Residents	6	.7593	.036
Daily activity choices	Residents	8	.7093	.023
Physician availability	Staff	14	.4675	.045
Privacy with physician	Staff	14	.7507	.001
Room cleanliness	Staff	15	.8507	.000
Bathroom cleanliness	Staff	15	.9024	.000
Strong administration	Staff	13	.6782	.005
Opportunity to practice religion	Staff	15	.5767	.012
Rights respected	Staff	15	.8047	.000
Community activities	Staff	15	.8308	.000
Problem resolution	Staff	15	.6660	.003

COMPARISON WITH NCCNHR STUDY

The rankings of the quality indicators' importance differed from the 1985 NCCNHR study results, which had a n=450. The NCCNHR study differed significantly and provided the foundation for this small study. Replication of this study is advised for further validation. Staff attitudes were very important to the residents in both studies. Some comments made by residents in the current study were "Tender loving care is very important," "Staff should like to take care of old people and not push you around," "Some are very good. Some don't care whether it comes off or not," and "I'd hate to have the job of hiring here."

Cleanliness, resident rights, and the opportunity to practice their religion were also ranked considerably higher by these residents. Several residents in one home reported that the cleaning was not as complete on the weekends. When considering residents' rights they said "Such as they are, I don't have many," "I won't answer," "We don't want to become nothings," and "They don't respect each other." These homes do have a strong religious foundation, which may be an influencing factor for the high ranking of opportunity to practice religion in these homes.

Having a broad range of activities available was much less important to these residents than to those in the NCCNHR study. Several of these residents seemed somewhat disengaged from the day-to-day activities, offering such comments as "I purposely don't get involved" and "I read a lot." The self-selection of the NCCNHR study residents may be the influencing factor for their perceived importance of the availability of activities.

SUGGESTIONS FOR FUTURE QUALITY ASSESSMENT RESEARCH

Upon admission to a nursing home, and periodically thereafter, residents could be asked to rank specific quality indicators. The nursing staff could also respond to the issue of quality indicators when hired and on a regular basis throughout their term of employment. The concern about repercussions against residents if they express dissatisfaction with the quality of care could be managed by careful administration of the quality indicator assessment tool. Using individuals who do not provide care on a regular basis to collect data—such as nursing students—would provide for confidentiality, as would ensuring that the interviews were conducted in an area where privacy could be maintained. In addition, it could serendipitously allow students to develop careers in gerontological nursing.

Residents' perceptions related to quality indicators need to be assessed in a wide range of nursing homes, especially those in rural and inner-city locations. Including residents of varying racial and ethnic mix and socioeconomic level would serve to provide a more thorough understanding of what is perceived as quality care in various settings. These specific findings could then be used by the facility staff to better serve individual residents.

Meister and Boyle revised and expanded the tool used in this researcher's study and measured the differences in perception of quality between residents, nursing staff, and families in a 387-bed geriatric hospital serving a Jewish catchment area in Montreal, Canada. Ethnicity appeared to play a role in the perceptions of quality care at this facility. The Jewish residents and families were closest in their ratings to the white nursing staff and in turn these groups thought differently from the black and Asian nursing staff. Also, the nursing staff members differed from each other on several of the ratings of the indicators based on ethnicity.[12] These results indicate the need to be sensitive to cultural concerns when the quality of nursing home care is evaluated as well as the need for replication of studies dealing with nursing home quality.

GERONTOLOGICAL NURSING IMPLICATIONS

The fact that the majority of 30 residents in two nursing homes considered these 17 quality indicators (see Table 4-2) to be important further validates them as markers of the quality of care in nursing homes. Quality indicators of nursing homes could be used to assist prospective residents and their families during the important, but stressful, time of choosing an appropriate nursing home.

Often this is a time when the elderly individual feels an impending sense of loss and the family members are experiencing guilt. At the time of nursing home selection, the elderly and their families could be presented a clear picture of what is available at their future home, compared to what they see as important. Nursing staff, operating from a base of honest and ethical behavior, can develop trust and respect for the individual's autonomy by encouraging involvement in the selection procedure.

In addition, the use of a comprehensive quality assurance process that includes some or all of these indicators for evaluating and improving care in nursing homes would demonstrate a commitment to quality, which is more than a response to external regulation. Nursing staff have a great deal of power over the very vulnerable residents to whom they provide care. It is essential that an environment be created in which not only the physical care of the residents is assured, but also where residents can maintain a degree of independence and dignity—and be treated with respect. Since prompt attention was ranked important as a quality indicator, staff should make every effort to respond quickly to residents' requests.

Staff attitude was considered very important by the residents and the staff of both homes, however, its frequency of occurrence was ranked highly only by the residents of one nursing home. It is important for administrators to assure that staff attitudes are assessed and that programs are available to attend to this important issue. Attitudes of caregivers can have a profound effect on nursing home residents. The residents in this study shared their need to be comforted and cared for by staff who value them as people.

Although these residents grew up in an era of modest homes and minimal material possessions, their homes were considered important and valuable. An RN shared that "residents must be able to maintain their dignity, individuality, control, and privacy. Institutional living is often a choice a person prefers not to make. However, if it is the only alternative, a home-like environment is important." The residents in both nursing homes rated home-like atmosphere as less important and occurring less frequently than the staff ranking. This seemed rather surprising but may be explained by residents who said that, although a home-like atmosphere is indeed important, they have left their homes—recreating them is not possible.

Older adults who are admitted to a nursing home expect their rights to be respected, especially the right of privacy. Health care facilities are busy places and, unfortunately, privacy can be overlooked. Residents of differing cultures may also have expectations and customs regarding privacy of which nurses may not be aware. It is incumbent upon the nurses caring for residents to determine culturally specific needs that residents have and attempt to meet them.

Nurses can grant the resident's right to privacy by the simple act of treating the resident's room as a place where staff are outsiders who must be invited in. The "token" knock on the door as the staff enters without waiting for a reply is not acceptable. Even the need for privacy while bathing, toileting, and dressing are often overlooked and create resident discomfort. Another privacy issue is the maintenance of boundaries around the residents' personal space. Nurses may overlook this personal space when they place their equipment and supplies on residents' tables, chairs, and beds. It is important to remember that the nurses' work site is where residents live and permission should be obtained before "invading" their space.

REFERENCES

1. Tellis-Nayak V. *Nursing Home Exemplars of Quality.* Springfield, IL: Charles Thomas; 1988.
2. Donabedian A. The quality of care: how can it be assessed? *JAMA.* 1988;260(12):1743-1748.
3. U.S. Congress. Omnibus Budget Reconciliation Act of 1987. Public Law 100-203. Washington, D.C.: U. S. Government Printing Office; 1987.
4. LeSage J, Barhyte DY. *Nursing Quality Assurance in Long-Term Care.* Rockville, MD: Aspen; 1989.
5. Morley JE, Kraenzle DM, Bible B, Bundren B. Perception of quality of life by nursing home residents. *Nursing Home Medicine.* 1995;3(8):191-194.
6. Merry MD. What is quality care? A model for measuring health care excellence. *Quality Review Bulletin.* 1987;September:298-301.
7. Davies AR, Ware JE. Involving consumers in quality of care assessment. *Health Affairs.*1988;Spring:34-47.
8. Kane RA, Kane RL. Long-term care: variations on a quality assurance theme. *Inquiry.* 1988;25:132-146.
9. Roberts KL, LeSage J, Ellor JR. Quality monitoring in nursing homes. *J Gerontol Nurs.* 1987;13(10):34-40.
10. Joint Commission on Accreditation of Hospitals. *Quality Assurance in Long-Term Care.* Chicago; 1986.
11. Kolata G. Life's basic problems are still top concern in the nursing homes. *New York Times.* January 19, 1989.
12. Meister C, Boyle C, Bliesmer M. Conducting a satisfaction survey as part of a quality improvement program. In: Miller T, Rantz M. *Quality Assurance for Long-Term Care* (Supplement #5). Rockville, MD: Aspen. In press.
13. National Citizens' Coalition for Nursing Home Reform. *A Consumer Perspective on Quality Care: The Residents' Point of View.* Washington, D.C.; 1985.
14. U.S. Department of Health and Human Services. *Personnel for Health Needs of the Elderly Through Year 2020.* [Report to Congress] (NIH Publication No. 87-2950). Bethesda, MD; 1987.
15. SPSS Inc. *SPSS User's Guide.* 2nd ed. Chicago; 1986.

Chapter 5

Patient Self-Determination Act: Implications for Long-Term Care

Susan K. Madson, RNC, MSN, and Joye A. Norris, EdD

OVERVIEW

The Patient Self-Determination Act (PSDA) has been law since 1991. PSDA was enacted to ensure that all newly admitted patients in health care institutions receiving any federal funds were advised of their right to complete an advance directive, thus avoiding complicated or contentious end-of-life decisions. The results have been mixed at best, with awareness increasing but behavior not changing. While intervention efforts have proven successful, patients still prefer deferring end-of-life decisions to family members. This chapter will examine the impact of PSDA to date, based on the experience of health care facilities. It will also look into the efficacy of various implementation strategies, the issues and concerns arising from PSDA, and provided gerontological nursing implications.

INTRODUCTION

The Patient Self-Determination Act (PSDA)[1] requires institutions receiving government insurance payments to inform incoming patients of their right to decide on life-preserving measures. Patients are to be given written information explaining right-to-die and other treatment options under state law, and to provide community and staff education on advance directives. The PSDA came on the heels of a landmark case involving Nancy Cruzan, who wanted to refuse medical treatment, including artificial nutrition and hydration. Left in a coma after an automobile accident, Nancy Cruzan lay in a vegetative state for 7 years. As she neared her 32nd birthday, her family petitioned the court to allow them to withdraw life support. Although approval was granted from the court, the case moved to the Missouri Supreme Court, which reversed the lower court order. The state believed it had the right to insist on proof of Ms. Cruzan's wishes before life support could be withdrawn. The United States Supreme Court upheld the Missouri decision, as well as the right of the state to require proof.[2] The Supreme Court recognized the constitutional right of a competent patient to refuse treatment and delegated regulation of this right to the states. Thus, the move toward advance directives, already generally available but widely unused, began in earnest. Congress clarified the role of the states. Specifically, health care facilities are required to do the following:

- Provide written information to patients about their right to make decisions concerning treatment by completing advance directives;
- Ensure compliance with the requirements of the law;
- Maintain written policies and procedures with respect to advance directives;
- Document in the individual's medical record whether or not the individual has executed an advance directive;
- Educate their staff and the communities they serve about state law governing advance directives;
- Avoid any impediments to the provision of care or otherwise discriminate against an individual based on whether or not the individual has executed an advance directive.[1]

An advance directive is a general term for oral and written instructions a person makes about his or her personal medical care in the event that he or she becomes unable to speak or communicate. "Advance directive" is generally an umbrella term for living wills and durable health care powers of attorney. A living will allows competent individuals to instruct their family, physicians, and others about their wishes for medical care should they be unable to communicate at the end of life.

A second type of advance directive is the durable power of attorney for health care. It is a document through which people appoint someone they trust to make medical care decisions for them should they not be able to execute this themselves. Other names for durable power of attorney for health care are health care proxy, appointment of a health care agent, or medical proxy. In many states, the person appointed as power of attorney for health care is authorized to speak for the patient any time that person is unable to make medical decisions, not just at the end of life. All 50 states and the District of Columbia have laws recognizing the use of advance directives.[3]

THE IMPACT OF PSDA

Prior to the 1991 implementation of PSDA, it was clear to researchers that the use of advance directives was in stark contrast to the number of people who said they desired them. Emanuel[4] found that just less than 10% of Americans had completed advance directives. Fifty-seven percent of the participants studied said they wanted some kind of document that specified care at the end of life, however only 7% had such a document. Gamble[5] interviewed 75 ambulatory senior citizens at a group dining hall. Eighty-six percent of them wanted only comfort care and pain management in a terminal illness. Surprisingly, not one of these senior citizens had actually signed a living will.

The passage of PSDA led to great expectations, beyond what was actually specified in the law. The obvious expectations would be that patients would become more aware of advance directives and subsequently more patients would complete them. A review of the literature after PSDA reveals an increased awareness of advance directives but not increased use. Park[6] investigated the impact of PSDA at hospitals in the state of Georgia. Hospital administrators were asked about present procedures for implementing the law and the perceived effect. Most of the responding hospitals complied with PSDA by providing patients with written explanations of state law regarding advance directives. They did not initiate discussions about the subject. Although not required by PSDA, 25% of the responding hospital administrators gave all patients forms for advance directives. One-third provided routine verbal explanations of advance directives. Seventy percent offered the patients an opportunity to ask questions. Another 10% provided their patients with a video explaining advance directives.

Admission was the most common time for patients to receive information on advance directives. No formal procedures existed that allowed staff to ascertain or evaluate if patients understood the material. The length of time taken to explain the information to each patient was approximately 10 minutes with 43% reporting that less than five minutes was taken. The hospital administrators also thought it was their role to inform patients about their rights to execute advance directives, however they did not see their role in education or in encouraging the use of advance directives. They were reluctant to go beyond the minimal legal mandate.

When asked about the number of advance directives in effect now versus prior to PSDA, respondents believed the percentage had gone from 3% to about 12%. Respondents were asked to choose the three major problems with PSDA. A list of eight problems were provided. The top choices were inappropriateness of the time of hospital admission for discussing advance directives and the difficulty in presenting information of this complexity to patients.

Robinson[7] also found a very low incidence of completion of advance directives. A telephone survey was administered to patients who had been hospitalized before PSDA and to patients hospitalized after PSDA. The questions probed patient knowledge about living wills and behavior toward obtaining living wills. The authors hypothesized that successful implementation of the PSDA should generate two measurable results: patients' knowledge about advance directives should increase if they were hospitalized after PSDA...and patient behavior should be affected.

Jacobson[8] learned that having completed an advance directive did not necessarily mean having an understanding of them. The researchers studied the awareness, understanding, and use of advance directives, using a 500-bed acute care hospital in Utah as their focal point. Interviews were completed with former patients hospitalized before PSDA (*n*=202) and patients hospitalized within the last 48 hours with PSDA implementation in effect. The researchers found no significant differences in the understanding of living wills and powers of attorney between the two groups. Before PSDA, 15% of the subjects interviewed reported having completed a living will and 5% a durable power of attorney for health care. After PSDA, the figures were 18% and 7% respectively. When knowledge of the documents was probed, patients who had completed advance directives showed no difference in understanding of their meaning than those who had not completed them. According to the researchers, 21% of all respondents thought physicians should ignore living wills or proxies if the physician or family members thought it was best. Another 15% were not sure.

INTERVENTION STUDIES

Several researchers have been interested in examining the effect of advance directive interventions. Sachs[9] tried an intervention with 48 non-demented outpatients aged 65 and older. Participants taking part in interviews about advance directives were given forms for preparing a living will and were also sent reminder cards. When compared after six months with a control group that did not receive the intervention, the experimental participants had not significantly increased completing advance directives.

In another study, High[10] tested the efficacy of various types of educational materials and provided free legal advice. Four hundred and thirty-one seniors were recruited from three different settings to serve as an experimental group. The experimental participants were divided into six groups. Group 1 received minimal educational materials, group 2 moderate materials, and group 3 maximum materials. The remaining three groups received materials in the same way, but also had the opportunity to attend a meeting about advance directives. A post-study examination revealed that knowledge of living wills did not significantly increase in the experimental group, but knowledge of choosing a health care surrogate decision maker did. When the six groups were compared in terms of the intervention, the only group showing a significant increase in completing advance directives was the group receiving moderate educational materials and a follow-up meeting.

Markson[11] looked at overcoming barriers to completing advance directives by focusing on physician intervention. A total of 10 physicians (six at a primary care physician home care service and four at a primary care nursing home service) were given a five-week course on the law relating to advance directives in their state. They were then asked to discuss advance directives with their newly enrolled patients and to assist those patients with completing the documents. In a two-month period, no new patients were approached by the doctors. The study was changed, therefore, to include all active patients. The physicians were given additional training that allowed them to observe, lead discussions, and answer questions about advance directives. Of the 116 patients approached by the physicians, 73% of them completed advance directives, with most of them choosing relatives as proxies. The authors concluded that teaching physicians about the law was not enough—they also had to be taught how to approach the subject and how to lead discussions.

Luptak[12] designed an intervention for elderly living in community dwellings who were identified as high risk for hospital admission. The participants were part of an experimental geriatric evaluation and management clinic. They were to receive comprehensive evaluation and treatment for 2 to 4 months at the experimental clinic and then return to their regular physicians. Thirty-four people received the intervention. First, a social worker conducted a face-to-face interview with the participants on their first visit to the clinic. The patients were given both verbal and written information about advance directives and also were given the appropriate forms. They were encouraged to ask questions, to take the material home to study, and to discuss it with their families. Dialogue about advance directives continued throughout the remaining clinic visits, with physicians involved along with other clinic staff. The total intervention took 60 minutes, longer if the patient requested help in preparing advance directives. The result was that 24 out of 34 patients recorded advance directives (70.6%). It appears that use of advance directives does increase when introduction to the subject goes beyond handing out information at admissions.

NURSING RESEARCH AND PSDA

Research reveals that nurses are more comfortable discussing advance directives and the requirements of PSDA than their physician colleagues.[13,14] Silverman,[15] in a qualitative study, examined nurses' attitudes and feelings about their role in implementing PSDA. Twenty nurses from a 750-bed acute care university hospital in Baltimore were interviewed about their perspectives on the hospital's PSDA program and their role in it. At this hospital, the nurses had the primary responsibility to implement PSDA. Specifically, they:

1. Asked adult patients if they had an advance directive prepared
2. Documented in the patient record
3. Provided patients with the hospital-developed brochure about advance directives
4. Offered the services of a social worker or chaplain in preparing advance directives.

The results of this qualitative study confirm the overall sentiment that admission is a poor time for discussing advance directives. The nurses were concerned about causing their patients unnecessary anxiety and quickly developed strategies to minimize it on their own. Although the nurses described several instances where raising the subject of advance directives was helpful to patients and their families, they were mostly skeptical about the benefit of the admissions intervention. It was felt that most patients were not interested in further information or discussions. One nurse claimed, "I think we're fulfilling the requirement that the government sets down, but I'm not sure what we're doing is adequate."[16]

The nurses believed the program had the potential to advance patient autonomy and to improve communication among patients, family members, and physicians regarding medical decisions. Since nurses often develop strong relationships with their patients and could better handle the emotional components, it was felt that they would be a likely professional to educate patients.

Nurses expressing a sense of responsibility for PSDA are supported by their professional association. Stepping out in front of PSDA early on, the American Nurses Association (ANA) took the position that nurses had a responsibility to play a primary role in PSDA implementation. The ANA felt it was imperative that the decision making that will fall to patients and their families as they make choices about end of life care be facilitated by nurses.[17] The ANA made it clear they supported the patients' rights to self-determination, the role of nurses in ensuring that right, and the need for more extensive education of nurses on the content and facilitation of advance directives.

CONCERNS AND CONSIDERATIONS

Health PSDAs are a continuing dilemma between care professionals and ethicists. A concern that has drawn attention in the literature is that families are systematically being discounted as capable decision makers and being removed from end-of-life decisions. Those patients who do complete advance directives overwhelmingly choose family members as surrogate decision makers, while those who do not complete advance directives also rely on family members to make end-of-life decisions. High believes this state of affairs is quite appropriate and badly undervalued in the name of patient autonomy.[16] According to High, "the rush to advocate advance written directives places the emphasis on legalistic solutions to what are primarily moral issues concerning a fundamental communication process involving patient, medical professional, and family relationships." People who complete advance directives, noted High, have little interest in the actual document. He cites evidence that elderly people overwhelmingly prefer informal practices of communication to the formality of written documents. High recommends increased examination of the family decision making process that occurs so that "we are no longer surprised and suspicious when an informal system of tradition and custom works well." The societal value placed on individual autonomy may be undermining the family in general, and quite specifically in the move toward advance directives. High believes gerontology professionals will be faced with the task of encouraging the elderly's link to family not only for caregiving but for surrogate decision making.

Emanuel[18] holds a different view towards leaving end-of-life decisions to the family and decries the traditional decision making process when families have to handle the situation. Problems with this approach include "chaotic, emotional decisions, family and medical team divisiveness, and, ultimately, decisions that may cause unnecessary suffering and fail to honor the patient's prior wishes." Zweibel[19] found that many elderly people rely on family members to make decisions about life sustaining treatment, but that few older people discuss their treatment preferences for end-of-life care with family or physicians. When asked, families made decisions opposite of what the patient wanted 24% to 50% of the time. The larger issue appears to be communication—or the lack of it—among patients, their families, and their medical professionals. There is little evidence that communication is improving after PSDA, which could ultimately minimize the need for advance directives in the first place.

GERONTOLOGICAL NURSING IMPLICATIONS

Most of the research shows a strong relationship between age and the completion of advance directives, which, while seeming obvious, has major implications for gerontological nurses. The most likely health care professionals dealing with PSDA will be nurses. They will be called upon to lead discussions about advance directives, initiate interactions with patients, physicians, and family, and at times the carrying out of advance directives. Nurses have already been shown to be more comfortable with the concepts, issues, and discussions about advance directives.

Nurses have an important role to play, regardless of approach to PSDA—from the need for legal documents to maintain autonomy and the right to die, to the need to improve communications among all parties involved. Nursing research supports the fact that information sharing at the time of admission is a poor and ineffective time for encouraging completion of advance directives and that patients rely heavily on family members to help with end-of-life decisions, preferring them to medical staff. Professional nurses know that completion of advance directives can be dramatically improved with interventions as simple as meetings and as complex as a 2- to 4-month team approach. Nurses can be the catalyst in improving communication between the physician and the family in order to promote a comprehensive approach to end-of-life decisions.

In order for nurses to expand their role in the implementation of PSDA, they will have to become more knowledgeable and practiced in several areas. One area in particular will be dealing with those patients who are not mentally competent to complete advance directives.[20,21] Working with families and institutional ethics committees will be an urgent priority. Nurses will also have to gain a better understanding of cultural differences and the varying roles of families. Especially critical will be their grasp of their respective states' laws about advance directives. Working with their own state nurses' associations (SNA) and other state associations, eg, the state hospital association and medical societies, will enhance their role. All of these various groups have an interest in PSDA and have spent time developing materials to help patients learn more about their role in PSDA. Nurses will be playing an increasing role in the development of policies and protocols for advance directives, an area already identified as problematic.[3] Communication will be the key to skill development and knowledge about PSDAs. Gerontological nurses are in a unique position to promote the health of their older patients and protect their wishes at the final stage of life.

REFERENCES

1. *Omnibus Budget Reconciliation Act of 1990*, P.L. 101-508,4206 and 4751, codified at 42 U.S.C. 1395 cc (a)(1)(Q), 1395 mm (c)(8), 1395 cc (f), 1396a(57), (58), 1396a(w).
2. Cruzan V. Director, Missouri Department of Health, 397 U.S. 261, 110 S. Ct. 2841, 1990.
3. Madson SK. Patient self determination act: Implications for long term care. *J Gerontol Nurs*. 1993;19(2):15-18.
4. Emanuel LL, Barry MJ, Stoeckle JD, Ettelson LM, Emanuel EJ. Advance directives for medical care: a case for greater use. *N Eng J Med*. 1991;324(13):889-895.
5. Gamble ER, McDonald PJ, Lichstein PR. Knowledge, attitudes, and behavior of elderly persons regarding living wills. *Arch Int Med*. 1991;151(2):277-280.
6. Park DC, Eaton TA, Larson EJ, Palmer HT. Implementation and impact of the patient self determination act. *South Med J*. 1994;87(10):971-977.
7. Robinson MK, DeHaven MJ, Koch KA. Effects of the patient self determination act on patient knowledge and behavior. *J Fam Prac*. 1993;37(4):363-368.
8. Jacobson JA, White BE, Battin MP, Francis LP, Green DJ, Kasworm ES. Patients' understanding and uses of advance directives. *West J Med*. 1994;160(3):232-236.
9. Sachs GA, Stocking CB, Miles SH. Empowerment of the older patient? A randomized, controlled trial to increase discussion and use of advance directives. *J Am Geriat Soc*. 1992;40(3):269-273.
10. High DM. Advance directives and the elderly: a study of intervention strategies to increase use. *Gerontologist*. 1993;33(3):342-349.
11. Markson LJ, Fanale J, Steel K, Kern D, Anna G. Implementing advance directives in the primary care setting. *Arch Int Med*. 1994;154(20):2321-2327.
12. Luptak MK, Boult C. A method for increasing elders' use of advance directives. *Gerontologist*. 1994;34(3):409-412.
13. Shore AD, Rubin HR, Haisfield ME. Health care providers and cancer patients' preferences regarding disclosure of information about advance directives. *J Psychosoc Oncol*. 1993;11(4):39-53.
14. Kelner M, Bourgeault IL, Hebert PC, Dunn EV. Advance directives: the views of health care professionals. *Can Med Assoc J*. 1993;148(8):1331-1338.
15. Silverman HJ, Fry ST, Armistead N. Nurses' perspectives on implementation of the patient self determination act. *J Clin Ethics*. 1994;5:30-37.
16. High DM. A new myth about families of older people? *Gerontologist*. 1991;31(5):611-617.
17. American Nurses Association. *Position Statement on Nursing and the Patient Self-Determination Act*. Washington, D.C.: American Nurses Association; 1991.
18. Emanuel L. Appropriate and inappropriate use of advance directives. *J Clin Ethics*. 1994;5(4):357-359.
19. Zweibel N, Cassel CK. Treatment choices at the end of life: a comparison of decisions by older patients and their physician-selected proxies. *Gerontologist*. 1989;29:615-621.
20. Janofsky JS, Rovner BW. Prevalence of advance directives and guardianship in nursing home patients. *J Geriatr Psychiatry Neurol*. 1993;6:214-216.
21. Emanuel L. Advance directives: what have we learned so far? *J Clin Ethics*. 1993;4(1):8-11.

Chapter 6

Gerontology, Spirituality, and Nursing

Richard Barry, MDiv, MLS, and Donald J. Joyce, OMI, MLS, MDiv

OVERVIEW

The nursing process operates beyond the biological and physical realities; it incorporates a holistic framework that also includes spirituality. By touching another human being, a unique encounter is established that is personal, intangible, transcendent, and spiritual. Dealing with abstract realities are difficult, yet spiritual caregiving involves a reality that exercises heart, hope, empathy, and silence. Encountering patients in a holistic manner provides enrichment for nurses and patients open to many possibilities. Spirituality is a unique individual coping mechanism that allows each of us to filter our experiences meaningfully. This chapter will alert and challenge nurses and institutions to assess for and provide spiritual care for their older patients.

INTRODUCTION

Glue is a familiar product that we are introduced to early in life. In childhood, it bonds together our material creations, the fruit of innate abilities. Spirituality is a glue that bonds together various dimensions of an individual personality. This spiritual glue also becomes familiar early in life. As children we ask, "why?" to everything, including the birth of siblings, death of pets, story characters, national civil holidays, blue sky, and green grass. Outlooks, opinions, values, moments of truth, decisions, and conclusions that make up an individual's understanding of the self, others, and the world constitutes an introduction to his or her spirituality. The trials and tribulations; successes and failures; joys and sorrows; boredom and excitement; and loneliness and friendship are experiences that help to form within each person an outlook on life, a personal philosophy, a spirituality.

How an individual perceives life happening for him or her is a dimension of spirituality. The level of meaning that an individual brings to each moment of existence and experience is part of spirituality. Acceptance or rejection of the facts of daily life constitute an individual's spirituality. Spirituality is a personal, unique part of personality. The beauty of something so personal is that aspects of individual spirituality are common to many. Nuances of meaning on the understanding of life and how each of us fits in, once shared and confirmed, bond us with one another to a power greater than ourselves, which empowers each of us in our own way.

Elderly people have had many life experiences upon which to craft a spirituality. It exists even if it is not named spirituality or exercised as a filter to draw meaning and value from the world. The elderly approaching the inevitability of death find death as a mirror allowing evaluation and reflection upon their individual journey. A particular health crisis or life-threatening disease shortens the path and intensifies the preparation. Vulnerability and a fragile sense of self are characteristic at such a time, calling for increased sensitivity and gentleness on the part of health care providers.

The ability to sense this dimension in individual patients is vital to nursing care. Florence Nightingale infused touching this core human reality into the art and care of nursing.[1] Not to know or be sensitive to this character dimension is like being with a patient who speaks a foreign language or has a different culture: genuine nursing care cannot be provided. Medical treatment attempts to eliminate disease, and nursing care incorporates the person's environment to achieve and sustain a healthy state. Attention to the intangible realities impacting upon health is that unique dimension of nursing and the unique quality of each and every nurse. Being sensitive to the spiritual dimensions of the patient is imperative to the healing process. Clearly, if the nurse does not recognize, assess for, or discuss spirituality with the patient, it will be missed and may interfere with the outcome of patient care.

Spirituality as discussed so far has not mentioned religion, since religion is part of spirituality. Religion involves the personal relationship of an individual to a deity. Religion's goal is to develop and fine tune the spiritual dimensions of life. Spirituality is a broad inclusive innate characteristic that allows individuals to interact with reality to understand it and give meaning to what is experienced. Spiritual development, like many other innate human qualities, is different for each person. There are no national standards set for spirituality, and each personal formulation is valid for that individual.

SPIRITUALITY IN NURSING

Florence Nightingale gave substance to the care of individuals, both physically and spiritually. *Notes on Nursing* and *Suggestions for Thought* contain within them her spiritual philosophy for herself personally, attitude toward patient care, and relationship to the world in general.[1] This touches upon the core elements of the abstract reality in which rational beings have some sort of relationship with self, the world, and a reality greater than the self.[2]

Diverse disciplines have looked into the phenomenon of spirituality in the healing relationship. Some research approaches it in a problem-solving fashion,[3] while others attempt to contain and classify the process.[4] Some lean toward the religious dimensions, others shy away, and the psychosocial approaches are available for those who desire them. The approach or framework seems to matter little in the long run, since each of these evolves to a similar reality: there is a transcendent value in life, and it is a part of the nursing process.[5,6]

The term spiritual well-being grew out of the 1971 White House Conference on Aging: "Spiritual well-being is the affirmation of life in a relationship with God, self, community, and environment that nurtures and celebrates wholeness."[7] The holistic nature of nursing practice led the North American Nursing Diagnosis Association (NANDA) to approve "spiritual distress" as a diagnostic category.[8] It is defined as "the state in which the individual experiences or is at risk of experiencing a disturbance in the belief or value system that provides strength, hope, and meaning to his life." Eliopoulos[9] discusses the causative factors:

- Health problems, which are the effects and care requirements of illness, that interfere with the practice of religious rituals or attendance at religious services.
- Hospitalization, institutionalization, which is the inaccessibility to one's religious organization, restrictions imposed by the plan of care, confinement, isolation, and embarrassment at practicing spiritual rituals in front of others. These can create barriers to fulfilling religious needs.
- Attitudes of others that may conflict between the patient's belief and what others see as good or reasonable. The patient, for example, or the family may oppose the patient's choosing prayer with a spiritual healer over surgical intervention.

These characteristics are triggers to alert the nurse in assessing for the spiritual needs of patients. Older people enter the health care environment in a fearful state, frequently not knowing what lies ahead. They have a foreshortened life span and are preoccupied with death.

Attention to patients with spiritual distress is not disputed. Taking this NANDA distress approach, though, may be operating from a perspective of crisis. That is to say until a patient is diagnosed with malnutrition we cannot feed them. Nourishment, in all of its forms, is an ongoing process. When we cannot nourish ourselves, we require the assistance of others. All patients need spiritual care, whose intensity varies with circumstances. Additionally, approaching patients to assess for spiritual distress implies the nurse can best address the situation. The nurse assesses, diagnoses, and treats many physical realities, however it is the chaplain or clergy person who must be called upon to decide what is best for the care of this spirit/soul.[3] This indicates the value of having community religious leaders as an integral part of the health care team. Involving these leaders in non-clinical discussions of the older patient's needs could provide needed sensitivity to the healing process.

ASSESSMENT

One of the very first components taught to student nurses in their classes on therapeutic communications is "to establish trust in the patient." This trusting relationship is very important while caring for the older adult and assessing for spiritual well-being. The priority given to assessing for this is often overlooked while the physiological and psychosocial assessment take precedence. Assessment can easily be accomplished and may significantly alter the physiological response of the individual and hasten recovery. There are many documented cases where patients have been ministered to by religious leaders. Afterwards, a peace and calm permeate their presence, and often a recovery results that was unjustified by any medical means. Nurses are challenged to assess for spiritual well-being, regardless of their own beliefs or bias about religion and its practices.

A case in point comes to mind from personal experience. A 63-year-old single man, Ron, had lost two of his close friends unexpectedly within a week of each other. Ron had a history of heart trouble. These deaths affected him tremendously. Ron took care of the affairs of the death of his first friend. Within a week, another friend, Frank, had a myocardial infarction.

The emergency response team worked on him on the way to the hospital where machines kept Frank alive. On the day chosen to remove Frank from life support, Ron woke up with severe chest pain. Ron went to the emergency room and told of his distress.

Shortly, Ron was on a gurney, and nurse Terry came to his side. She asked the usual questions and was busy setting up the EKG. Following the EKG and no evidence of a heart attack, Terry questioned Ron as to what may have triggered this chest pain. Ron told of his distress, the loss of such a good close personal friend a week ago, and the imminent demise of another after life support is removed.

Terry immediately assessed that Ron had a "broken heart." Terry gave Ron a hug and said, "Honey, the only thing wrong with you is you have a broken heart. You have lost people you love, and you are hurting." Ron cried uncontrollably for a very long time. After the sobbing stopped, a sense of peace prevailed. Needless to say, nurse Terry was right on target. Terry perceived the whole person, the spiritual and emotional need, and responded. A satisfactory outcome was achieved through listening attentively and establishing a trusting relationship, both critical to providing spiritual care. Nurses often touch the spirit of their patients and may not fully realize they are delivering spiritual care.

Like nurse Terry, conversation must be initiated on the issue, and the patient given an opportunity to clarify fundamental beliefs that illness may bring into question. "Why did God allow this to happen to me?" is often heard and is a point for initiating dialogue. The inner turmoil can be uncovered and a foundation can be laid for follow-up with a clergyperson. Murray[8] suggests using certain questions to address the general areas of strength, hope, and meaning:

- What is your typical response to fearful situations?
- How easy is it for you to feel hopeful when you face uncertainty or loss?
- What inspires you?
- Do you participate in any formal or informal spiritual practices that have been interrupted by illness?

The health history always lists religion, and that is often a point of reference for the nurse to ask if they would like a visit from their religious leader. Table 6-1 lists some criteria and interventions to be considered while planning the care of the older patient and attempting to meet his or her need for spiritual wholeness.

SPIRITUAL CAREGIVING

Evidence suggests that spirituality is an important medical tool that could be incorporated when developing a therapeutic regimen.[10] Spiritual caregiving, minimally, is touching, empathy, understanding, listening, presence, and support. These are the elements of caregiving on a spiritual plane. Spiritual needs are identified as religious, values, relationships, transcendence, affective feeling, and communication.[4] The dynamic recognition of the spirit can open providers to ponder previous personal experiences of their patients and lead to establish productive positive behaviors; better understand life's struggles as well as reliance on others for support.[2,11]

Studies have indicated that nurses and patients alike find spiritual care appropriate and welcome.[11,12] For spiritual care to happen, the institutions governing nursing practice need to acknowledge this type of care through policies and procedures, including the need to report and document it.[13] Nurses need to be educated regarding the type and form of spiritual care they can provide and maintain those skills through continuing education. Personal awareness on the part of the nurse regarding comfort level dealing with these issues and an ability to acknowledge this to staff and patients is vital. Not everyone can or chooses to relate on a spiritual level. This is true for patients and health care providers alike.

TABLE 6-1

Assessing and Intervening in Spiritual Distress

ASSESSMENT	INTERVENTIONS
Brief history: • Losses • Challenged belief • Separation from religious and cultural ties • Death • Personal and family disasters	• Create a therapeutic environment • Assess support systems • Assess past methods of decreasing distress (ie, prayer, imagery, healing, memories/reminiscence therapy, medication, relaxation)
Symptoms (defining characteristics): • Unmet needs • Threats to self • Change in environment, health status, self-concept, etc. • Seeking spiritual assistance • Questioning meaning of own existence • Depression • Feelings of hopelessness, abandonment, fear	• Determine environmental changes needed to enhance functioning • Assess and assist implementation of coping mechanisms • Refer to clergy • Evaluation of effects of nursing interventions
Assessment of etiology of spiritual distress: • Depletion anxiety • Helplessness/hopelessness • Perceived powerlessness • Medication reactions • Hormonal imbalances	• Evaluation of medications and their interactions • Activation and evaluation of appropriate community referrals • Techniques to assist client and family in reducing spiritual distress

Used with permission. Ebersole P, Hess P. Transcendence: death, dying, grief, and legacies. *Toward Healthy Aging*, St. Louis: Mosby Year Book, Inc; 1994:739.

GERONTOLOGICAL NURSING IMPLICATIONS

Viewing the daily caring for patients and families as opportunities for spiritual insight and growth can lend personal meaning to the work-a-day world of nursing.[11] Spirituality is not only a part of nursing care, but also an integral dimension of every health care encounter. Personal fulfillment through a nursing career is achieved one patient at a time, one day at a time. Anyone can do for another, yet nursing's spiritual dimension is being with another,[11] fully present, responsive, interested while providing nursing care. Spirituality is a coping mechanism that allows each of us to filter our experiences meaningfully. Being with patients, and others being with us, enriches us, opens us to wisdom, if we allow it to happen.

Illnesses that interrupt routine, retirement, or loss of independence are conditions that put the individual experiencing them in a reflective stance. Removing daily distractions focuses attention on more transcendent issues. Facing terminal illness, knowing that death is closer now than ever, elevates awareness of the grand scheme of life. These factors precipitate a vulnerable, fearful demeanor in patients. There are wounds that can be seen only with the eyes of the heart. Spiritual caregiving is an exercise of the heart and intuition in harmony with knowledge and experience. Silent presence, touching, supportive smiles, and genuine interest all demand of health care providers a level of personal involvement beyond biological orientation to infection and trauma.

Awareness and knowledge of spiritual issues are a nursing concern that demand quality education. Questions of human suffering, weakness, pain, and relationship to deity (in all traditions) are a required awareness. Nurses study many human conditions in which they will never fully participate so also studying the spiritual dimensions of humanity doesn't require participation, it does however require knowledge. This should be seen as another necessary tool to providing quality care to all patients.

Work place managers and supervisors should provide sufficient time for spiritual caregiving procedures. Essential physical and psychological care are integrated with spiritual care. Denominational affiliation is one aspect of a vast range of points of interaction that should be charted on the patient's record. As health care providers take the time to personally regroup after a particularly difficult experience, so also the patient care team needs to provide professional interpersonal support to those who encounter patients with deep spiritual need. Nurses' own fears, guilt, vulnerability, and unanswered questions about the meaning of life and death are important continuing education topics.

There is much research to be accomplished in this area as contemporary health care awakens to the power of the spirit in the healing process. Holistic health includes integration, balance, and harmony of one's mental, physical, emotional, and spiritual components.[14] Research needs to focus on the outcomes achieved when spiritual care is rendered. Including the clergy as team members and developing a research protocol can provide invaluable findings. Research can focus upon health care environments that seem to be attentive to issues beyond the biological. This may indicate positive, supportive health care teams facilitating shorter lengths of stay.

Assessment tools for spiritual issues need to be more readily available and used. They should be incorporated into existing intake assessment and routine follow-up procedures. Research is needed to develop these tools and find those that are most appropriate for nursing.[15]

Awe, wonder, and mystery surround birth and death. Gerontological nursing is part preparation for the mystery of the life stage known as death. Often, we are the last people that patients talk with or see. Each passing is as unique as the person experiencing this life event. Reducing pain through medication or listening are part of the preparation. The ability to have experienced this individual, listened to his or her story, participated in his or her journey impacts our own preparations and our own journey. Spiritual caregiving makes demands on our person, as well as time, knowledge, and skill. Much like nursing itself, spiritual caregiving can be rewarding personally, taking the time and effort to hold a hand, rub a shoulder, help with a shoe, offer a hug, and listen in the silence.

Gerontology is about the finite. Spirituality is about the infinite. These two realities uniquely blend when nursing is added to these elements of life. Gerontological nurses participate in a life stage where the wisdom of generations can be experienced. Gerontological spiritual nursing is an expanse of timeless encounters of the human spirit, the depth of personal character, enduring values, and essential life forces. Synthesizing these dimensions as a health care provider harmonize with the true aspects of holistic care of the older person.

REFERENCES

1. Macrae J. Nightingale's spiritual philosophy and its significance for modern nursing. *Image*. 1995;27(1):8-10.
2. Forbes EJ. Spirituality, aging, and the community-dwelling caregiver and care recipient. *Geriatric Nurs*. 1994;15(6):296-301.
3. Berggren-Thomas P, Griggs MJ. Spirituality in aging: spiritual need or spiritual journey? *J Gerontol Nurs*. 1995;21(3):5-10.
4. Emblen JD, Halstead L. Spiritual needs and interventions: comparing the views of patients, nurses, and chaplains. *CNS*. 1993; 7(4):175-182.
5. Miller MA. Culture, spirituality, and women's health. *JOGNN*. 1995; 24(3):257-263.
6. Price JL, Stevens HO, LaBarre MC. Spiritual caregiving. *J Psychosocial Nurs*. 1995;33(12):5-9.
7. Thorson JA, Cook TC. *Spiritual well being of the elderly*. Springfield, IL: Charles C. Thomas, 1980.
8. Murray CK. Addressing your patient's spiritual needs. *AJN*. 1995;95(11):16N-16P.
9. Eliopoulos C. *Caring for the Elderly in Diverse Care Settings*. New York: J.B. Lippincott, Co.; 1990.
10. Marwick C. Should physicians prescribe prayer for health? *JAMA*. 1995;273(20):1561-1562.
11. Stiles MK. The shining stranger. *Cancer Nurs*. 1990;13(4):235-245.
12. Zerwekh J. Transcending life: the practice wisdom of nursing hospice experts. *Am J Hospice Palliative Care*. 1993;10:26-31.
13. Taylor EJ, Amenta M, Highfield M. Spiritual care practices of oncology nurses. *ONF*. 1995;22(1):31-9.
14. Scaward BL. Reflections on human spirituality for the worksite. *Am J Health Promotion*. 1995;9(3):165-68.
15. Brennan MR. Spirituality in the homebound elderly. *Dissertation*. Catholic University of America, Washington, D.C.; 1994.

Chapter 7

Care of the Older Adult With Diabetes

Martha Mitchell Funnell, MS, RN, CDE,
and Jennifer Hayden Merritt, MSN, RN, CDE

OVERVIEW

Healthy People 2000[1] identifies objectives for improving the health and longevity of people in this country older than 65 and those with diabetes. Because of the prevalence of diabetes among older adults, the goals for the two groups overlap and compliment each other. In fact, it is unlikely that the goals for either group can be attained until diabetes care is addressed by geriatric health care providers and geriatric care is addressed by diabetes providers.

There are four diabetes-specific *Healthy People 2000* objectives identified as particularly relevant for older adults.[1] Two of these objectives are the reduction in mortality and the prevalence of diabetes and its complications, and an increase in the number who receive self-management education. Many of the objectives directed toward the elderly population are especially applicable for people with diabetes. Among objectives identified for all older adults are, in particular, reduction in significant visual impairment, increase in years of healthy life among black and Hispanic Americans, and increase in personal care independence and activity level are of concern for people with diabetes. These cannot be achieved unless their diabetes is effectively treated.

This chapter will address the extent of the problem of diabetes among older adults, available treatment and educational strategies to decrease morbidity and improve quality of life, and the role of nurses in the attainment of these objectives.

INTRODUCTION

Diabetes is almost 10 times as common among adults older than 65 as those in the 20 to 44 age group[2] and affects 9.6% of all people in the U.S. older than 65.[3] Undiagnosed diabetes is estimated to exist in 10% to 20% of the population older than 50, with higher estimates among minority people.[4] Noninsulin-dependent diabetes mellitus (NIDDM) may begin up to 12 years before diagnosis. This lack of detection poses a significant health risk for older adults as microvascular and macrovascular complications begin to occur, which increase morbidity and mortality.[3]

Prevalence of NIDDM varies by race, with prevalence rates of 50% higher among blacks than whites.[4] Among Hispanic Americans the rate is even higher.[5] Black women show the highest prevalence with a rate of 21%, and among black women older than 75, almost one in four has diabetes.[4]

IMPACT OF DIABETES

Diabetes is not only common, it is serious. Because of the asymptomatic nature of diabetes, health professionals and patients often underestimate its seriousness. However, all people with diabetes are at risk for long-term complications, and these can be devastating to the older adult's functional ability, independence, quality of life, and psychosocial status. Diabetes has a significant impact on the development and progression of cardiovascular disease, the major cause of death among people older than 65.[6] Compared to those without diabetes, people with diabetes are 25 times more likely to become blind, 17 times more likely to develop kidney disease, 20 times more likely to develop gangrene, 15 times more likely to require amputation, and twice as likely to have a cerebrovascular accident or myocardial infarction. The risk for developing long-term complications of diabetes increases with longer duration of diabetes. Hospitalization, rehospitalization rates, and nursing home admissions are significantly higher for people with diabetes when compared to those without diabetes.[5,7,8] Diabetes is the fifth ranking cause of death for Americans older than 65[9] and reduces the life expectancy by 7 years for women and 9 years for men. It was estimated that the total health care costs for people with confirmed diabetes in 1992 was $85.7 billion, excluding nursing home costs.[10]

Given the prevalence of diabetes among older adults and its negative impact, the question often arises: what can be done to reduce its associated morbidity and mortality? The first step is early diagnosis, followed by individualized care, and self-management education. These are essential components of diabetes care for all older adults regardless of the care delivery setting.

DIAGNOSIS OF DIABETES

Among individuals without diabetes, biochemical and hormonal mechanisms balance glucose and insulin to maintain normoglycemia, usually around 70 to 115 mg/dL in the fasting state. With aging, there is often an impairment in these mechanisms that result in elevated glucose levels, particularly after eating. Blood glucose ranges above normal but below values diagnostic of diabetes are considered impaired glucose tolerance (IGT). In the past, IGT was considered by some to be a normal aging phenomena or was called "borderline diabetes." However, since increases in macrovascular disease are associated with IGT among older adults,[11] interventions such as weight reduction and exercise are encouraged to decrease the risk of progression to NIDDM.

The diagnosis of IGT and diabetes are based on the National Diabetes Data Group criteria.[12] The screening test of choice for older adults is fasting glucose levels.[13] Two fasting blood glucose readings of greater than 140 mg/dL are required for the diagnosis of diabetes, unless the individual is symptomatic and has a random glucose value of greater than 200 mg/dL. Age-specific screening criteria are not warranted,[14] and oral glucose tolerance tests are generally not needed for the elderly.[13]

Diabetes may present atypically in older adults so that the usual symptoms of polyuria, polyphagia, polydipsia, fatigue, and rapid weight loss may be either masked or nonexistent. Among older adults, blurred vision, increased nocturia or urinary incontinence, gradual weight loss, and symptoms of diabetes complications should signal nurses to screen for diabetes.

The vast majority (>99%) of older adults have NIDDM.[15] The development of NIDDM in later life is associated with hypertension, vascular disease, elevated very-low-density lipoprotein cholesterol, use of diuretics, obesity, positive family history, and sedentary lifestyle.[16] While many older adults have improved glycemia with diet, weight correction and/or oral hypoglycemic agents, others with NIDDM require insulin to maintain desired metabolic control.

The Diabetes Control and Complications Trial (DCCT) established the value of intensive therapies to decrease the risk for complications in insulin-dependent diabetes mellitus (IDDM).[17] Among older adults, poor glucose control is predictive of the progression of retinopathy.[18] While the link between glucose control and the other long-term complications has not been established in the elderly, their impact on morbidity and mortality means that nurses who work with older adults who have NIDDM cannot ignore this issue if the objectives of *Healthy People 2000* are to be met.[19,20]

LONG-TERM COMPLICATIONS

Older adults are at risk for all of the long-term complications of diabetes, which include neuropathy, retinopathy, nephropathy, and macrovascular disease. The results of the DCCT indicate that intensive management of diabetes can decrease the risk for retinopathy up to 76%, nephropathy up to 56%, and neuropathy up to 60% in patients with IDDM.[17] Therefore, prevention efforts are primarily aimed at blood glucose control and the reduction of other risk factors (eg, smoking, blood pressure control).

Other efforts are focused on early detection and treatment when the complications are most amenable to intervention. Complications screening guidelines developed for NIDDM apply to older adults as well as younger.[26] Because NIDDM is often present for many years, initial screening for complications should occur upon diagnosis. Recommended initial and annual evaluations include dilated retinal examination, ECG, lipid profile, and evaluation of renal function. Self-management education for people with diabetes must include information about the prevention, early detection, and treatment of each of these complications, including the need to request screening if it is not ordered. Assisting primary care providers to make needed referrals and to monitor these parameters is also an important role for a gerontology nurse case manager.

In the elderly, the presentation of a complication may be atypical, misinterpreted, or overshadowed by other illnesses. As examples, neuropathy may be confused with "rheumatism," cerebral or myocardial infarcts may occur "silently" and be diagnosed only during physical exam, and retinopathy missed in an older adult with dense cataracts. Coronary artery disease remains the number one cause of death in people older than 65. Coronary artery disease is more common among older people with diabetes, which compounds the risk for myocardial infarcts and stroke. Patients and providers need to treat both diseases effectively in order to decrease mortality rates among older adults. The incidence of high blood pressure increases with age, particularly among blacks. Hypertension alone increases the risk for renal, cardiovascular, and cerebrovascular disease; diabetes compounds these risks. Treatment of hypertension can be problematic in older adults with diabetes since diuretics and beta blockers need to be used with caution. Angiotensin converting enzyme (ACE) inhibitors are the preferred treatment as they may also protect the kidneys and have few side effects. Generally, the earlier an ACE inhibitor is used, the better its nephroprotective effect.[21]

The vascular disease prevalent with diabetes often leads to amputation. Amputations are costly to the health care system through hospitalizations, nursing home care, and rehabilitative services, and to individuals and their families through personal suffering, loss of independence, and decreased quality of life. Amputations, however, are largely preventable with appropriate foot wear and foot care by the person with diabetes.[22] Self-management education must include information about foot care skills and provide patients with the opportunity to practice necessary skills. Because older adults have difficulties with foot care, a thorough assessment of patient skills and if needed teaching significant others or providing home care support is an important part of preventive care.[23]

TREATMENT OPTIONS FOR DIABETES

The available treatment options are the same for the older adults as for other persons with IDDM and NIDDM. These include medical nutritional therapy, weight control, exercise, and oral medications or insulin. The treatment options selected should be based on blood glucose goals and priorities established by the patient and his or her family or caregivers in collaboration with the nurse and other members of the geriatric and diabetes care teams. The goals selected provide a rational basis for decision-making and determining treatment options. Based on the goals, a program of either basic or more intensive diabetes care should be initiated with clear guidelines for moving to the next stage in therapy. Basic diabetes care is designed to prevent symptomatic hyperglycemia by maintaining fasting blood glucose levels at less than 200 mg/dL. Treatment programs often include meal planning, exercise, and the addition of an oral medication if this goal is not met. Intensive diabetes care is designed to prevent the long-term complications by maintaining fasting blood glucose levels at less than 140 mg/dL, post-prandial glucose levels of less than 180 mg/dL, and glycosylated hemoglobin levels of about 1% to 2% above the normal range. Insulin is often used along with diet, exercise, and home blood glucose monitoring. Regardless of the therapy selected, older adults with NIDDM should be offered an individualized program that includes education, medical therapy, nutrition counseling, an exercise program, and oral medications or insulin as needed.[24]

MEAL PLANNING

Medical nutritional therapy is a major component in the treatment of all types of diabetes and for all age groups. Dietary recommendations for older adults are the same as those for other adults with diabetes, although individual and age-related health concerns and goals need to be taken into account.[25] Meal planning has become increasingly individualized with recommendations based on assessed needs and existing eating habits, rather than specific guidelines or standard meal plans.

Individual meal plans for older adults may include dietary recommendations for blood glucose control, achievement of an ideal or reasonable body weight, a decrease in the intake of saturated fats and cholesterol, and a nutritionally adequate and balanced diet.[23] Meal planning may also need to accommodate dietary interventions for concomitant illnesses or other concerns common among the elderly (eg, poor dentition). The interventions may be based on a specific meal pattern or behavioral strategies. Major dietary changes are difficult at any age and may negatively affect quality of life and increase social isolation among the elderly. For many older adults, eating similar amounts of food at regular times throughout the day may be adequate for glucose control.[27] Those who are more than 20% above desirable body weight often significantly decrease glucose levels with reduced calorie intake or a modest amount of weight loss.[28] Referral for dietary counseling is recommended at diagnosis and annually thereafter.[29]

EXERCISE

Exercise may not only be effective in preventing NIDDM,[30] but is generally part of the treatment plan for diabetes. Benefits include improved insulin action and glucose utilization, cardiovascular status, toning, appetite and bowel function, preservation of joint mobility and range of motion, sleep patterns, and sense of well-being. Overall health and diabetes status need to be assessed through a history, physical, and exercise stress test before older adults initiate an exercise program.[31] Exercise is particularly important for the elderly who have been sedentary for many years as they may have significant vascular narrowing that becomes symptomatic only with aerobic exercise.

ORAL DIABETIC AGENTS

Diet and exercise are generally considered to be the first line of treatment for NIDDM among the elderly. If these strategies are inadequate to achieve target glucose levels after 3 to 6 months, medication should be added to the regimen. Of the sulfonylureas, both glyburide and glipizide may be effective to achieve target blood glucose levels and are generally tolerated by older adults.[32]

Two additional oral agents have been approved for the treatment of NIDDM. Metformin is a biguanide that inhibits hepatic glucose production, increases insulin sensitivity, decreases lipid levels, and promotes weight loss. Metformin alone or in combination with a sulfonylurea has been shown to be effective in improving blood glucose control and lipid concentrations among people with NIDDM.[33] Older adults who take this medication need frequent evaluation of liver and kidney function. Because lactic acidosis is a potential side effect, patients should be taught symptoms (eg, respiratory or abdominal distress) and to seek medical care if they occur.

Acarbase inhibits the uptake of carbohydrates thus preventing post-prandial increases in blood glucose concentrations and is recommended as an adjunct to dietary or sulfonylurea therapy. Side effects include gastrointestinal disturbances such as bloating and gas caused by undigested carbohydrates emptying into the large intestine. These effects generally disappear after 6 months of use. The potential for interactions with other drugs needs to be assessed prior to initiation of any oral agents (see Chapter 19, *Screening for Polypharmacy in a Nursing Home Care Unit*).

INSULIN

If blood glucose levels do not improve after 3 to 6 months of maximum dose therapy with oral agents, insulin is considered as the next line of therapy. BID's therapy, which is the combination of insulin and oral sulfonylureas, is sometimes implemented, particularly among people with insulin resistance. While BID's therapy may improve glucose control,[34] it increases regimen complexity and possibly costs, and its usefulness must be individually evaluated for older adults.

Insulin treatment allows dosage adjustments that can be individualized to meet the patient's glucose goals. Because hypoglycemia awareness may diminish with aging, the ability to recognize and manage insulin reactions is an important treatment and educational consideration.[35] Other considerations include the patient's ability to draw-up and administer insulin, monitor blood glucose levels, cognitive function, visual acuity, manual dexterity, and family support. Some older adults can reach their glucose goals with one or two shots per day of an intermediate-acting insulin, although others need additional short-acting insulin. More than two insulin injections per day are rarely needed by the elderly.[13]

More intensive regimens are feasible in older adults but may require additional office or home care visits, support, and education. Gradual adjustments in insulin doses and frequent contact with the health care team can facilitate the intensification process. As part of initial education, older adults who are candidates for this type of therapy should be informed of this option and potential advantages and disadvantages.

MONITORING

Home blood glucose monitoring and testing of glycosylated hemoglobin levels are recommended to determine treatment efficacy. Home blood glucose monitoring is useful to determine glucose patterns and stability, detect hypoglycemia and hyperglycemia, and determine the impact of food, exercise, stress, and medications on glucose levels. Many blood glucose meters are available that are accurate and easy for older adults to use. Recommendations for testing frequency are based on individual goals, treatment regimen, and glycemic stability.[36] Monitoring records should be easy for older adults to use and facilitate both patients and professionals to make modifications in the treatment plan. Glycosylated hemoglobin measurements provide information about the average glucose control for the previous 6 to 8 weeks. It is recommended that this test be done every 6 months in patients with NIDDM.[29]

GERONTOLOGICAL NURSING IMPLICATIONS

The acute and chronic complications that can occur in diabetes are a serious concern for older adults. Gerontological nurses have a challenge to prevent these concerns and develop a self-care strategy for care of the older diabetic. The acute complications of diabetes include hypoglycemia, hyperglycemia, and hyperosmolar hyperglycemic nonketotic syndrome (HHNS). Diabetic ketoacidosis (DKA) is rare in older adults. Low blood glucose reactions can occur among people taking insulin or sulfonylureas. Patients who are diet controlled or taking only Metformin are not usually at risk. The adrenergic symptoms of hypoglycemia, which result from the release of epinephrine (shaking and nervousness), may be blunted or absent with aging. Hypoglycemia unawareness is blood glucose levels of less than 60 mg/dL with no symptoms to prompt treatment. Left untreated, a mild reaction can then progress to the point where assistance is needed or loss of consciousness occurs. Because this is not only frightening but may threaten independence, patients tend to overtreat hypoglycemia and health professionals may be hesitant to treat asymptomatic hyperglycemia. Since many elderly have few symptoms of hyperglycemia, they are then at increased risk for the acute and chronic complications of diabetes. Self-management education about prevention, recognition, and appropriate treatment for hypoglycemia may help to increase the likelihood that blood glucose levels are more reasonably controlled.

Diabetes self-management education is effective in improving diabetes knowledge and metabolic control.[37] While diabetes educational programs developed specifically for older adults, particularly those that include elements of support, result in improvements in self-care behavior or glycemia,[38-40] older adults are less likely to receive diabetes education than younger adults. In a study of 2268 subjects with NIDDM, only 41% of insulin taking and 21% of noninsulin taking subjects 65 or older had ever attended a class or program about diabetes.[41] Gerontological nurses have a unique opportunity through self-care management training to not only prevent the complications of diabetes but also restore a sense of control to the older person.

Content areas for diabetes education are established,[42] and specific topics and objectives within each area delineated.[43,44] The content areas relevant for the elderly are diabetes overview; stress and psychosocial adjustment; family involvement and social support; nutrition; exercise and activity; medications; monitoring and use of results; relationships among nutrition, exercise, medication, and blood glucose levels; prevention, detection, and treatment of acute complications; prevention, detection, and treatment of chronic complications; foot, skin, and dental care; behavior change strategies, goal-setting, risk factor reduction, and problem solving; benefits, risks, and management options for improving glucose control; and use of health care systems and community resources.

While these content areas are considered essential components of a diabetes education curriculum, an individualized program should be developed for each patient based on a needs assessment. Assessment and individualized instruction is particularly important for older adults who often have special educational needs as a result of the aging process, long-term complications of diabetes, or other medical problems. Outpatient diabetes education programs are available in most areas and are often reimbursed by Medicare if criteria are met for American Diabetes Association Recognition or state certification. These programs are taught by nurses and dietitians who are also Certified Diabetes Educators (CDE). The gerontology nurse is an important member of the education and care team who participates in assessment, referral, and follow-up for the patient with diabetes. The initial assessment must include functional abilities, knowledge and beliefs about diabetes, physical ability, cognitive ability, literacy, emotional status, social and care support, culture and ethnicity, financial status, and readiness to learn. Patients and their families should be given the opportunity to express their thoughts and feelings about diabetes, the intensity of the treatment program, and the educational process. Because health and functional status of older adults may change frequently, assessment needs to occur at every interaction with the patient.

The content of educational sessions should be tailored for type of diabetes, stated interest, treatment plan, and personal goals. Because older adults may require more time to process new information, initially focusing on survival skills and presenting additional information in manageable sections over a period of time will assist them to learn and apply the information.

Ongoing education provides the opportunity to answer questions, reinforce previous content, and give feedback on self-care strengths. Asking patients what they are doing to care for their diabetes and observing self-care skills, such as insulin administration, blood testing, and foot inspection, are useful indicators of both functional abilities and current care practices. This information can be used to tailor the educational session by offering recommendations or content in areas of self-management deficits. Patients may also need assistance in coordinating several complex treatment programs for other acute or chronic conditions. Motivation for self-care is often overlooked, yet plays a significant role in chronic illness. If the patient seems less willing to assume responsibility for care, it may be appropriate to investigate possible reasons.

The purpose of diabetes education is to provide the information needed by the patient to make informed decisions about the personal consequences of non-treatment, benefits of treatment options, and appropriate blood glucose levels.[45] Self-management education that includes problem-solving, goal-setting, assertiveness training, and other behavioral strategies will empower patients with the knowledge, skills, and self-awareness needed to influence their own behavior to manage diabetes and become active participants in their own care.[45,46]

Gerontology nurses need to be aware of the risk of HHNS and provide education about sick day care to patients and their families. Self-management includes frequent blood glucose testing during illness, infection, or high stress, the need to maintain adequate fluid intake, and to report any trends in hyperglycemia with accompanying weakness or changes in level of consciousness. Nursing home residents are a high-risk population for HHNS, and nurses need to monitor these patients closely.

REFERENCES

1. Department of Health and Human Services. *Healthy People 2000: National Health Promotion and Disease Prevention Objectives.* (DHHS publication no. (PHS) 91-50212) Washington, D.C.: U.S. Government Printing Office; 1991.
2. Barrett-Connor E. Commentary. *Diabetes Spectrum.* 1989;2:164-166.
3. Harris MI. Epidemiology of diabetes mellitus among the elderly in the United States. *Clin Geriatr Med.* 1990;6(4):703-729.
4. U.S. Department of Health and Human Services. *Diabetes Surveillance 1993.* Atlanta, GA: Centers for Disease Control; 1993.
5. Harris MI. Undiagnosed NIDDM: clinical and public health issues. *Diabetes Care.* 1993;16(4):642-652.
6. Davidson MB. The impact of diabetes in the elderly. *Diabetes Educator.* 1983;8:10, 65.
7. Boult C, Dowd, B, McCaffrey D, Boult L, Hernandez R, Krulewitch H. Screening elders for risk of hospital admission. *J Am Geriatr Soc.* 1993;41(8):811-817.
8. Polin SS. Paying for health care: the high cost of diabetes. *Clinical Diabetes.* 1985;3:108-116.
9. U.S. Department of Health and Human Services. *Diabetes in the United States: A Strategy for Prevention.* Atlanta, GA: Centers for Disease Control; 1993.
10. Rubin RJ, Altman WM, Mendelson DN. Health care expenditures for people with diabetes mellitus. *J Clin Endocrinol Metab.* 1994;78(4):809A-809F.
11. Harris MI. Impaired glucose tolerance in the U.S. population. *Diabetes Care.* 1989;12:464-474.
12. National Diabetes Data Group. Classification and diagnosis of diabetes mellitus and other categories of glucose intolerance. *Diabetes.* 1979;28:1039-1057.
13. Morrow LA, Halter JB. Treatment of the elderly with diabetes. In: Kahn CR, Weir GS, eds. *Joslin's Diabetes Mellitus.* (13th ed.) Philadelphia: Lea & Febiger; 1994.
14. Blunt BA, Barrett-Connor E, Wingard DL. Evaluation of fasting plasma glucose as a screening test for NIDDM in older adults. *Diabetes Care.* 1991;14(11):989-993.
15. Wingard D, Sinsheimer P, Barrett-Connor E, McPhillips J. Community based study of prevalence of NIDDM in older adults. *Diabetes Care.* 1990;13(Suppl 2):3-8.
16. Wilson PW, Anderson KW, Kannel WB. Epidemiology of diabetes in the elderly. The Framingham Study. *Am J Med.* 1986;80(5A):3-9.
17. The DCCT Research Group. The effect of intensive treatment of diabetes on the development and progression of long-term complications in insulin-dependent diabetes mellitus. *N Engl J Med.* 1993;329:977-986.
18. Morisaki N, Watanabe S, Kobayashi J, et al. Diabetic control and progression of retinopathy in elderly patients: five year follow-up study. *J Am Geriatr Soc.* 1994;42(2):142-145.
19. American Diabetes Association. Position statement: implications of the diabetes control and complications trial. *Diabetes Care.* 1993;16:1517-1520.
20. Halter JB, Christensen NJ. Introduction: diabetes mellitus in elderly people. *Diabetes Care.* 1990;13(Suppl 2):1-2.
21. White JR Jr. Angiotensin converting enzyme inhibitors, their potential role in diabetes care. Research to practice: introduction and conclusion. *Diabetes Spectrum.* 1993;6:169-20.
22. Haas LB. Lower extremity amputations: strategies for prevention: from research to practice. *Diabetes Spectrum.* 1995;8:230-232.
23. Thomson FJ, Masson EA. Can elderly diabetic patients cooperate with routine foot care? *Age Aging.* 1992;21(5):333-337.
24. Henry RR, Edelman SV. Advances in treatment of type II diabetes mellitus in the elderly. *Geriatrics.* 1992,47(4).24-30.
25. Franz MJ, Horton ES, Bantle JP, et al. Nutritional principles for the management of diabetes and related complications: a technical review. *Diabetes Care.* 1994;17(5):490-518.
26. American Diabetes Association. Position statement: nutrition recommendations and principles for people with diabetes mellitus. *Diabetes Care.* 1994;17:519-922.
27. Rost FM, Flavin KS, Schmidt LE, McGill JB. Self-care predictors of metabolic control in NIDDM patients. *Diabetes Care.* 1990;13(11):1111-1113.
28. Reed RL, Mooradian AD. Nutritional status and dietary management of elderly diabetic patients. *Clin Geriatr Med.* 1990;6(4):883-901.
29. American Diabetes Association. Position statement: standards of medical care for patients with diabetes mellitus. *Diabetes Care.* 1995;17(Suppl 1):8-15.
30. Helmrich SP, Ragland DR, Leung RW, Paffenbarger RS. Physical activity and reduced occurrence of non-insulin-dependent diabetes mellitus. *N Engl J Med.* 1991;325(3):147-52.
31. Graham C. Exercise and aging: implications for persons with diabetes. *Diabetes Educator.* 1991;17:189-195.
32. Rosenstock J, Corrao PJ, Goldberg RB, Kilo C. Diabetes control in the elderly: a randomized, comparative study of glyburide versus glipizide in non-insulin dependent diabetes mellitus. *Clinical Therapeutics.* 1993;15:1031-1040.
33. DeFronzo RA, Goodman AM. Efficacy of metformin in patients with non-insulin-dependent diabetes mellitus. Multicenter metformin study group. *N Engl J Med.* 1995;333(9):541-549.
34. Pugh JA, Wagner ML, Sawyer J, Ramirez G, Tuley M, Friedberg SJ. Is combination sulfonylurea and insulin therapy useful in NIDDM patients? A meta-analysis. *Diabetes Care.* 1992;15(8):953-959.
35. Meneilly GS, Cheung E, Tóukko H. Counterregulatory hormone responses to hypoglycemia in the elderly patient with diabetes. *Diabetes.* 1994;43(3):403-410.
36. American Diabetes Association. Consensus statement: self-monitoring of blood glucose. *Diabetes Care.* 1994;17:81-86.

37. Brown SA. Effects of educational interventions and outcomes in diabetic adults: a meta-analysis revisited. *Patient Education and Counseling*. 1990;16:189-215.
38. Gilden JL, Hendryx S, Casia C, Singh SP. The effectiveness of diabetes education programs for older patients and their spouses. *J Am Geriatr Soc*. 1989;37:1023-1030.
39. Gilden JL, Hendryx S, Clair S, Casia C, Singh SP. Diabetes support groups improve health care of older diabetic patients. *J Am Geriatr Soc*. 1992;40(2):147-150.
40. Glasgow RE, Toobert DJ, Hampson SE, Brown JE, Lewinson PM, Donnelly J. Improving self-care among older patients with type II diabetes: the sixty... something study. *Patient Education and Counseling*. 1992;19:61-64.
41. Coonrod BA, Betschart J, Harris MI. Frequency and determinants of diabetes patient education among adults in the US population. *Diabetes Care*. 1994;17(8):852-858.
42. American Diabetes Association. National standards for diabetes self-management education. *Diabetes Care*. 1995;18:141-143.
43. Funnell MM, Haas LB. National standards for diabetes self-management education programs: technical review. *Diabetes Care*. 1995;18(1):100-116.
44. Brink SB, Siminerio L, Hinnen-Hentzen D, et al. *Diabetes Education Goals*. Alexandria, VA: American Diabetes Association; 1995.
45. Funnell MM, Anderson RM, Arnold MS, et al. Empowerment: an idea whose time has come in diabetes patient education. *Diabetes Educator*. 1991;17:37-41.
46. Anderson RM, Funnell MM, Butler PM, Arnold MS, Feste CC. Patient empowerment: results of a randomized controlled trial. *Diabetes Care*. 1995;18(11):943-949.

Chapter 8

Cardiac Assessment in Gerontology

Marycarol McGovern, PhD, RN,
and Janet Kwaiser Kuhn, EdD, RN

OVERVIEW

The process of aging affects all body organs and systems, and their functioning can become less competent. Cardiac function is no exception. In fact, half of all adults older than age 65 have heart disease, and the number of elderly patients experiencing acute myocardial infarction is growing rapidly.[1] This chapter discusses thorough cardiac assessment and physical examination. It includes an overview of the relevant issues, a review of the basic techniques of cardiac assessment, and a discussion of implications for gerontological nursing practice, education, and research.

INTRODUCTION

The elderly in America are the fastest growing segment of the population and have a higher incidence of coronary disease than younger groups.[2] Although heart disease remains the leading cause of death in the United States, mortality has declined during the past 30 years.[3] The factors contributing to the reduction in mortality include improved cardiac life support and emergency care, advanced diagnostic and therapeutic technology, and an increased public awareness of health seeking behaviors that reduce or modify those risk factors associated with cardiac disease and disability.

OVERVIEW OF THE ISSUES

RISK FACTORS

Factors that are associated with an increased incidence of heart disease are commonly classified as non-modifiable or modifiable. Non-modifiable factors, those that cannot be changed, include age, family history, and male gender (or females after menopause). Modifiable risk factors that have been shown to be directly related to coronary artery disease are cigarette smoking, hypertension, hyperlipidemia, diabetes, and a history of occlusive peripheral vascular disease. Other factors associated with an increased risk of heart disease include obesity, sedentary lifestyle, and stress. Risk is magnified when more than one risk factor is present.[3-5] Studies have shown that risk reduction programs that focus on regular exercise, a lower fat diet, blood lipid treatment, smoking cessation, and weight loss can reduce the incidence of heart disease or slow the progression of coronary atherosclerosis in patients with known coronary artery disease.[6,7] One of the aims of nursing intervention is to educate clients about their risk of heart disease and encourage them to modify those factors that can be changed. Another purpose is to identify those patients who show signs of cardiac dysfunction and arrange for appropriate treatment and cardiac rehabilitation services.

TABLE 8-1

Healthy People 2000: Risk Reduction Objectives Related to Cardiac Health in U.S. Populations

- Reduce incidence of being overweight
- Increase regular physical activity (30 minutes/day)
- Adopt sound dietary practices (reduce dietary fat)
- Reduce cigarette smoking
- Reduce prevalence of hypertension
- Reduce mean serum cholesterol
- Preserve function and independence

Health Promotion/Illness Prevention

The key to optimal health and to the reduction of illness and disability is to recognize, control, or alleviate modifiable risk factors. Many of the health status objectives and priorities identified in *Healthy People 2000* are related to cardiac health and to the reduction of cardiac risk factors (Table 8-1). This discussion will focus specifically on the prevention of cardiac disease and disability in individuals, families, and communities.

> Since the interaction of heredity, behavior, and environment is a dynamic process that can be altered to some degree, prevention offers a promising approach for decreasing the prevalence of chronic illness, particularly in the middle and older adult years.[8]

Prevention is an important responsibility of nurses in all practice settings. Particularly with the movement from acute, episodic intervention to a continuum of services that address issues related to both health and illness. This is congruent with the historical essence of professional nursing intervention, which has always been to prevent illness by promoting health and to assist the person who has experienced illness to return to his or her maximum functional level. The goals of both *Healthy People 2000* and *Nursing's Agenda for Health Care Reform*[9] are to improve people's health status by recognizing at-risk populations and reducing that risk by promoting access to the full range of health care services. This front-line intervention can make a difference in the health of the nations elderly through programs in cardiovascular risk reduction and by timely and comprehensive restorative programs that are designed to return the elderly to their highest functional level.

With the change from fee-for-service to a managed care system of health care financing, patients are discharged from acute care settings quicker and sicker. Most hospital protocols, for example, now allow only 4 days for in-hospital care for coronary artery bypass grafts. This allows little time to determine individual and family needs and to teach patients about risk factor reduction strategies, safe medication use, and appropriate follow-up care. Elderly patients may also need in-home and caregiver support systems, but there is little time for comprehensive assessment to elicit that information. There may be a need for nutritional or psychological counseling. Patients may need to become aware of resources available for meals, transportation, and rehabilitation services.

Nurses can provide more cost-effective, comprehensive, patient and family centered services. *Nursing's Agenda for Health Care Reform* proposes a continuum of care design, which would guarantee preventive, restorative, and rehabilitative services to elders who are at risk or who have experienced coronary disease. It further recommends that in order to reduce fragmentation of those services, nurses function as case managers to coordinate care.

CARDIAC ASSESSMENT

A thorough cardiac assessment can help determine if changes in activity tolerance or other signs that often occur with age are musculoskeletal or neurological in origin, or if they indicate serious heart disease or cardiovascular conditions that would respond to treatment or lifestyle modifications. Before beginning the initial cardiac examination, it is important to have the proper equipment available. This includes a stethoscope with a double chestpiece, a marking pencil for indicating auscultation sites, and a quiet, well-lit environment.

Follow the usual sequence of physical examination: history, inspection, palpation, percussion, and auscultation. A common error is to listen to the heart sounds first. This may miss important clues that will help interpret heart sounds in terms of past history and lifestyle. Explain to the patient that a thorough cardiac assessment might take as long as 10 minutes and that the amount of time spent does not necessarily indicate a serious problem. Because a thorough cardiac exam requires the patient to assume a number of different positions, the nurse may need to slow the pace of the exam or alter the sequence for the older patient. Monitoring the elderly patient's level of comfort and breathing pattern is important throughout the exam.

HISTORY

The first step is to elicit a relevant health history (Table 8-2). In addition to eliciting symptoms of cardiac disease, it is important to determine and discuss cardiac risk factors. Does the patient understand these factors? Do physical or cognitive limitations exist that would interfere with the ability to learn and implement risk reduction practices such as dietary modification or increased exercise? Are there family support and resources available to begin or maintain a cardiac risk reduction or rehabilitation program?

A dietary history will help to determine whether there is evidence of malnutrition. An exercise program to decrease cardiac risk will be unsuccessful and dangerous for the elderly patient with inadequate caloric and protein reserves. This is particularly important in older women, who lack adequate calcium and vitamin D to prevent bone degeneration and injury. The nurse should ask about episodes of fatigue, restlessness, syncope, or confusion that may be due to oxygen deprivation and can be an early sign of congestive heart failure or myocardial infarction.

TABLE 8-2

Health History

- Ask the client if there is any history of heart attack, chest pain, or irregular heartbeat.
- Is anything specified associated with the onset of symptoms or alleviation of them?
- Does the client have cardiac risk factors, such as diabetes, high cholesterol or triglyceride levels, hypertension, obesity, sedentary lifestyle, smoking, or high levels of stress?
- Is there a decrease in activity tolerance, or is the client unable to continue normal activities of daily living?
- Does the client report "spells" that are indicative of transient ischemic attacks?
- Have there been any episodes of fatigue, restlessness, syncope, or confusion?
- Does the client take any medications, especially such things as nitroglycerin, digoxin, diuretics, beta blockers, or antihypertensives?
- Be alert for symptoms of:
  Digitalis toxicity (anorexia, nausea, vomiting, headache, dysrhythmias)
  Low potassium level (weakness, fatigue, muscle cramps, dysrhythmias)
  Elevated potassium level (weakness, bradycardia, hypotension)

It is a good practice to have patients show you any medications that they are taking or "sometimes" take, and to check that the medications are taken as prescribed. If the patient does not have the medications on hand, have the patient or family bring them to you. Evaluate how long the person has been taking the medication, whether it is taken as ordered, and whether there are inconsistent or incompatible combinations of drugs being taken. Nurses, as holistic health care providers, are in a position to comprehensively evaluate a patient's medication regimen and to implement appropriate patient and family teaching to maximize the therapeutic effect of prescribed medications and to minimize the chances for potential side or toxic effects.

INSPECTION

The next component of the cardiac examination is inspection, which provides clues to the size of the heart and the effect of ventricular contraction on the precordium. Look at the anterior chest with the patient supine for visible pulsations, lifts, or heaves. Visualization is best if the light source is from the side.

The apical impulse, or point of maximal impulse (PMI), is a visible pulsation caused by left ventricular contraction that is synchronous with S_1 (the first heart sound) and the carotid impulse. Its location provides a clue to cardiac size because it is near the apex of the heart. Nearly half of all normal adults will not have a visible apical impulse. It may become visible when the patient sits up and the heart is closer to the chest wall. The presence or absence of a visible apical impulse can be affected by the shape of the chest wall, obesity, or the amount of air or fluid through which the impulses must pass. When the apical impulse is present, it should be located near the mitral site, which is also the site for taking an apical pulse. It should be present in only one intercostal space. Describe the location according to both the intercostal space and the midclavicular line. In a patient with an enlarged heart, the apical impulse may be displaced distally or laterally. In elderly patients, however, the PMI can be displaced due to kyphosis or scoliosis and not necessarily be indicative of cardiac enlargement.

When cardiac function is abnormally forceful, the pulsation is readily visible even when the patient is supine. The ribs may appear to lift as the heart beats, suggesting the presence of a cardiac problem; document this as a lift or heave and note the location. It is also important to document the appearance of cyanosis, venous or abdominal distention, capillary refill, skin temperature, shortness of breath, or coughing. Each of these can assist in determining the adequacy of cardiac function.

PALPATION

Palpate the precordium systematically, making sure your hands are warm. Use the proximal half of the four fingers or your palm. Apply gentle pressure so that you can detect movements rising up against your hand. An impulse that is more forceful than anticipated can be characterized as a lift or a heave. A heave will be noted near the sternum if the patient has increased pressure or enlargement of the right ventricle. Problems in the left ventricle will be detected near or lateral to the apex of the heart. If you note either, check to see if the patient has signs of congestive heart failure. Right-sided failure will result in venous and abdominal distention; left-sided failure will result in congestion in the lungs.

A thrill has been described as a palpable heart murmur and will be felt as a vibration. If you detect a thrill, be alert for a murmur when you auscultate. Note the location of any lists or thrills, using the intercostal spaces and midsternal or midclavicular lines as landmarks.

PERCUSSION

Percussion to estimate the size of the heart or to define the cardiac borders by identifying areas of dullness is less reliable than chest x-ray or other diagnostic studies. Sufficient preliminary information can be obtained by inspection and palpation.

TABLE 8-3

Overview of the Examination of the Heart

Examine each site (aortic, pulmonic, tricuspid, and mitral) during each step of the cardiac assessment. Inspect and palpate the precordium for:

- Apical impulse
- Pulsations
- Lifts or heaves
- Thrills

Auscultate systemically with the patient supine, sitting, leaning forward, and left side-lying for:

- S_1 and S_2
- Split sounds
- S_3 and S_4
- Murmurs

EXAMINATION—AUSCULTATION SITES

Certain landmarks on the chest wall determine where cardiac function can be assessed most accurately. Heart sounds result from the closing of the four valves in the heart. They can be auscultated over the entire precordial area, but the sound produced by each of the valves can be heard best at specific locations on the chest. That location is not directly over the valve, but away from it in the direction of blood flow.

In the second intercostal space at the right sternal border, you will hear the aortic (A) valve best. Right across from it at the left sternal border, you will hear the pulmonic (P) valve best. The best place to hear the tricuspid valve (T) is in the fifth intercostal space at the left sternal border. The mitral valve (M) can be heard best at the fifth intercostal space at the midclavicular line. The mitral area is also the site used to assess the apical pulse because it lies over the apex of the heart. It may be helpful in the beginning to mark the chest wall with an X at each site or a small A, P, T, M over the appropriate area.

Just as various locations enhance certain sounds, varying the patient's position may elicit certain signs, such as pulsations on the chest wall, or allow you to hear other sounds, such as murmurs. Examine each of the four sites with the patient supine, then go through the entire sequence again with the patient sitting erect, leaning forward, and finally in a left side-lying position (Table 8-3).

AUSCULTATION

Becoming skillful at auscultating heart sounds takes concentration and practice. If you are a beginner, practice on family members, friends, and colleagues. The more familiar you become with normal heart sounds, the more adept you will become at hearing variations. Listen to as many elderly people as possible to differentiate nominal changes associated with the aging heart (eg, occasional extra beats) from pathologic ones.

NORMAL HEART SOUNDS

Normal heart sounds are produced by the closing of the valves of the heart. The first sound, S_1, results from the closure of the atrioventricular (AV) valves, the mitral and tricuspid. The closure of the AV valves and S_1 mark the beginning of systole, the period of maximal contraction and pressure. The second heart sound, S_2, results from the closure of the semilunar valves, the aortic and pulmonic. S_2 marks the end of systole and the beginning of diastole, the period during which the heart muscle is relaxed. Diastole is normally of longer duration than systole. Normal heart sounds are produced when the valves and the heart muscle are working efficiently.

Begin auscultation with the patient lying on his or her back, or with the head elevated 300 to 450 if the patient is short of breath. Auscultate from the right side if you are right-handed, the left side if left-handed. Begin either at the mitral or aortic area, but use the same sequence with each patient. Listening systematically will improve your skill in interpreting the sounds. Use both the diaphragm and the bell to listen in each area. The diaphragm is best for picking up the higher pitches sounds of S_1 and S_2 and split sounds and should be applied firmly to the chest. The bell is best for picking up the lower pitches sounds of S_3 and S_4 and should be applied lightly to the chest.

Focus on one sound at a time, blocking out other heart sounds, breath sounds, and room noises. This is important because even at a heart rate of 60 beats per minute, all of the events in the cardiac cycle occur within a second. Elderly patients frequently have more rapid, less distinct heartbeats. Listen for the normal heart sounds (S_1 and S_2, "lub-dub") first. Tune in to S_1 first ("lub"). Because this results from the closure of the mitral and tricuspid valves, the intensity will be greatest in those areas and loudest at the mitral valve (the apex). To ensure you are listening to S_1, check if the carotid pulse is in synchrony with the sound. Inch the stethoscope from site to site, listening at each place to the characteristics of S_1.

Make another round of the auscultation sites, listening this time for S_2 ("dub"). It will be heard best at the pulmonic and aortic areas, but loudest at the aortic. After identifying normal heart sounds, note the location of greatest intensity. Greater intensity may be heard in other than the usual site if the heart is enlarged or if normal blood flow is altered. Also listen to whether the intensity seems diminished or muffled or if it varies from beat to beat, which may suggest heart block. Note the rate (usually between 60 and 90 beats per minute) and the rhythm. Atrial fibrillation and infrequent ectopic (extra) beats are fairly common in the elderly, but any irregularity should be documented and reported. Always refer patients with irregular rhythms that occur without a pattern.

Split Sounds

After listening to the first and second heart sounds, listen for split sounds. They are usually heard best on the right side (the pulmonic and tricuspid sites). The left valves usually close before the right, but the timing is so close that no split is detected. When the timing widens, each sound is heard. A split S_1 sounds like **t-lub-dub**. If the split S_2 is heard only during inspiration or disappears when the patient sits up, it may be normal or physiologic. If it is unaltered by breathing or position, it is not normal and could indicate right ventricular failure or other cardiac disease.

Extra Heart Sounds

Although many practitioners consider the presence of extra heart sounds to be abnormal in adults, the presence of S_3 or S_4 does not necessarily indicate cardiac pathology but must be evaluated in light of other heart sounds and diagnostic clues. It is important, however, for the nurse to be aware that S_3 or S_4 may be the earliest signs of heart failure and may need to be brought to the attention of a nurse practitioner or a physician.

S_3 and S_4 occur during diastole and are best heard with the bell of the stethoscope with the patient in the left side-lying position. S_3 occurs early in diastole and sounds like **lub-dub-dee**. In the elderly, it is generally considered pathologic and is usually due to left ventricular failure. If S_3 is heard, auscultate the lungs for crackles, which indicate that fluid is collecting in the respiratory system, perhaps due to left ventricular failure. S_4 occurs late in diastole and sounds like **dee-lub-dub**. When either sound becomes intense, the heart rhythm sounds like a gallop. This occurs frequently in geriatric patients because the heart muscle has become less compliant. Gallops should always be reported.

Describe the location, timing, and characteristics of the patient's heart sounds. The nurse may be uncertain as to what is causing the extra or different sounds, but you can learn to hear them and to document your findings. Report what is heard even if you are unable to distinguish, for example, between a split S_2 or an S_3.

Murmurs

A murmur is heard as a relatively prolonged swishing sound between normal heart sounds and is the result of turbulent or backward flow of blood through the heart. After S_1 and S_2

(systole) there should be a silent interval (diastole) until the next cardiac cycle. As a person ages, the heart valves become thicker, more rigid, and do not shut as effectively. The turbulence of the blood flow around these valves produces a heart murmur, which sounds like a hum. Not all murmurs are the result of valvular defects. Other causes could include diminished strength of myocardial contraction or a condition in the major vessels near the heart. Remember that the presence of a murmur does not necessarily indicate cardiac disease and, conversely, cardiac disease can be present without evidence of a murmur. Murmurs are usually heard best with the patient in the left lateral position.

A murmur should be documented by location (where on the chest wall it is loudest), quality (harsh, blowing, musical), loudness or intensity (using a grading system such as in Table 8-4), radiation, and timing. Murmurs are described by the location on the chest where they sound loudest. The point on the chest wall where a murmur is best heard may not correspond to the valve site because of the transmission of sound. Murmurs of the aortic valve frequently radiate to the third intercostal space at the left midsternal line. This site is known as Erb's point and is frequently recommended as an additional inspection/auscultation site. In addition to documenting the location at which the murmur sounds loudest, describe the radiation of the sound. Specific information can be helpful in diagnosis: murmurs of mitral origin frequently radiate to the axilla, whereas aortic murmurs radiate to the carotid arteries. It is important to note the timing of the murmur. Does it occur during systole (systolic murmur) or diastole (diastolic murmur)? Early, soft systolic murmurs are fairly common in the elderly. If a murmur is heard best in midsystole, it is termed an ejection murmur. If loudness is equal throughout systole, it is called a pansystolic murmur. Diastolic murmurs are usually associated with valvular abnormalities. Early diastolic murmurs that fade out in late diastole are described as decrescendo; late diastolic murmurs that become louder toward S_1 are termed crescendo.

Although some murmurs may be benign, or functional, the discovery of a heart murmur requires careful assessment. It is important to describe and document what is heard. Physical examination alone cannot always identify the cause of the murmur, but it can narrow the possibilities so that the patient can be referred for appropriate diagnostic follow-up.

SPECIAL CONSIDERATIONS

Individual differences in the patient's age, build, and state of health will affect the visibility, palpable force, and sounds of the heart's action. In general, heart sounds are not as loud in the elderly as they are in younger patients. Findings in patients with thin, non-muscular chests may be clearer or louder than in muscular or obese patients. In these patients, visible or palpable pulsations and heart sounds may be more difficult to elicit. Changes in the anteroposterior diameter of the chest related to aging or emphysema can alter the location of the pulsations and make heart sounds more difficult to hear (eg, kyphosis can alter the location of heart sounds and of the apical impulse). Nurses in all phases of the health care continuum have the opportunity to provide professional intervention, which will enhance cardiac health in the geriatric population. All practice settings afford nurses the opportunity to educate about cardiovascular risk reduction, to evaluate progress, and to monitor for extension of cardiac disease or return to functional capacity. This can only be accomplished by eliciting and interpreting appropriate relevant patient information through an understanding of cardiac assessment techniques.

TABLE 8-4

Six-Point Grading Scale of Heart Murmurs

- Grade 1—Very soft
- Grade 2—Easily heard
- Grade 3—Moderately loud
- Grade 4—Loud
- Grade 5—Loud (heard with stethoscope barely on chest)
- Grade 6—Heard with stethoscope off chest

GERONTOLOGICAL NURSING IMPLICATIONS

Nurses, as individual practitioners, can affect positive outcomes in elderly patients by providing access to professional services that reduce the risk and enhance the quality of life for those with cardiac risk factors and disease. There are numerous opportunities for nursing practice, education, and research to promote cardiac health in the geriatric population.

PRACTICE

Nurses come into contact with elders who may require primary, secondary, and tertiary prevention of cardiac disease or disability. They encounter elderly patients during wellness screening or ambulatory visits to physicians or advanced practice nurses, in acute care settings for both cardiac and other illnesses, in extended care facilities, cardiac rehabilitation programs and other outpatient services, as well as in adult day care centers and home care. A prerequisite for cardiac health is a commitment to a healthy lifestyle, which reduces or modifies coronary risk factors. People need information in order to make informed decisions about behaviors that result in cardiovascular risk reduction; therefore, a fundamental nursing activity is patient, family, and caregiver education. Studies of cardiac patient education programs demonstrate their positive impact on behavioral and physiologic parameters such as blood pressure, exercise, and diet.[10]

The educational process begins with assessment and the identification of risk factors, then the nurse and patient work together to establish goals for lifestyle changes and the means to evaluate those changes. For any educational intervention, the issue of patient adherence is the true test of the effectiveness of teaching. It is important to attend to the emotional, physical, social, and environmental barriers to cardiovascular risk reduction behaviors.[11] In any teaching/learning interaction, the issue of motivation to initiate and sustain behavioral change must be considered in developing a teaching plan. Patients must feel that they have some control over their decisions about behavioral change. It is important to work with the elderly person to establish realistic goals and priorities. Physiologic and behavioral milestones should be established to serve as a motivator and a means of evaluation. Give the patient or family the responsibility for self-monitoring and self-reporting: Did I lose one pound this week? Is my cholesterol lower than it was 6 weeks ago? Did I walk for 30 minutes three times this week? Did I reduce or eliminate the number of cigarettes smoked this week? Do I have more strength and endurance?

The physical symptoms and limitations imposed by acute and chronic illness can be a barrier to motivation, especially to physical exercise.[11] It is important to work with the patient to determine the best type of exercise, the best time of day, and the method of symptom management (eg, control of joint pain or shortness of breath). Acknowledging the existence of these factors and being flexible in adapting risk reduction behaviors to the realities of the patient's life can improve the chances for successful and permanent change.

Patients should be encouraged to share their experiences about environmental and social situations that influence them to continue high-risk behaviors or that work against their risk modification efforts. Perhaps family members may not be supportive of their efforts to change or, conversely, are overprotective to the point that the patient feels powerless. An atmosphere of trust must be created in order for patients to discuss why they did not continue with dietary, exercise, and other lifestyle modifications.

Providing a continuum of care that is competent, cost-effective, and accessible, nurses must be proactive in the redesign of nursing services in a restructured health care environment. Managed care will be the prevailing mode of health care delivery and financing,[12,13] with more Medicare patients enrolled in managed care plans. Managed care is not just a system of financing but of organizing health care.[14] Nurse case managers can facilitate access to and coordination of comprehensive services across the continuum from wellness/prevention, illness, and rehabilitation in a health care environment in which early discharge from acute care settings increases the need for appropriate teaching and follow-up with elders who are learning to live with cardiac risk reduction and rehabilitation interventions. Nurse-managed health care programs can be cost-effective alternatives to more expensive physician and specialty based practice. Recent studies have demonstrated that people will seek alternative, non-physician treatment for numerous medical conditions and health promotion services and that patients express equal or greater satisfaction with nurse-provided versus physician-provided services. In addition, patient adherence and knowledge about their illness and plan of care is enhanced by nursing's holistic, comprehensive approach to patient care services, yet, in some studies, the average cost per visit to a nurse practitioner is 39% less than the fee for a physician visit.[15,16] It is the responsibility of the individual practitioner to develop and maintain the skills of cardiac assessment that will enable them to make decisions about the appropriate care and management of elderly patients.

EDUCATION

Educators must maintain a commitment to developing comprehensive health assessment skills, including specific variations for the geriatric population. Nurse educators must prepare nurses to work in a reformed health care system by increasing students' exposure to community-based and diverse populations. Students should understand the concept of a collaborative model of health care delivery in which the nurse is one of a group of providers who can offer primary, secondary, and tertiary services for the cardiac patient. Gerontological nursing should be discussed as a viable and growing area of professional specialization. The needs of the elderly cardiac patient are similar to other age groups, but there are specific and important differences related to physiological, emotional, and psychosocial parameters.

The shift to home- and community-based care demands more reflective and independent decision making and a conscious attention to the process of learning. Educators should incorporate varied perspectives while teaching a skill such as cardiac assessment since sociocultural values affect lifestyle and communication. Activities that require critical thinking should become a part of all class sessions and assignments.

Graduate programs that prepare expert clinicians to deliver primary health care and other essential health care services must continue to increase the number of advanced practice nurses who can provide a full range of services to the elderly, particularly in community-based and cardiac rehabilitation programs.

In line with changes in national priorities away from disease and illness and toward health and wellness, there have been profound changes in funding for research, which reflect a health rather than disease emphasis. Many of the risk factors associated with cardiac disease and disability in the elderly have been identified, and studies have demonstrated that risk reduction programs can have a positive outcome. If nursing is to be considered a legitimate provider of health care services, then we need to study how nursing intervention affects patient behaviors and health care outcomes. Further research is needed into what specific nursing interventions are effective in fostering compliance in cardiovascular risk reduction behaviors and how nursing care makes a difference in the patient's cardiac status. Nurses should seek opportunities to submit proposals for community-based health promotion/illness prevention projects,[8] which can demonstrate the effectiveness of nursing intervention in the reduction of coronary disease and disability in the elderly.

The roles of both gender and age in cardiac disease is a prime area for research. Heart disease is reaching epidemic proportions in women; in fact it is the leading cause of death among postmenopausal older women, yet females have historically been underrepresented in cardiac research.[2,17,18] One important field for study is the role of hormone replacement therapy (HRT) in the prevention of cardiac disease in postmenopausal women. Studies on the use of estrogen (in some cases combined with progestin) in postmenopausal women suggest that HRT is associated with a 40% reduction in the risk of coronary heart disease.[19,20] The role of HRT in the prevention of injury and disability related to osteoporosis is being investigated as well. It is important that nurses be aware of the risks and benefits of HRT and present this information to their female patients so that they are prepared to make informed choices about the use of HRT to prevent heart disease and other illnesses related to postmenopausal longevity.

The effect of exercise on cardiac rehabilitation in patients older than 65 has not been studied as comprehensively as in other age groups; men have been studied more extensively than women, but data show that both male and female elderly patients with known cardiac disease can benefit from the effects of exercise on cardiac work load and functional capacity.[2] Nurses should investigate the role of gender and age in risk reduction, and study the effects of exercise on elderly cardiac patients. In addition, they should encourage elder participation in cardiac rehabilitation programs. Through practice, education, and research, nurses can make significant contributions to the health and wellness of elderly people by skillful cardiac assessment and an ongoing investigation of the effectiveness of illness prevention and cardiac rehabilitation efforts by nurses.

REFERENCES

1. Behar S, Gilat D, Reicher-Reiss H, Kaplinsky E, Zion M, Mandelzweig L, Goldbourt U. Myocardial infarction in patients older than 75 years of age: the short- and long-term prognosis in 653 consecutive patients. *Cardiology in the Elderly.* 1993;1:103-111.
2. Hellmann E, Williams M. Outpatient cardiac rehabilitation in elderly patients. *Heart and Lung.* 1994;23:506-512.
3. American Heart Association. *1990 Heart and Stroke Facts.* American Heart Association: 1990.
4. National Cholesterol Education Program: *Detection, Evaluation and Treatment of High Blood Cholesterol in Adults.* Bethesda, MD: NIH Publication No. 88-2926, 1987.
5. Hopkins P, Williams R. Identification and relative weight of cardiovascular risk factors. *Cardiol Clin.* 1986;4:3.
6. Stovsky B. Nursing interventions for risk factor reduction. *Nurs Clin North Am.* 1992;27:257-270.
7. Haskell W, Alderman E, Fair J, et al. Effects of intensive multiple risk factor reduction in coronary atherosclerosis and clinical events in men and women with coronary artery disease: the Stanford Coronary Risk Intervention Project (SCRIP). *Circulation.* 1994;89:975-990.
8. Pender N. *Health Promotion in Nursing Practice.* 2nd ed. Norwalk, CT.: Appleton & Lange; 1987.
9. American Nurses Association. *Nursing's Agenda for Health Care Reform.* Washington, D.C.: American Nurses Association; 1991.
10. Mullen P, Mains D, Velez R. A meta-analysis of controlled trials of cardiac patient education. *Patient Educ Couns.* 1992;19(2):143-162.
11. Biggs J, Fleury J. An exploration of perceived barriers to cardiovascular risk reduction. *Cardiovas Nurs.* 1994;30:41-46.
12. Packard N. The price of choice: managed care in America. *Nursing Administration Quarterly.* 1993;17:8-15.
13. Friedman E. Managed care: where will your hospital fit in? *Hosp.* 1993;67(7):18-23.
14. Himali U. Managed care: does the promise meet the potential? *Am Nurse.* 1995;27(6):1,14,16.
15. Eisenberg D, Kessler R, Foster C, Norlock F, Calkins D, Delbanco T. Unconventional medicine in the United States: prevalence, costs, and patterns of use. *N Engl J Med.* 1993;328(4):246-252.
16. The American Nurse. Study shows nurse practitioner care may rival physician primary care. *Am Nurse.* 1993;25(2):3.
17. Holm K, Penckofer S, Keresztes P, Biordi D, Chandler P. Coronary artery disease in women: assessment, diagnosis, intervention, and strategies for lifestyle change. *Clin Issues Perinat Women's Health Nurs.* 1993;4(2):272-285.
18. Deshotels A. Male and female perceptions of quality of life in cardiac rehabilitation programs. *Heart Lung.* 1992;21(3):287.
19. Nabulsi A, Folsom A, White A, et al. Association of hormone-replacement therapy with various cardiovascular risk factors in postmenopausal women. The atherosclerosis risk in communities study. *N Engl J Med.* 1993;328:1069-1075.
20. Rosenberg L, Palmer J, Shapiro S. A case-control study of myocardial infarction in relation to use of estrogen supplements. *Am J Epidemiol.* 1993;137:54-63.

Chapter 9

Self-Care Interventions for Congestive Heart Failure

Frances Kathleen Bushnell, RNC, EdD, MPH

OVERVIEW

Congestive heart failure (CHF) affects approximately 2.5 million elderly patients in the United States and is the cardiac problem most frequently encountered by gerontological nurses.[1] Although mortality from cardiovascular disease has declined in the past two decades, it continues to be the leading cause of death. The prevalence of CHF has increased. CHF occurs in 3 million Americans or approximately 1% of the population with 400,000 new case presentations each year.[2] CHF is also the most common hospital discharge diagnosis in patients older than 65 years. More than 500,000 CHF patients are discharged annually, which is increasing and may be due to the aging population and improvement of other forms of cardiovascular disease.[3] This chapter discusses self-care teaching for patients with CHF.

INTRODUCTION

In our aging society, preventive nursing interventions for congestive heart failure (CHF) patients can improve quality of life, decrease mortality and morbidity, and reduce health care costs. Nursing recently has turned increasingly to the social and behavioral sciences for a better understanding of the forces shaping lifestyles. The application of positive health habits, promoting the diffusion of health knowledge, and providing support or pressure for the adoption of healthy and unhealthy behavior has positioned nurses as key players in the prevention of disease. CHF is one disease that lends itself to modifications rooted in patient changes in lifestyle.

The framework found in the literature for behavior change include the process of change, health-related behavior life transitions requiring adaptations of health behavior, and policies for health behavior change. For our purposes, CHF self-care practice is used synonymously with CHF health promotion, which is any combination of health education and related organizational, economic, and environmental supports for individual, group, and community behavior conducive to health.[4]

LITERATURE REVIEW

There are only four studies in the literature that study CHF and self-care.[1,4-6] Cintron found that when CHF patients received education concerning their medications prior to discharge from the hospital, they returned to the hospital with significantly reduced rates than patients who did not receive such instruction.[7] Another study with 100 CHF elderly patients found those with knowledge about the condition and the perceived benefits of treatment complied with dietary adherence, medication adherence, smoking cessation, and stress avoidance.[8] The third research study concluded that elderly CHF patients who received home teaching concerning CHF had significantly fewer readmissions to acute care hospitals than those who did not receive additional instruction.[1] The fourth study researched patients' CHF disease knowledge and compliance with instructions for medications, a low-salt diet, and self-care activities.[5] The patient pool consisted of 41 patients with chronic CHF as the primary diagnosis. All chronic CHF patients who met the criteria for hospitalization were invited to participate in the study. Exclusion criteria included a history of myocardial infarction. All chronic CHF patients admitted to these units were offered self-care nursing intervention.

Studies of the incidence and prognosis of cardiac failure in the general population are quite sparse. The Framingham Heart Study is one of the few clinical research studies that provide data on CHF.[9] After three decades of follow-up with 5209 subjects, the Framingham Study developed criteria to define cardiac failure. CHF increased annually among subjects: from 3 per 1000 between the ages 35 and 64 to 10 per 1000 between ages 65 and 94. Sixty percent of CHF patients had additional chronic debilitating illnesses. In addition to CHF, 14% of men and 26% of women had diabetes. About half of those diagnosed with CHF had a history of coronary heart disease. Cardiac failure continues to be a lethal end-stage cardiovascular disease. According to the criteria established in 1987, cardiac mortality rates are little better than cancer mortality rates. Within 5 years, about half the CHF patients die.

The degree of compliance with a therapeutic regimen is negatively correlated with its complexity.[10,11] Patients often comply with regimens in varying degrees. According to recent studies, medicinal compliance was not directly related to the extent of a patient's knowledge about his or her illnesses and treatments. However, compliance increased when patients believed they were susceptible to serious problems. Rideout explains that patients must understand the nature of their illness, why they are being treated, how long the treatment will last, and the results of treatment in order to comply.[12]

SAMPLE DESCRIPTION

The focus of the current study was to measure the knowledge of CHF patients admitted to acute care hospitals in the following areas: CHF symptoms, medication regimen, diet, activities of daily living, and self-care activities. A self-care program was implemented for a subset of the hospitalized patients.

TABLE 9-1

Self-Care Lesson Plan

Gerontological nurses teach CHF patients self-care in hospitals, long-term care facilities, clinics, or private homes. After nursing instruction, patients can do the following:

CHF

- Identify CHF and problems related to cardiac reserve to decrease the heart workload.

Weight

- Weigh in every morning before eating, wearing the same clothes and using the same scale.
- Report a weight gain of more than 3 pounds to the primary care provider (physician or nurse practitioner) if diet has not changed.

Nutrition

- Identify high- and low-salt foods.
- Keep a daily journal of foods for the gerontological nurse to reinforce a low-salt diet.

Symptoms

- Identify CHF symptoms (eg, weight gain, shortness of breath, exercise intolerance, edema, sensation of heart pounding, increased fatigue, confusion, polyuria, and stomach ache).
- Report any of these symptoms to the primary care provider.

Medication Regimen

- Identify all prescribed medications, discuss the reasons why they were prescribed, side effects, and identify the correct dosage.
- Take medications as prescribed, and document information on a self-care medication sheet (drug name, dosage, and time and date taken).
- Report drug side effects to the primary care provider (MD or NP).

Activity Tolerance

- Identify activity level (eg, number of stairs or blocks walked without experiencing CHF symptoms).
- Identify ways to conserve energy (eg, dress in the bathroom after a shower rather than in the bedroom).
- Set limits to decrease cardiac workload.

The mean age for the sample was 71 years of age. The sample consisted of 23 men (58%) and 18 women (42%). Thirty-one participants were white (75%), seven were black (17%), and three were Hispanic (8%). Thirty-one (75%) attended high school or college; 10 achieved less than a grade-school education. Thirteen (35%) participants were married, 16 (40%) were widowed, seven (17%) were separated or divorced, and five (8%) were never married. Eight

(20%) participants were currently employed, while 14 (34%) were not working because of poor health, and 19 (46%) were retired. Almost all participants (92%) earned $20,000 or less annually, and 8% earned more than $20,000. Fifty-one percent of the participants were on Medicare, one fourth were on Medicaid, and the remaining fourth were covered with private insurance. Nearly half (20%) of the participants lived alone, while 11 (27%) lived with spouses, and 10 (24%) lived with others including children and siblings. Some people reported needing assistance in performing multiple activities of daily living. These included dressing (14 patients or 29%), bathing (13 patients or 35%), walking (four patients or 9%), and grooming (four patients or 9%). Others reported needing assistance with the instrumental activities of daily living, such as taking medication (11 or 28%), planning meals (16 or 38%), grocery shopping (27 or 66%), cooking (23 or 58%), cleaning (25 or 60%), and driving (19 or 46%).

INTERVENTION

The nurse researcher gave the patient a CHF self-care booklet to read. The booklet contained information developed from the American Heart Association. In 24 hours the nurse researcher returned to question the patient about the content of the booklet. If the patient answered the questions correctly, the nurse researcher taught the patient about self-care procedures regarding medications, diet, activity level, and symptom recognition. The nurse researcher reviewed this information with the patient until the patient could verbalize it and demonstrate sufficient knowledge. The researcher then directed the hospital pharmacy to place the patient's medications at the bedside. The nurse researcher also informed the primary care physician and staff nurses about the self-care medicine regimen. If the patient did not know the medication regimen, the nurse researcher taught the patient, who was then retested in 24 hours. After implementing this self-care medication regimen, the pharmacist placed a sufficient amount of medication for 1 week at the bedside. The patient had the self-care medicine sheet at the bedside and was expected to take the medicine as directed. The staff nurse checked on the patient 15 minutes after the medication was to be taken in order to verify that indeed it had been taken. This procedure was followed throughout the patient's hospital stay.

In order to develop additional self-care responsibility, patients also ordered their own meals. They weighed in daily before breakfast and informed the staff nurse of any identifiable CHF symptoms such as weight gain or shortness of breath. This procedure was followed until discharge.

Upon release from the hospital, the nurse researcher followed the research sample. At 3- and 6-month intervals, the nurse researcher documented hospital readmissions and verified continued adherence to the medication regimen, diet, daily weigh-ins, and CHF symptom control. The dependent variables were 3- and 6-month acute hospital readmission rates. Another dependent variable was the ability to follow the self-care protocol. Three months after hospital discharge, 16% had two or more hospital readmissions, 26% had one readmission, and 58% had no readmissions. Six months after hospital discharge, 25% had one or more readmissions. Approximately one third (34%) of participants died before the study was completed.

The self-perceived reasons for hospitalization included shortness of breath (79%), swelling of limbs (58%), exercise intolerance (54%), increased fatigue (50%), cough (38%), inability to buy medication (29%), diet noncompliance (27%), polyuria (27%), sensation of pounding heart (27%), stomach ache (21%), medication noncompliance (15%), and confusion (14%). Ninety-seven percent of participants could not define CHF correctly; only 6% could partially define their condition. The majority (76%) of the participants in the study could identify one to three CHF symptoms while 16% could identify four symptoms. The remaining 8% could not identify any symptom related to their CHF disease.

When asked about medication history before the intervention, 82% of participants were compliant more than half the time, 9% were compliant less than half the time, and 9% never took their medications. When asked to identify their prescribed medications, 42% could identify all of their medications, 19% were able to identify all but one or two, 22% misidentified three to five medications, and 17% misidentified six or more medications.

In reference to diet, 71% participants weighed in less than weekly, 17% weighed in weekly, and only 12% weighed in daily. Before self-care instructions, 73% of participants correctly identified five or more high-salt foods, 18% identified two to four high-salt foods, and 9% identified one or more high-salt foods. Sixty-five percent of participants followed the low-salt diet more than half the time, 16% followed the diet less than half the time, and 19% never followed the low-salt diet.

FINDINGS

Sixteen patients were able to follow the self-care intervention during their hospital stay. It is difficult to compare this group to those who did not carry out the self-care intervention due to differences in age, education, gender, and income. Those who did follow self-care intervention were older, less educated, more often widowed, less wealthy, and more often lived alone. Past research indicated that to successfully care for CHF patients, nurses must identify patients' self-care deficits. In order to do this, nurses must teach self-care practices related to specific illnesses (Table 9-1).

GERONTOLOGICAL NURSING IMPLICATIONS

Gerontological nurses have a unique responsibility to teach self-care practices to elderly, chronic CHF patients. These patients can participate in their health care, which may improve quality of life.[11,13] Nursing interventions with chronic CHF patients in the home and clinic have significantly decreased re-hospitalization rates.[14] Thus, chronically ill CHF patients may need continued follow-up and re-education to stay out of the hospital. Self-care practices include a number of activities that significantly give patients responsibility for their health. These are managing diet, exercise, and recognition of symptoms, in addition to medication administration. Future nursing studies need to compare nursing interventions in acute care and clinical settings to study the effect of patients' self-care behavior on mortality, morbidity, and quality of life. As the population expands, so will the problem of chronic CHF in the elderly. Thus gerontological nurses must provide high-quality, scientifically based clinical care for these patients. This clinical care encompasses not only acute care but also community care. Office nurses, occupational health nurses, clinic and home care nurses all need to incorporate self-care plans into their practice. The more knowledge a nurse can give to a patient concerning CHF, the more responsibility the patient may take to promote his or her own healthy lifestyle (Table 9-2).

TABLE 9-2

Self-Care Activities for CHF Patients

- Weigh myself daily upon wakening before breakfast, in the same clothes and using the same scale.
- If I have gained more than 3 pounds in a week and have not changed my diet, call my health care provider and report the weight gain.
- I will maintain a low-salt diet. I will know the foods low in salt. I will include them in my diet. I will avoid foods high in salt.
- I will take all medications as prescribed and know the names, dosages, side effects, and action of each medication.
- I will call my health care provider and report any side effects or problems with my medication.
- I will know the symptoms of CHF and if I have shortness of breath, increased fatigue, swelling, having to go to the bathroom frequently, or frequent colds, I will not wait, but call the health care provider as soon as possible.
- I will conserve energy and think about what I will be doing and plan ways to save my heart from having to work hard. I will ask others to help me if needed.

REFERENCES

1. Singh P. Managing chronic congestive heart failure in the home. *Home Health Care Nurse.* 1995;13(2):11-15.
2. Edwards VL. Recognition and management of heart failure in the primary care setting. *Nurse Practitioner Forum.* 1991;2(1):42-47.
3. Stearns SC. Hospital discharge decisions, health outcomes, and the use of unobserved information on case-mix severity. *Health Services Research.* 1991;26(1):26-46.
4. Hagenhoff BD, Feutz C, Conn VS, Sagehorn KL, Moranville-Hunziker M. Patient education needs as reported by congestive heart failure patients and their nurses. *J Adv Nurs.* 1994;19(4):685-690.
5. Bushnell K. Self-care teaching for congestive heart failure patients. *J Gerontol Nurs.* 1992;18(10):27-32.
6. Cintron G, Bigas CA, Linares E, Aranda JM, Hernandez E. Nurse practitioner role in a chronic congestive heart failure clinic: in-hospital time, costs, and patient satisfaction. *Heart Lung.* 1983;12(3):237-240.

7. Schaefer KM, Shober MJ. Fatigue associated with congestive heart failure: use of Levine's conservation model. *J Adv Nurs.* 1993;18:260-268.
8. Lacy AL. *Health Beliefs and Health Behaviors in Elderly, Chronically Ill Males.* Rush University, College of Nursing, DNSc; 1988.
9. Kannel WB, Seidman JM, Fercho W, Castelli WP. Vital capacity and congestive heart failure: the Framingham Study. *Circulation.* 1974;49:1160-1167.
10. Gold ME. Pharmacology of nitrovasodilators. *Nurs Clin N Am.* 1991;26(2):437-451.
11. Jessup M, Lakatiu EC, Leier C, Santin AI. Managing CHF in the older patient. *Patient Care.* 1990;7(3):55-58,61,62,65,67.
12. Rideout E. Chronic heart failure and quality of life: the impact of nursing. *Canadian J Cardiovas Nurs.* 1992;3(1):4-8.
13. Wingate S, Leach SP, Michell SM, Dudas GM. Case study in perioperative right heart failure. *J Cardiovas Nurs.* 1991;6(1):80-86.
14. Smith T, Kelly RA. Therapeutic strategies for CHF in the 1990's. *Hosp Prac.* 1991;26(11):127-150.

Chapter 10

Osteoporosis Prevention in Menopausal and Elderly Women

Nagia S. Ali, PhD, RN

OVERVIEW

Osteoporosis among menopausal and elderly women is a major public health problem. It predisposes individuals to fractures of the spine, wrist, and hip with minimal or no trauma. Prevention of osteoporotic fractures includes adequate calcium intake, regular exercise, and taking estrogen/hormone replacement therapy. This chapter discusses the risk factors, prevention, and treatment of osteoporosis in elderly women.

INTRODUCTION

Osteoporosis is a major health problem mainly afflicting menopausal and elderly women. Osteoporosis predisposes individuals to fractures of the spine, wrist, and hip with minimal or no trauma. The overall cost of care for osteoporotic patients with hip fractures is $10 billion annually.[1] Since the world population is aging, the number of osteoporotic fractures is expected to increase dramatically in the next 50 years.[2] In addition to the economic costs of hip fractures, other outcomes include pain, functional limitations, reduced quality of life, hospitalization, loss of independence, and caregivers' difficulties.[2]

Risk factors for the development of osteoporosis include two groups: those factors that women cannot control and those factors that women can control. Factors that women cannot modify include female sex, white or Asian race, thin build, premature menopause by bilateral oophorectomies, maternal history of osteoporosis, presence of concomitant diseases (ie, hyperthyroidism and hyperparathyroidism), and chronic use of some medications (ie, dilantin, glucocorticoids, thyroxine, and furosemide [lasix]).[3-7] Factors that women can modify include cigarette smoking, alcohol use, chronic inadequate calcium intake, and decreased physical activity.[3,8-11]

EFFECTS OF CALCIUM, EXERCISE, AND HORMONE THERAPY ON BONE MASS

Bone mass, as measured by bone mineral density (BMD), is inversely related to the incidence of osteoporotic fractures.[1] Research studies in perimenopausal, menopausal, and elderly women support the influence of adequate calcium intake and participation in regular, moderate, weight-bearing and/or resistant training exercise. Additional studies have supported hormone replacement therapy (HRT) usage, avoidance of smoking, and moderate consumption of alcohol influence BMD positively and prevent osteoporosis.[3,4]

Perimenopausal women need 1000 mg of calcium daily and menopausal women need 1500 mg if they are not receiving HRT.[7,12] Oral calcium supplements are essential for perimenopausal women to overcome inadequate dietary calcium and for menopausal and elderly women to compensate for inadequate intestinal absorption and rapid excretion of calcium through the kidneys.[12] Positive effects of calcium supplements on BMD are attributed to their effects on inhibiting bone turnover. Many clinical trials and correlational studies conducted in menopausal women supported liberal amounts of dietary and/or supplemental calcium; significantly maintained bone mass; reduced further bone loss from the femoral neck, femur, radius, spine, wrist, and total body; and reduced the number of hip fractures.[10,13-19]

Bone mineral density diminishes with physical inactivity and increases with regular exercise, either weight-bearing or resistant training or a combination of both.[20-22] Stressed bones have an increased level of BMD and, consequently, are less prone to osteoporotic fractures. Additionally, exercise improves muscle strength and flexibility, both of which help maintain balance and decrease the risk and impact of falls and possible fractures. Effective weight-bearing exercise, such as walking, stair climbing, household chores, playing tennis, dancing, bowling, light aerobics, or jogging, should be maintained for 30 to 60 minutes a day for 3 to 5 days a week.[10] Resistant training exercises, such as use of exercise machines and weight lifting, are only effective if performed in three sets of eight to 12 repetitions.[22] Regular low-impact moderate exercise, in combination with calcium supplements, will maintain appropriate BMD values.

One study examined the efficacy of weight-bearing exercise intervention on BMD and found that exercise significantly reduced bone loss in the arm and wrist of the intervention group at a higher rate than for the control group.[23] Likewise, correlational studies supported a significant association between an increase in caloric expenditures on physical activity and an increase in BMD at the spine, distal, and mid-radius sites.[10,20,24] When weight-bearing was combined with resistant training exercise in an intervention study, a significant increase in spinal BMD in the experimental group was observed at a higher rate than for the control group.[25]

Hormone usage, either by estrogen replacement therapy (ERT) or HRT, is proposed to be the most therapeutic strategy in preventing further loss of bone mass after menopause and reducing the incidence of fractures for elderly women.[26-29] Hormone usage continues to be effective as long as the treatment is used, but once stopped, subsequent bone loss may be substantial.[27] Clinical trials of the effects of HRT found that hormone usage significantly increased BMD in lumbar spine, femoral neck, Ward triangle, and forearm of users at a higher rate for the experimental group than for the control groups.[13,30] Correlational studies also supported significant associations between HRT usage and increase in BMD at different body sites and subsequent reduction in the risks of fractures in the wrist and hip.[10,31,32] The researchers suggested HRT should be initiated soon after menopause and continued for at least 7 years for women who are candidates to receive the therapy.[31,32]

Despite the major benefit of hormones for the prevention of osteoporosis, ERT has been linked with the risks of breast and uterine cancers.[33] Researchers report the increased risk of breast cancer found in previous studies is attributed to the effect of taking higher doses of hormone therapy for prolonged periods of time.[33] The risk of uterine cancer can be eliminated by taking progestin concomitantly with estrogen either in a cyclic or a continuous pattern for women with an intact uterus.[28] Therefore, ERT is recommended safely for women without a uterus. This regimen continues to be studied and researched for effects on women's health.

OSTEOPOROSIS PREVENTIVE BEHAVIORS AND ATTITUDINAL VARIABLES

Despite the close association between adequate calcium intake, regular exercise participation, HRT usage and the increase in BMD and the subsequent prevention of osteoporotic fractures, studies of menopausal women showed inadequate performance of the recommended behaviors.[10,14,15,20,32,34-36] Inadequate performance of behaviors may be attributed to some attitudinal variables. For example, some studies found perceptions of benefits and barriers to calcium intake, exercise participation, and HRT usage significantly explained behavior performances.[34-36] Perceptions of greater benefits and fewer barriers to calcium intake, exercise participation, and taking HRT explained greater behavior performances. Qualitative assessment of women's perceptions about the recommended behaviors revealed lack of knowledge and a variety of beliefs.[35,36] Some of these beliefs were that menopausal and elderly women reported that milk is not necessary for them as they get older; exercise is only beneficial for their hearts, control of blood pressure, diabetes mellitus, and reduction of cholesterol; and hormone therapy is unnecessary treatment that needs to be taken for the rest of their lives.[35,36]

Menopausal women who exhibited greater knowledge of preventive behaviors reported significantly greater practice of health promotion and osteoporosis preventive behaviors.[34] Women with an increased level of education exhibited a significantly greater tendency to practice osteoporosis preventive behaviors, greater knowledge of the recommended preventive behaviors, and perceived fewer barriers to calcium intake than women with a lower level of education.[34] In another study, women who reported greater exercise participation also exhibited a significantly higher level of general self-efficacy and perceived themselves to have better health status.[36] Furthermore, women who used hormone therapy reported higher calcium intake and greater exercise participation than non-hormone users, however, the difference was not significant.[36]

GERONTOLOGICAL NURSING IMPLICATIONS

Gerontological nurses have an important role in educating menopausal and elderly women about strategies to prevent osteoporosis. Women should be counseled and encouraged to be active participants in their individualized plan of care. A teaching program including the need for calcium supplementation, physical activity, and the role of hormone therapy will be discussed. Before developing an individualized teaching plan, the nurse must be aware of all the medications that patient is currently taking in order to avoid drug interactions.[37] For example, calcium supplements interfere with iron absorption and should be taken at a different time.

Promoting adequate calcium intake in menopausal and elderly women is a nursing responsibility. A teaching plan should include the following:

- The need for calcium supplements and the need for Vitamin D to increase calcium absorption.
- Education about the benefits of calcium for bones, muscles, heart, nerves, and blood clotting.
- Instruction about the need to drink 6 to 8 ounces of fluid per day, if possible, in order to enhance solubility and absorption of calcium supplements as well as the need to avoid the use of laxatives, which can promote calcium loss through the GI tract.
- Education about calcium-rich foods and written material about calcium contents of foods and dairy products.
- Instruction about avoiding excessive amounts of caffeine, protein, and salt when ingesting calcium-rich foods, since they hinder the absorption of calcium.
- Suggestions about calcium-fortified foods, such as some fruit juices, cereals, and breads for women who have problems with the taste of dairy products.
- Instruction about milk alternatives available for women with lactose intolerance.

PHYSICAL ACTIVITY

Physical activity plays an important role in prevention of osteoporosis and its chronic debilitating effects. Nurses need to consider not only the benefits of physical activity for those women with osteoporosis but also the contraindications that exist for patients with this disease. Patients should first consult with their physician before beginning a program or initiating a change from their normal exercise routine. Gerontological nurses should:

- Instruct the patient about weight-bearing and resistant training exercise and the different activities in each.
- Advise about frequency, intensity, and duration of exercise.
- Advise the patient to consult with an exercise specialist who can assist with the setting of reasonable and achievable goals.
- Advise to stop exercise if there is any experience of chest pain or other problems.
- Encourage the patient to incorporate walking into activities of daily living to make it a habit.
- Encourage the patient to exercise with a spouse or a friend.

HORMONE THERAPY

HRT has been debated for a number of years. In order to counsel older women regarding the potential hormone therapy usage, nurses have the responsibility to:

- Advise women to consult with their physician or primary care provider about BMD measurement, which predicts potential osteoporotic fractures.
- Emphasize that hormone therapy is not recommended for every woman. For example, estrogen should not be used in women with known or suspected breast cancer, estrogen-dependent neoplasia, abnormal genital bleeding, and active thrombophlebitis.
- Educate women about the short-term benefits of hormones that include relief of hot flashes, night sweats, and irritability; prevention of urogenital atrophy with reduction of episodes of cystitis and dyspareunia; and improvement in libido and cognitive and affective behavior.
- Instruct women about the long-term benefits of hormones, which include prevention of bone loss and subsequent osteoporotic fractures and improvement in quality of life.
- Discuss potential risks to hormone usage, including endometrial and breast cancers, cholelithiasis, and thromboembolic disorders.
- Inform women about potential side effects of the therapy, such as menstrual-like bleeding, breast tenderness, and edema.
- Advise women to practice health promoting behaviors such as breast self-examination and a yearly mammogram.
- Explain the need for prolonged use of hormone therapy.

Because of the chronic effects of a preventable disease, gerontological nurses can extend their practice into the community and provide local churches and college settings with programs. This is one disease that is potentially easy to prevent. The cost in human life and suffering is worth the effort.

REFERENCES

1. Lindsay R. The burden of osteoporosis: cost. *Am J Med.* 1995;98:2A-9S-2A-11S.
2. Barrett-Connor E. The economic and human costs of osteoporotic fractures. *Am J Med.* 1995;98:2A-3S-2A-8S.
3. Consensus Development Conference. Prophylaxis and treatment of osteoporosis. *Am J Med.* 1991;90:107-110.
4. Cummings SR, Black D. Bone mass measurements and risks of fracture in Caucasian women: a review of findings from prospective studies. *Am J Med.* 1995;98:2A-24S-2A-28S.
5. Weinstein R, Bell N. Diminished rates of bone formation in normal black adults. *N Engl J Med.* 1988;319:1698-1701.
6. Ribot C, Tremolliers F, Pouilles J. Can we detect women with low bone mass using clinical risk factors? *Am J Med.* 1995;98:2A-52S-2A-55S.
7. Allen S. Primary osteoporosis: methods to combat bone loss that accompanies aging. *Postgrad Med.* 1993;93:43-55.
8. Kiel D, Baron J, Anderson J, Hannah M, Felson D. Smoking eliminates the protective effect of oral estrogen on the risk for hip fractures among women. *Ann Intern Med.* 1992;116:617-721.
9. Krall E, Dawson-Hughes B. Smoking and bone loss among postmenopausal women. *J Bone Min Res.* 1991;6:331-338.
10. Bauer D, Browner W, Cauley J, et al. Factors associated with appendicular bone mass in older women. *Ann Intern Med.* 1993;118:657-665.
11. Bikle D, Genant H, Cann C, Recker R, Halloran B, Strewler G. Bone disease in alcohol abuse. *Ann Intern Med.* 1985;103:42-48.
12. Heaney R. Thinking straight about calcium. *N Engl J Med.* 1993;328:503-505.
13. Aloia J, Vaswani A, Yoh J, Ross P, Flaster E, Dilmania F. Calcium supplementation with and without hormone replacement therapy to prevent postmenopausal bone loss. *Ann Intern Med.* 1994;120:97-103.
14. Reid I, Ames R, Evans M, Gamble G, Sharpe S. Effects of calcium supplementation on bone mass in postmenopausal women. *N Engl J Med.* 1993;328:460-464.
15. Reid I, Ames R, Evans M, Gamble G, Sharpe S. Long term effects of calcium supplementation on bone mass and fractures in postmenopausal women: a randomized controlled trial. *Am J Med.* 1995;98:331-335.
16. Chapuy M, Arolot M, Duboeuf F, et al. Vitamin D3 and calcium to prevent hip fractures in women. *N Engl J Med.* 1992;327:1673-1642.
17. Andon M, Smith K, Bracker M, Sartoris D, Saltman P, Strause L. Spinal bone density and calcium intake healthy postmenopausal women. *Am J Clin Nut.* 1991;54:927-929.

18. Dawson-Hughes B, Dallal G, Krall E, Sadowski L, Sahyoun N, Tannenbaum S. A controlled trial of the effect of calcium supplementation on bone density in postmenopausal women. *N Engl J Med.* 1990;323:878-883.
19. Elders P, Netelenbos J, Lips P, et al. Calcium supplementation reduces vertebral bone loss in perimenopausal women: a controlled trial in 248 women between 46 and 55 years of age. *J Clin Endoc Metab.* 1991;73:533-540.
20. Zhang J, Feldblum P, Forteny J. Moderate physical activity and bone density among perimenopausal women. *Am J Public Health.* 1992;82:736-738.
21. Block J, Smith R, Block D, Grenant H. Does exercise prevent osteoporosis? *JAMA.* 1987;257:3115-3117.
22. Campbell W. Can resistant training maintain physical function? *Contemp Intern Med.* 1994;6:26-37.
23. Smith E, Gilligan C, McAdam M, Ensign C, Smith P. Deterring bone loss by exercise intervention in premenopausal and postmenopausal women. *Calc Tissue International.* 1989;44:312-321.
24. Michel B, Block D, Fries J. Weight-bearing exercise, over exercise, and lumbar bone density over 50 years. *Arch Intern Med.* 1989;149:2325-2329.
25. Dalsky G, Stocke K, Ehsani A, Slatopolsky E, Lee W, Birge S. Weight-bearing exercise training and lumbar bone mineral content in postmenopausal women. *Ann Intern Med.* 1988;108:824-828.
26. Barret-Connor E. Estrogen and estrogen-progestogen replacement therapy and cardiovascular disease. *Am J Med.* 1993;95:40S-43S.
27. Belchetz P. Hormonal treatment of postmenopausal women. *N Engl J Med.* 1994;330:1062-1071.
28. Lindsay R. Hormone replacement therapy for prevention and treatment of osteoporosis. *Am J Med.* 1993;95:37S-39S.
29. American College of Physicians. Guidelines for counseling postmenopausal women about preventive hormone therapy. *Ann Intern Med.* 1992;117:1038-1041.
30. Prince R, Smith M, Dick I, et al. Prevention of postmenopausal osteoporosis: a comparative study of exercise, calcium supplementation, and hormone replacement therapy. *N Engl J Med.* 1991;325:1189-1195.
31. Felson D, Zhang Y, Hannah M, Kiel O, Wilson P, Anderson J. The effect of postmenopausal estrogen therapy on bone density in elderly women. *N Engl J Med.* 1993;329:1141-1146.
32. Cauley J, Seeley D, Ensurd K, Ettinger B, Black D, Cummings S. Estrogen replacement therapy and fractures in older women. *Ann Intern Med.* 1995;122:9-16.
33. Steinberg K, Thacker S, Smith S, et al. Meta-analysis of the effects of estrogen replacement therapy on the risk of breast cancer. *JAMA.* 1991;265:1985-1990.
34. Ali N, Bennett S. Postmenopausal women: factors in osteoporosis preventive behaviors. *J Gerontol Nurs.* 1992;18:23-32.
35. Ali N, Twibell R. Barriers to osteoporosis prevention in perimenopausal and elderly women. *Geriat Nurs.* 1994;15:201-206.
36. Ali N, Twibell R. Health promotion and osteoporosis prevention among postmenopausal women. *Prev Med.* 1995;24:528-534.
37. Ali N. Teaching osteoporosis prevention. *Adv Clin Care.* 1991;6:32-33.

Chapter 11

Breast Cancer Screening in Older Women

Marge Drugay, ND, RN, C

OVERVIEW

Breast cancer is the second leading cause of cancer mortality in women older than 55. In 1995, 182,000 women are expected to be diagnosed with the disease, and 45% of those will be older than 65. Yet breast cancer screening, especially mammography, is underutilized by older women, particularly black or poor women. Nurses are positioned to educate women and other health care providers about potentially life-saving screening strategies, regardless of the practice setting. Nurses also have the opportunity to improve practice through clinical research and utilization activities.

INTRODUCTION

The thought of breast cancer strikes fear in the hearts and minds of many women. Aside from gender, the single most reliable risk factor for developing this disease is advancing age, yet it has been shown that most women older than 50, and particularly those older than 65, do not take advantage of regular screening mammography.[1-3]

Table 11-1 details the objectives specific to the older woman as they relate to breast cancer. Programs to improve early detection of breast cancer through mammography have been conducted across the country under the leadership of the American Cancer Society. Much work remains to be done, however. Nurses, regardless of their practice setting, are positioned to educate women about the benefits of breast cancer screening strategies, particularly mammography.

BREAST CANCER SCREENING STRATEGIES

There is no way to prevent breast cancer, but there are three screening strategies for the secondary prevention or early detection of breast cancer:

- Breast self-examination
- Clinical breast examination by a health professional
- Mammography.

Used together, they provide powerful tools for cancer detection at the earliest stages of the disease, when the probability of cure is greatest and the extent of intervention is potentially the least. An unreserved recommendation for periodic clinical breast examination and mammography screening for older women is supported in the literature.[5-8]

TABLE 11-1

Healthy People 2000: Objectives Targeting Breast Cancer Control in Older Adults

(16.3)	Reduce breast cancer deaths to no more than 20.6 per 100,000 women. (Age adjusted baseline: 22.9 per 100,000 in 1987.)
(16.11)	Increase to at least 80% of the proportion of women aged 40 and older who have ever received a clinical breast examination and a mammogram, and to at least 60% those aged 50 and older who have received them within the preceding 1 to 2 years. (Baseline: 36% of women aged 40 and older "ever" in 1987; 25% of women aged 50 and older "within the preceding 1 to 2 years" in 1987.)

BREAST SELF-EXAMINATION

Breast self-examination (BSE) is a standardized technique performed by the client at monthly intervals to identify changes in the breast appearance, configuration, or structure. In a study reported in 1991, less than 47% of women older than 50 performed regular BSE.[9] This may be due in part to embarrassment, lack of understanding of age-related risk for breast cancer, lack of knowledge of the procedure or the need to perform BSE, cultural or religious inhibitions, or it may be associated with functional limitations such as arthritis or sensory deficits. Older women in particular may not accept the practice readily[10] and may not exhibit proficiency or consistency for numerous reasons. It must also be stressed that the present day older population may not feel comfortable with BSE.

CLINICAL BREAST EXAMINATION

Clinical breast examination by a health care professional is recommended on an annual basis for women older than 40. Barriers to routine health care preclude this possibility for many women. Isolated, homeless, or institutionalized women may be the "forgotten" women, with little or no opportunity for preventive care.[11] It has also been found that age itself may be a factor in not receiving certain screening services such as breast examinations and Pap smears.[2,12]

MAMMOGRAPHY

This simple x-ray procedure of the breast can detect minute cancers, long before they are discovered by palpation. **Screening mammography** is a term used to indicate two views of each breast taken in asymptomatic women. **Diagnostic mammography** is the term used to indicate views taken to evaluate breast tissue for suspected pathology. It is generally indicated for women with symptoms such as a palpable lump, recent visible changes in the breast (dimpling or asymmetry), nipple discharge, or to follow up on inconclusive or suspicious screening films. Compression or magnification views may also be requested for more definitive information.

Mammography usually takes 10 to 20 minutes to complete, plus additional time to view the x-rays for the presence of motion, artifacts, or suspicious areas. This does not include the time it takes for the radiologist to interpret the films, and extra views may be requested, which requires additional time. The procedure may be considered uncomfortable due to the compression of the breast, but it should not be painful. The use of deodorant, perfumes, or powders may produce artifacts on the x-ray and are discouraged.

Most technologists performing mammography are women, which should help to eliminate the embarrassment some clients may experience regarding the procedure. In addition, if the technologist appears empathetic and knowledgeable, it may encourage some women to ask questions regarding the procedure, thereby reducing their anxiety about additional views or the amount of time required.

MAMMOGRAPHY QUALITY

The Mammography Quality Standards Act[13] went into effect in October 1994, designed to impose national standards on facilities that provide mammography services. The Act covers personnel qualifications and training, equipment, quality assurance and reporting, and criteria for Food and Drug Administration certification and annual inspection of facilities that receive federal monies such as Medicare. Information that a facility is accredited must be prominently displayed, and the information should be available to consumers on request. As of mid 1995, more than 8000 mammography units in almost 7000 facilities have been accredited by the American College of Radiology and have received a certificate from the FDA.

In 1995, the *Quality Determinants of Mammography Clinical Practice Guideline* was disseminated under the auspices of the Agency for Health Care Policy and Research.[14] The stated purpose of the guideline is "to improve the quality and delivery of mammography." The guideline addresses all elements of high-quality mammography, from personnel qualifications and responsibilities to hardware requirements, adverse consequences and problems, and the expected communication among and between providers and clients.

To that end, a comprehensive approach was undertaken that evaluated all aspects of mammography services, from the initial contact to schedule a mammogram, through tracking, monitoring, and follow-up with the client. Information and recommendations specifying roles and responsibilities of all involved health care providers, as well as the facility, person scheduling appointments, receptionist, and service personnel are addressed. It is a document that nurses should be aware of, and related documents for consumers are available to educate them about quality mammograms.

CONSIDERATIONS IN BREAST CANCER TREATMENT IN OLDER WOMEN

The treatment of cancer in the aging population is an issue that is beginning to be recognized and discussed by major groups of health care providers, including the American Medical Association and Oncology Nursing Society.[15,16] In acknowledging the present patterns of treatment, it is now recognized that aggressive breast cancer treatment in older women should not be discounted on the basis of response to treatment or anticipated toxic effects.[17,18] This message should be a heartening one for older women who frequently have received less dramatic treatment as they age.

Frequently, the only treatment option offered to older women has been mastectomy, with little discussion of surgical, medical, and/or radiation alternatives. Nurses working with older women need to be aware of the array of current treatment possibilities available for breast cancer management. This is particularly important for nurses who do not specialize in oncology, as they may be less cognizant of advances and changing priorities in that field.

GERONTOLOGICAL NURSING IMPLICATIONS

Every nurse who works with older women, regardless of the setting, should be aware of the three primary breast cancer screening strategies available. Breast cancer is an issue that should be discussed in both lay and professional education sessions, and can be introduced in the community, home care, and institutional settings. Physician offices, worksites, clinics, senior centers, adult day centers, retirement communities, park districts, correctional facilities, mental health settings, shelters, churches, libraries, and long-term care facilities are all appropriate areas in which to conduct health care education.

Sensitivity to culture, ethnicity, lifestyle, sexual orientation, language, and literacy needs will reduce resistance and improve communication between the nurse and client. Individualized interventions for older women and minority women have demonstrated improved use of mammography in these groups.[19] Older lesbian women may not have had the opportunity to learn BSE at an earlier point, as they often receive less preventive health care services than women seeing providers for reproductive health care needs. They are also frequently at a higher risk for developing the disease if they have never been pregnant.[20]

When teaching the BSE procedure, take into consideration any functional limitations the woman may have, and alter the procedure to accommodate those requirements. Arthritis in the hands, visual difficulties, or lack of touch sensitivity may dissuade a woman from the routine practice of BSE and deprive her of a simple opportunity for self-care.

The easiest and most fundamental of the screening strategies is the regular performance of BSE. When conducting an assessment of client health practices, this area should not be neglected. Older women can and should be taught the simple procedure for self-examination, and they should be encouraged to alert their physician or primary care provider when changes are noted. An easily remembered day of the month—such as the date of birth, first day of the month, or day the Social Security check arrives—can be used as the regular date to perform the examination.

The ideal technique may not be employed by all older women, but BSE can be done standing, seated, lying down, or a combination of these, and should be taught in a manner that will improve the probability of adherence. The assistance of a partner to compensate for particular deficits may also be considered. BSE should take only 10 minutes a month, but can mean a difference in the quality of life for an older woman if a cancer is detected in early stages.

BSE is not universally advocated as a screening measure; studies have found that the mere performance of BSE may not be related to proficiency in detection of lesions.[21] In addition, BSE has not been shown to have an impact on mortality.[22] In contrast to these findings, women who conducted monthly BSEs and detected their own cancers found much smaller lesions than women who never examined themselves, or did so only on an intermittent basis.[23] Therefore, it would be prudent for nurses to continue to teach and recommend BSE as an appropriate self-care behavior and as part of an individual health maintenance plan.

While health promoting self-care behaviors such as cancer screening have been correlated with higher socioeconomic and educational levels, women who perform regular BSE may be more highly motivated to also comply with recommendations for clinical breast examinations and mammography, regardless of their educational or socioeconomic level. We should give all women the opportunity to learn more about health promotion and disease prevention, emphasizing the positive outcomes not only for themselves but for their families as well. This may be especially fruitful in cultures that emphasize care of family health issues over personal health concerns.

The second screening strategy to encourage is clinical breast examination, and this should be a part of any routine physical examination. It should not be deferred based on age or potential embarrassment to the client, and should be as expected a procedure as the recording of blood pressure or pulse rate. Individuals conducting clinical breast examinations should be qualified to do so, by virtue of specific training. The American Cancer Society has been instrumental in educating providers in proper technique for this aspect of physical assessment. Providers may be accredited to train other providers.

Mammography is the single most effective weapon in detecting breast cancer and must be an accessible strategy for all older women. The cost of the procedure should be less of a barrier for older women, now that screening mammography, as well as diagnostic mammography, are benefits covered by Medicare. This change went into effect in January 1991, but many women are unaware of the scope of their Medicare benefits. In 1995, only 40% of the 10 million Medicare beneficiaries took advantage of this benefit. Nurses can advocate for this. Other third-party payers (including CHAMPUS) reimburse the cost of screening mammography, and multiple low-cost mammography projects exist. Cost alone should no longer be an insurmountable obstacle for older women. Women who are still employed may be covered for screening by their employers.

Women of all ages need to be educated to request and expect routine health promotion services. Older women in particular may need coaxing to request the procedures their physicians may neglect to recommend, as many women were socialized in an era that dictated unquestioning acceptance of medical authority. A study published in 1994 supports the concept that personal decision making may be less important than recommendations from health professionals for older women.[24]

TABLE 11-2

Breast Cancer Advocacy Groups and Health Promotion Resources

ORGANIZATION	ADDRESS	PHONE
American Cancer Society		800-ACS-2345
Office of Minority Health Resource Center	PO Box 37337 Washington, DC 20013-7337	800-444-MHRC
National Cancer Institute	Office of Cancer Comm. 9000 Rockville Pike Building 31, Room 4843 Bethesda, MD 20892	301-496-6792
Y-Me	National Office 212 West Van Buren Street Chicago, IL 60607	800-221-2141
National Alliance of Breast Cancer Organizations (NABCO)	1180 Avenue of the Americas 2nd Floor New York, NY 10036	
National Eldercare Institute on Health Promotion (AARP)	601 E Street NW 5th Floor B Washington, DC 20049	202-434-2200
Breast Cancer Action	PO Box 460185 San Francisco, CA 94146	415-922-8279
Agency for Health Care Policy and Research (AHCPR)	Quality Determinants of Mammography Clinical Practice Guidelines AHCPR Publications Clearinghouse PO Box 8547 Silver Spring, MD 20907	800-358-9295
Clinician's Handbook of Preventive Services	Superintendent of Documents PO Box 371954 Pittsburgh, PA 15250-7954	202-512-2250

Significant opportunities exist to educate providers regarding the need for regular, ongoing mammography screening for older women. It has been noted that physician-related barriers, such as lack of understanding about effectiveness, may affect mammography utilization more so than patient-related barriers, such as cost.[25] Nurses too have been less aggressive in patient teaching about mammography because of feeling unqualified to do so.[26] The American Cancer Institute and the National Cancer Institute both provide free information for providers and patients.

Older women should be encouraged to explore their options for treatment if cancer is detected, and a second opinion may be indicated. Other factors besides age and stage of the disease should be considered. General physical condition, cognitive status, co-morbidity, and personal beliefs should be deliberated, and women should have a range of treatment modalities available. Mastectomy should not be acceptable as the only option under consideration, and pros and cons of all possibilities must be weighed.[27]

The American Cancer Society and breast cancer advocacy groups such as Y-Me can provide resources, referrals, and direction for women and their families. Centers specializing in the treatment of breast diseases are becoming more common, and most medical centers in urban areas can refer women for additional resources (Table 11-2).

Research opportunities for nurses abound, from the development of original research to the replication of research as utilization projects. Clinical research to improve practice and the delivery of preventive services has resulted in system alterations to improve physician recommendations for mammography and to stimulate client compliance with the recommendation.[25,28-34] In one study, eligible women receiving a mammogram within the previous 12-month period rose from 47% to 72% after using a manual clinician reminder system.[29] Another study using a similar system improved physician recommendation rates for mammography in eligible women older than 50 from 52% to 81%, and improved compliance in women who received the recommendations from 43% to 71%.[31] These studies demonstrate that even simple, manual interventions can improve the probability that a woman will receive a mammogram—and approach the goals set out in *Healthy People 2000.*

Large-scale national efforts are also underway to recruit women into clinical trials for numerous research studies. These include massive studies like the Breast Cancer Prevention Trial that is investigating the use of tamoxifen citrate (Nolvadex) to prevent the development or recurrence of breast cancer. Older women are specifically being recruited for these investigations, since they have been underrepresented in previous studies. The Women's Health Initiative is another longitudinal study designed to investigate osteoporosis and cardiac disease as well as other conditions that affect older women.[35]

Since the multiple advances that have been made in breast cancer detection and treatment, women no longer need to live with the paralyzing fear of undergoing radical, disfiguring surgery immediately following a biopsy. As nurses engaged in a profession dominated by women, we owe it to our clients, mothers, sisters, daughters, partners, and to ourselves to learn those strategies that will improve early detection of breast cancer. In 1995, breast cancer will be diagnosed in 182,000 women, 81,900 of whom will be older than 65 years.[36] As nurses with a special interest in gerontological nursing care, we have an obligation to the older women in our care now and in the future.

REFERENCES

1. Thompson GB, Kessler LG, Boss LP. Breast cancer screening legislation: a commentary. *Am J Pub Health.* 1989;79(11):1541-1543.
2. Calle EE, Flanders WD, Thun MJ, Martin LM. Demographic predictors of mammography and Pap smear screening in U.S. women. *Am J Pub Health.* 1993;83(1):53-60.
3. Rimer BK. Improving the use of cancer screening for older women. *Cancer.* 1993;72(Suppl 3):1084-1087.
4. Public Health Service: U.S. Department of Health and Human Services. *Healthy People 2000.* Boston, MA: Jones & Bartlett; 1990.
5. Beers MH, Fink A, Beck JC. Screening recommendations for the elderly. *Am J Pub Health.* 1991;81(9):1131-1140.
6. Yancik R, Ries LG, Yates JW. Breast cancer in aging women. *Cancer.* 1989;5:976-981.
7. Faulk RM, Sickles EA, Sollitto RA, Ominsky SH, Galvin HB, Frankel SD. Clinical efficacy of mammographic screening in the elderly. *Radiology.* 1995;194:193-197.
8. Costanza ME. Breast cancer screening in older women: overview. *J Gerontol.* 1992;47(Special Issue):1-3.
9. Kaplan KM, Weinberg GB, Small A, Herndon JL. Breast cancer screening among relatives of women with breast cancer. *Am J Pub Health.* 1991;81(9):1174-1179.
10. Sawyer PF. Breast self-examination: hospital based nurses aren't assessing their clients. *Oncol Nurs Forum.* 1986;13:44-48.
11. Drugay M. Battling breast cancer in older women: where do we stand? *Geriatr Nurs.* 1992;13(5):240-244.
12. Steiner CB. Access to cancer prevention, detection, and treatment. *Cancer.* 1991;67(Suppl 6):1736-1740.
13. Mammography Quality Standards Act of 1992. October 27, 1992, P.L. 102-539. USCS 201 nt.
14. Public Health Service:U.S. Dept of Health and Human Services. Agency for Health Care Policy and Research. *Quality determinants of mammography: Clinical Practice Guidelines AHCPR.* Publication number 95-0632, 1994.
15. Harris JE. The treatment of cancer in an aging population. *JAMA.* 1992;268(1):96-97.
16. Boyle DM, Engelking C, Blesch KS, Dodge J, Sarna L, Weinrich S. Oncology Nursing Society position paper on cancer and aging: the mandate for oncology nursing. *Onc Nurs Forum.* 1992;19(6):913-933.
17. Christman K, Muss HB, Case D, Stanley V. Chemotherapy of metastatic breast cancer in the elderly. *JAMA.* 1992;268(1):57-62.
18. Crowe JP Jr, Gordon NH, Shenk RR, Zollinger RM Jr, Brumberg DJ, Shuck JM. Age does not predict breast cancer outcome. *Arch Surg.* 1994;129(5):483-488.
19. Rimer BK. Interventions to increase breast screening: lifespan and ethnicity issues. *Cancer.* 1994;74(Suppl 1):323-328.
20. Denenberg R. Report on lesbian health. *Womens Health Initiative.* 1995;5(2):81-91.
21. Stefanek ME, Wilcox P. Breast self-examination among women at increased risk: Assessment of proficiency. *Cancer Prevention.* 1991;1(2):79-83.
22. Scanlon EF. Secondary prevention of cancer. Human behavior and cancer risk reduction, Part II. *Cancer Prevention.* 1990;1(2):115-116.
23. Foster RS Jr, Lang SP, Costanza MC, Worden JK, Haines CR, Yates JW. Breast self-examination practices in breast cancer stage. *N Engl J Med.* 1987;229(6):205-270.
24. Champion V. Relationship of age to mammography compliance. *Cancer.* 1994;74(Suppl 1):329-335.
25. Taylor VM, Montano DE, Koepsell T. Use of screening mammography by general internists. *Cancer Detect Prev.* 1994;18(6):455-62.
26. Fischera S, Frank DI. Attitudes, practices, and role of nurses in the use of mammography. *Cancer Nurs.* 1994;17(3):223-228.
27. Satariano WA. Comorbidity and functional status in older women with breast cancer: Implications for screening, treatment and prognosis. *J Gerontol.* 1992;47(Special Issue):24-31.
28. Kohatsu ND, Cramer E, Bohnstedt M. Use of a clinician reminder system for screening mammography in a public health clinic. *Am J Prev Med.* 1994;10(6):348-352.
29. Taplin SH, Anderman C, Grothaus L, Curry S, Montano D. Using physician correspondence and postcard reminders to promote mammographic use. *Am J Pub Health.* 1994;84(4):571-574.
30. Drugay M. Prompting for Mammography: Effects on Physician Recommendation and Patient Compliance in Women Over 50 Years of Age. Chicago: Rush University; 1993. Unpublished doctoral study.
31. King ES, Rimer BK, Seay J, Balshem A, Engstrom PF. Promoting mammography use through progressive interventions: is it effective? *Am J Pub Health.* 1994;84(1):104-106.
32. Gann P, Melville SK, Luckmann R. Characteristics of primary care office systems as predictors of mammography utilization. *Ann Intern Med.* 1993;118(11):893-898.
33. Schoen RE, Marcus M, Braham RL. Factors associated with the use of screening mammography in a primary care setting. *J Community Health.* 1994;19(4):239-252.
34. Yarnall KS, Michener JL, Broadhead WE, Tse CK. Increasing compliance with mammography recommendations: health assessment forms. *J Family Practice.* 1993;36(1):59-64.
35. Office of Research in Women's Health. Overview Statement, Women's Health Initiative. Bethesda, MD: National Institutes of Health, 1994.
36. American Cancer Society. *Cancer statistics.* 1995.

Chapter 12

Cervical Cancer Screening Among the Elderly

Joyce White, DrPH, CRNP, Lisa Begg, DrPH, FAAN, and Nancy Wieler Fishman, RN, MPH

OVERVIEW

Screening for early disease detection is one strategy for decreasing morbidity and premature mortality and enhancing quality of life.[1,2] Although there has been some controversy about the value of screening for cervical cancer among elderly women, there is current evidence of its value especially among those older women who have not previously received regular, periodic screening.[3] This chapter describes the development of cervical cancer, risk factors associated with its development, and the value of screening for the premalignant changes characterizing its early stages. It concludes with recommendations for nursing interventions to increase screening for cervical cancer.

INTRODUCTION

Cervical cancer develops slowly, progressing from mild dysplasia (also referred to as cervical intraepithelial neoplasia [CIN]; CIN I and low-grade squamous epithelial lesion; LSIL) to moderate to severe dysplasia (CIN II or high-grade squamous epithelial lesion; HSIL) to carcinoma in situ (CIS) to invasive carcinoma. It is a disease that can easily be prevented by routine, periodic screening because detection of premalignant changes before symptoms develop permits appropriate treatment, thus preventing progression to malignancy.

Cervical cancer is primarily a disease of squamous epithelium. The ratio of incidence of squamous cell carcinoma and adenocarcinoma (which represents the other histologic cervical cancer type) is reported as between 2:1 and 6.5:1. Prognosis and survival do not vary significantly according to histological type,[4] and Pap smear testing is a useful screening procedure for both. Most cervical cancers arise from the transformation zone of the cervix, the area where the squamous epithelium that covers the ectocervix and the columnar epithelium that lines the endocervical canal meet.

Cervical cancer occurs most frequently in those who begin sexual intercourse early and who have multiple sexual partners; it is decreased by the use of barrier methods of contraception and occurs rarely in those who are lifelong celibates. Seminal work in this regard is that of Kessler[5] who found that second wives of men whose first spouse had cervical cancer had an increased risk of developing the disease themselves.

It seems likely that Human Papilloma Virus (HPV) is associated with the development and progression of cervical cancer. Certain HPV types are implicated in higher grade lesions and others are involved in lower grade lesions. HPV types 16, 18, 31, and 33 are implicated in the most severe lesions with 95% of invasive cervical cancers containing these virus types.[6] Parity, nutrition, and cigarette smoking also have been implicated as factors that affect the development and/or progression of cervical intraepithelial abnormalities.[7]

The rate of progression from earliest lesion to invasive carcinoma is unknown as is the degree to which progression is affected by the age of the patient and by other factors. Different approaches to estimating the duration of each premalignant stage yield different estimates, so that the duration of CIS has been variously estimated as from 1 to 17 years.[8]

LITERATURE REVIEW

Research has shown that the stage at which cervical carcinoma is detected is a function of the age and race of the woman in whom it is discovered and that mortality is related to the stage at diagnosis.[9] Grover[10] found, in the review of data on tumor development among white women taken from the Connecticut Tumor Registry, that 98% of cervical cancer was diagnosed at a localized stage when patients were between the ages of 26 and 34 and only 59% was diagnosed at this early stage when patients were older than 65 years of age. Norman,[11] using data from the Pennsylvania Cancer Registry, found that only 11% of all in situ cancers were diagnosed in women 50 years of age and older. Conversely, 74% of all stage 3 (regional) and 4 (distant) cervical cancers were diagnosed in this age group. Forty-one percent of deaths from invasive cervical cancer occur among women 65 and older.[12]

Race is also related to the diagnosis of cervical cancer. A disproportionate number of cervical carcinomas among black women are diagnosed at more advanced stages. In analyzing cancer registry data for black and white women, Norman[11] found 80% of CIS cases in white women and 20% in black women while 69% of invasive cancer was found in white women and 31% in black women, a difference that is statistically significant. While these differences held true across all age groups, the largest difference was seen among women 50 to 64 years of age. The interaction of race and age was also found by Mandelblatt.[13] Also using cancer registry data, these investigators found that older black women in public hospitals were 2.54 times more likely to have late stage cervical cancer than were younger white women in non-public hospitals. Chen[14] found that the percentage of early stage cervical cancer diagnoses was significantly lower among blacks and Hispanic whites than among non-Hispanic whites.

The stage at diagnosis is extremely important because there is a marked, inverse relationship between stage at diagnosis and the 5-year survival rate.[15] The failure to detect disease in its earlier, more curable stage inevitably results in the higher rates of death from cervical cancer seen among the elderly. When cervical cancer is diagnosed at the in situ stage, 5-year survival is virtually 100%.[11] Survival decreases to 88% when cervical cancer is diagnosed at localized invasive stage, to 51% with regional invasion, and to only 14% with distant spread.[16]

SCREENING FOR CERVICAL CANCER

The single most important risk factor for the development of invasive cervical cancer is failure to receive routine, periodic screening. The recognition of this fact has led to the adoption of goals for screening in order to reach the national goal of reducing deaths from cancer of the cervix described in *Healthy People 2000*.[17] These goals are to reduce deaths from cancer of the uterine cervix to no more than 1.3 per 1 million women, increase to at least 95% the proportion of women aged 18 and older with uterine cervix who have ever received a Pap test, and to at least 85% those who received a Pap test within the preceding 1 to 3 years.

Because baseline participation in cervical cancer screening varies according to population subgroups, nursing interventions should be targeted at specific groups to yield the greatest improvement. These groups include black women, the poor, and the elderly. While 90% of all white women were found by the 1987 National Health Interview Survey to have ever received a Pap test, only 88% of black women, 76% of women older than 70, and 80% of women with a family income of less than $10,000 had ever participated in this screening. Rates for routine screening within the previous 3 years were even lower: 76% for white women, 80% for black women, 44% for women 70 and older, and 64% for low-income women.[17] Most, if not all, of the excess mortality due to invasive cervical cancer among elderly women and black women can be attributed to this low rate of participation in cervical cancer screening in comparison with that of younger white women.[18]

Celentano[18] found that more than 50% of elderly women who were diagnosed as having cervical cancer reported that they had never had a Pap test. Mandelblatt[12] reported that 75% of the elderly women in their study had not had prior regular screening and 25% had never been screened. Elderly black and Hispanic women have been found to have lower rates of participation in Pap smear testing than white women.[19] Baquet[20] found that 68% of elderly black women living in non-metropolitan areas had never had Pap smears. Norman[21] found that 66% of Pennsylvania women aged 65 and older reported having their first Pap tests at the time their invasive cervical cancer was diagnosed.

There is also a relationship between race and income. Ackermann,[22] using data from the Behavioral Risk Factor Surveillance System reported during 1987, 1988, and 1989, found that a higher proportion of blacks than whites obtained Pap tests but that receiving Pap smear testing was negatively associated with age and positively associated with income. In analyzing National Health Interview Survey data, Harlan[23] found that Hispanics, especially those who spoke only or mostly Spanish, were the least likely to have ever heard of Pap smear testing.

Responding to this documented need, the United States Congress enacted the Breast and Cervical Cancer Mortality Prevention Act (Public Law 101-354) in August of 1990. State health departments were provided with grants to increase breast and cervical cancer screening among underserved women, especially women who are elderly, have low incomes, or are members of racial/ethnic minority groups. A 1994 update of the program reported that women aged 60 and older were successfully recruited for cervical cancer screening (24% of the total women screened). The rates of abnormal results, especially high-grade squamous epithelial lesion, were similar in women aged 40 to 59 and aged 70 and older.[24] Two reports from state health departments participating in this program confirm the relationship of cervical cancer screening with older women less likely to report recent (within previous 2 years) screening.[25,26] Katz, in comparing screening rates of Canadian women, found that elderly Canadian women were even less likely than their American counterparts to undergo screening.

BARRIERS TO PAP SMEARS IN THE ELDERLY

There are a number of factors that influence the lower participation of elderly and minority women in routine Pap smear screening. One is a cohort effect. Although the usefulness of Pap smear was discovered in the 1930s, Pap testing did not become a routine part of gynecologic care in the United States until 1960.[18] Being widowed, not having a telephone or access to a telephone, and having no family history of cancer were found to be important predictors of nonparticipation in cervical cancer screening.[27]

In a review of studies of barriers to obtaining Pap smears, Coyne[28] found that lack of physician recommendation, in addition to factors such as lack of knowledge of the need for and value of Pap smears, cost, fear of finding cancer, and embarrassment, was a barrier among women aged 50 and older. Lichtman[29] found that middle-aged and elderly women with cervical cancer were significantly less likely to have ever visited a gynecologist or to have reported a physician visit in the 3 years before the diagnosis.

Some women, however, have had recent physician contact and still have not received timely Pap smear testing. In a survey of 114 residents of high-rise apartments for the elderly, 95% of the elderly women residents had visited a physician within the previous 3 years but no more than two-thirds had received Pap tests during that period.[30] Others have noted the same disparity between physician visits and participation in cervical screening. Makuc[31] found that 82% of older women who had never had a Pap smear have had recent contact with a physician. Harlan[23] found that 90% of women who reported (as part of the 1987 National Health Interview Survey) that they had never heard of or never had a Pap smear had seen a physician within the previous 5 years. Norman[21] found that there is a decline in Pap testing with age in spite of continued contact with physicians. Indeed, more than 90% of women with both in situ and invasive disease reported having a usual source of medical care.

This disparity, a "missed opportunity" to screen, may be due, at least in part, to the division between reproductive and non-reproductive care that has developed in our traditional medical care system. With age, women are more likely to need the care provided by specialists, such as internists.[32] With their reproductive years behind them, they may infrequently seek the care of a gynecologist in the absence of gynecologic problems. Unfortunately, internists and family physicians are less likely than are gynecologists to include routine gynecologic screening measures into ongoing care.[29] In addition, there appears to be some gender bias in physicians' recommending Pap smears. Franks[33] found that women who had a female physician as their usual provider were less likely to be deficient in Pap smear testing.

Adequate Pap smear testing in the elderly is made more difficult by the effects of the aging process on the female reproductive system. Sampling of the transformation zone is considered essential for accurate Pap smear testing but this becomes more difficult as the vagina narrows, the cervix undergoes atrophic changes, and the transformation zone moves up into the endocervical canal.[34] Pap smear specimens from older, postmenopausal women are less likely to contain endocervical cells,[35] which often leads to laboratory reports that the specimen is "less than adequate" for evaluation. While using a cytobrush for sampling the endocervical canal has been shown to increase the yield of endocervical cells,[36] fewer endocervical cells are found in women older than 50.[37] More research must be carried out to more completely understand the relationship of smears with no endocervical cells to adequate sampling in the elderly.

Women who report having had hysterectomies should be examined to determine the need for Pap testing. Hysterectomy is the most commonly performed major surgical procedure in the United States; by age 60, 37% of all American women have had hysterectomies.[38] Many older women who have had hysterectomies have intact cervices. One-third of patients who reported having had hysterectomies had intact cervices.[12,30] It has been estimated that between 4% and 8% of cervical cancers arise in these stumps.[39] Decreased estrogen levels may result in mild abnormalities leading to the recommendation that estrogen treatment precede diagnostic testing.[40]

GERONTOLOGICAL NURSING IMPLICATIONS

In addition to recognizing the value of Pap smears among the previously unscreened or inadequately screened elderly, nurses should be aware of previous work that has demonstrated the ability to increase Pap smear screening among this group. These successful efforts can be categorized as public education campaigns to ensure that women request screening, professional education campaigns to ensure that primary health care workers offer screening, and efforts combining these two approaches, neither of which may be as effective when offered separately.[41]

When older women in Melbourne, Australia, were exposed to a 4-week community campaign and/or were personally invited to participate in such screening, their participation increased significantly. Combined strategies were found to be more effective than single strategies.[42]

The ability of routine Pap tests to decrease in situ and invasive cancers when their accessibility to poor, predominantly black, urban women was enhanced was demonstrated in Newark, New Jersey. Data from Newark hospitals before, during, and after the 5-year program demonstrated that the ratio of in situ to invasive cancer increased and decreased in a "striking parallel with the provision and subsequent cessation of (program) funding." The program demonstrated the value of both publicizing the value of Pap testing and making the testing easily available.[43]

Nurses working with the elderly should optimize the clinical visit and screen for cervical cancer. The Harlem Study demonstrated a significantly increased rate of cervical cancer screening when a nurse practitioner offered such screening to women within the context of their visits. Screening rates were still, however, below nationally targeted levels.[44] Ward[45] found that even brief advice regarding the desirability of adding the screening procedure to the routine consultation visit was effective in increasing the percentage of women screened. It is important for nurses to acknowledge that older women may not be familiar with the concept of secondary screening in general and that Pap smears may be new to them.

The use of a lifestyle assessment/risk appraisal inventory is an important nursing tool to identify the need for routine screening within the context of the clinical visit. Pap smears may not be indicated in women older than 65 who have had several negative smears in the previous 10 years and no positive smear,[46] but they are indicated in women who have not received periodic screening. In addition, the regular use of a risk appraisal increases the possibility that factors that increase the likelihood of cervical cancer, such as poor nutrition, cigarette smoking, and risky sexual practices, will be identified.

Providing an appropriate and comfortable environment during the clinic visit will enhance repeat screenings. Nurses can take an active role in making the procedure more comfortable. There are several approaches that may be taken to improve patient comfort during the clinical exam. Difficulties associated with age-related changes can be overcome by using metal speculums lubricated with warm water, using pediatric-sized narrow speculums, and offering assistance with positioning and support during the examinations. These techniques made it possible to adequately examine even those with advanced osteoarthritis and other disabling conditions.[30]

Nurses must target programs to specific populations based on evidence that cancer models held by specific patient populations differ from those held by clinicians. Different populations may respond differently to interventions, with some approaches being more effective than others.[47,48] A coordinated, community-based approach to empowering women to accept responsibility for and control over their own health is imperative,[49] but there is need for continued research to determine the best ways to recruit women from different cultural backgrounds and of different ages.

Public information campaigns and individual patient consultations can do much to decrease embarrassment and increase the likelihood that older women will ask their clinicians for routine Pap smear testing. While younger women may have Pap smears on the recommendation of their physicians, the burden of initiating such screening may fall to older women themselves.[50] Nurses are ideally suited to discuss these intimate matters with their patients and participate in mass campaigns.

REFERENCES

1. U.S. Preventive Services Task Force. *Guide to Clinical Preventive Services.* Baltimore: Williams and Wilkins; 1989.
2. Valanis B. *Epidemiology in nursing and health care.* Norwalk, CT: Appleton-Century-Crofts; 1986.
3. Oddone E, Feusser J, Cohen H. Can screening older patients for cancer save lives? *Clin Geriatr Med.* 1992;8(1):51-67.
4. Anton-Culver H, Bloss J, Bringman D, Lee-Feldstein A, DiSaia P, Manetta A. Comparison of adenocarcinoma and squamous cell carcinoma of the uterine cervix: a population-based epidemiologic study. *Am J Obstet Gynecol.* 1992;166(5):1507-1514.
5. Kessler I. Human cervical cancer as a venereal disease. *Cancer Research.* 1976;3(6):783-791.

6. Cuzick J, Terry G, Ho L, Hollingworth T, Anderson J. Type-specific human papillomavirus DNA in abnormal smears as a predictor of high-grade cervical intraepithelial neoplasia. *Br J Cancer.* 1994;69(1):167-171.
7. Burger M, Hollema H, Gouw A, Pieters WJ, Quint WG. Cigarette smoking and human papillomavirus in patients with reported cervical cytological abnormality. *BMJ.* 1993;306(6880):749-752.
8. Mandelblatt J, Schechter C, Fahs M, Muller C. Clinical implications of screening for cervical cancer under Medicare. *Am J Obstet Gynecol.* 1991;164(2):644-651.
9. Samelson E, Speers M, Ferguson R, Bennett C. Racial differences in cervical cancer mortality in Chicago. *Am J Public Health.* 1994;84(6):1007-1009.
10. Grover S, Cook E, Adam J, Coupal L, Goldman L. Delayed diagnoses of gynecologic tumors in elderly women: relation to national medical practice patterns. *Am J Med.* 1989;8(6):151-157.
11. Norman S, Weinberg G, Powell K, Marconi K. Cervical cancer study using the cancer registry. *Penn Med.* 1989;92(12):42-46.
12. Mandelblatt J, Gopaul I, Wistreich M. Gynecologic care of elderly women: Another look at pap smear testing. *JAMA.* 1986;25(6):367-371.
13. Mandelblatt J, Andrews H, Kerner J, Zauber A, Burnett W. Determinants of late stage diagnosis of breast and cervical cancer; the impact of age, race, social class and hospital type. *Am J Public Health.* 1991;81(5):646-649.
14. Chen F, Trapido E, Davis K. Differences in stage at presentation of breast and gynecologic cancers among whites, blacks, and Hispanics. *Cancer.* 1994;73(11):2838-2842.
15. National Cancer Institute. *Cancer Statistics Review, 1973-1986.* Rockville, MD: U.S. Department of Health and Human Services, National Institutes of Health; 1985.
16. National Cancer Institute. *Cancer Statistics Review 1973-1986.* Bethesda, MD: National Cancer Institute NIH publication # 89-2789; 1989.
17. *Healthy People 2000: National Health Promotion and Disease Prevention Objectives.* Washington, D.C., U.S. Department of Health and Human Services DHHS Publication # PHS 91-50212; 1991.
18. Celentano D, Klassen D, Weisman C, Rosenshein N. Cervical cancer screening practices among older women: results from the Maryland cervical cancer case-control study. *J Clin Epidemiology.* 1988;41:531-541.
19. U.S. Department of HHS, NIH, NCI, Division of Cancer Prevention and Control, *Cancer Statistics Review 1973-1986.* Bethesda, MD: NCI. 1989.
20. Baquet C, Dingen K. Health policy: gaps in access, delivery and utilization of the pap smear in the United States. *Milbank Quarterly.* 1987; 65 supplement #2:322-347.
21. Norman S, Talbott E, Kuller L, et al. The relationship of Papincolaou testing and contacts with the medical care system to stage at diagnosis of cervical cancer. *Arch Intern Med.* 1991;151(1):58-64.
22. Ackermann S, Brackbill R, Bewerse CN, Sanderson L. *Cancer screening behaviors among US women: breast cancer, 1987-1989, and cervical cancer, 1988-1989.* MMWR CDC Surveillance Summaries. 1992;41(2):17-25.
23. Harlan L, Bernstein A, Kessler L. Cervical cancer screening: who is not screened and why? *Am J Public Health.* 1991;81(7):885-890.
24. Taft T, Cardillo R, Letzer D, Kaufman D. Results from the national breast and cervical cancer detection program. *MMMWR.* 1994;29:530-534.
25. Kottke T, Trapp M, Fores M, et al. Cancer screening behaviors and attitudes of women in southeastern Minnesota. *JAMA.* 1995;273(14):1099-1105.
26. Katz S, Hofer T. Socioeconomic disparities in preventive care persist despite universal coverage: breast and cervical cancer screening in Ontario and the United States. *JAMA.* 1994;172(7):530-534.
27. Weinrich S, Coker A, Weinrich M, Eleazer G, Greene F. Predictors of Pap smear screening in socioeconomically disadvantaged elderly women. *J Am Geriatr Society.* 1995;43(3):267-270.
28. Coyne C, Hohman K, Levinson A. Reaching special populations with breast and cervical cancer public education. *J Cancer Ed.* 1992;7(4):293-303.
29. Lichtman S. Geriatric oncology: cervical cancer screening in elderly women. *NY State J Med.* 1991;91(4):147-149.
30. White J, Begg E, Fishman N, Guthrie B, Fagan J. Increasing cervical cancer screening among minority elderly: education and on-site services increase screening. *J Gerontol Nurs.* 1993;19(5):28-34.
31. Makuc DM, Freid VM, Kleinman JC. Trends in the use of preventive health care. *Am J Public Health.* 1989;7(9):21-26.
32. Gluck M, Wagner JL, Duffy BD. The use of preventive services by the elderly. Preventive Health Services under Medicare #2. *OTA*, Washington, D.C.; Government Printing Office; 1989.
33. Franks P, Clancy D. Physician gender bias in clinical decision making: screening for cancer in primary care. *Medical Care.* 1993;31,3:213-218.
34. Hamblin JE, Brock CD, Litchfield L, Dias J. Papanicolaou Smear adequacy: Effect of different techniques in specific fertility states. *J Fam Prac.* 1985;20:257-260.
35. Allingham J, King A. Patient characteristics and endocervical cell recovery on Papanicolaou smears. *J Fam Prac.* 1985;20:185-190.
36. Helderman G, Graham L, Cannon D, Waters K, Feller D. Comparing two sampling techniques for endocervical cell recovery on Papanicolaou smears. *Nurse Pract.* 1990;15(11):30-32.
37. Ginsberg C. Exfoliative cytologic screening: the Papanicolaou test. *JOGNN.* 1991;20(10):39-46.
38. Pokras B, Hufnagel V. Hysterectomy in the United States, 1965-1984. *Am J Public Health.* 1988;78:852-853.
39. Sala JM, Diaz deLeon AD. Treatment of carcinoma of the cervical stump. *Radiology.* 1983;81:300-306.
40. Mueller C, Mandelblatt J, Schectu C. Cost and effectiveness of cervical cancer screening in elderly women. Preventive Health Services under Medicare #4. *OTA*-BP-H-65, Washington, D.C.: Government Printing Office; 1990.
41. Ponten J, Adami H, Bergstrom R, Dillner J, Friberg LG, Gustafsson L, Miller AB, Parkin DM, Sparen P, Trichopoulos D. Strategies for global control of cervical cancer. *Int J Cancer.* 1995;60(1):1-26.
42. Mitchell H, Hirst S, Cockburn J, Reading D, Staples M, Medley G. Cervical cancer screening: a comparison of recruitment strategies among older women. *Med J Australia.* 1991;155(2):79-82.
43. Holland B, Foster J, Louria D. Cervical cancer and health care resources in Newark, New Jersey, 1970 to 1988. *Am J Public Health.* 1993;83(1):45-48.
44. Mandelblatt J, Traxler M, Lakin P, Thomas L, Chauhan P, Matseoane S, Kanetsky P. A nurse practitioner intervention to increase breast and cervical cancer screening for poor, elderly black women. The Harlem Study Team. *J Gen Int Med.* 1993;8(4):173-178.
45. Ward J, Boyle K, Redman S, Sanson-Fisher R. Increasing women's compliance with opportunistic cervical cancer screening: a randomized trial. *Prev Med.* 1991;7(5):285-291.
46. Fahs M, Mandelblatt J, Schechter C, Muller C. Cost-effectiveness of cervical cancer screening for the elderly. *Ann Intern Med.* 1992;117(6):520-527.
47. Rudolph A, Kahan V, Bordeu M. Cervical cancer prevention project for inner city black and Latina women. *Public Health Reports.* 1993;108(2):156-160.

48. Yancey A, Walden L. Stimulating cancer screening among Latinas and African-American women: a community case study. *J Cancer Ed.* 1994:9(1):46-52.
49. Curry R, Moen J, Morris S, Scheivelhud L. Community-directed cancer screening program. *Cancer Practice.* 1994;4:256-263.
50. Eardley A, Elking A, Spencer B, Hobs P, Pendleton L, Haran D. Attendance for cervical screening—whose problem? *Social Science and Medicine.* 1985;20:955-962.

Chapter 13

Clinical Practice Guideline: Prediction and Prevention of Pressure Ulcers

Brenda Bergman-Evans, PhD, RN, CS, Janet Cuddigan, PhC, RN, and Nancy Bergstrom PhD, RN, FAAN

OVERVIEW

Pressure ulcers are not inevitable. Prevention, as well as effective early treatment and intervention, provides an opportunity for both reducing financial costs and improving the quality of life for older individuals. The Agency for Health Care Policy and Research (AHCPR) has developed clinical practice guidelines concerning the prevention and treatment of pressure ulcers. The *Guidelines* target four overall goals:

- Identify at-risk individuals who need prevention and the specific factors that place them at risk.
- Maintain and improve tissue tolerance to pressure in order to prevent injury.
- Protect against the adverse effects of external mechanical forces (pressure, friction, shear).
- Reduce the incidence of pressure ulcers through educational programs.

The guidclincs set the precedent for prevention of pressure ulcers—the focus of this chapter.

INTRODUCTION

Whether at home, in the hospital, or in a nursing home, a patient confined to a bed or chair is vulnerable to a potentially dangerous complication: pressure ulcers. Fortunately, most pressure ulcers can be prevented and Stage I ulcers (nonblanchable erythema of intact skin) need not worsen. When pressure ulcers do develop, prevention strategies are critical to healing existing ulcers and preventing formation of additional ulcers.[1]

Prevention and effective early treatment provides an opportunity for both reducing financial costs and improving the quality of life for the patients involved. Therefore, the Public Health Service's Agency for Health Care Policy and Research (AHCPR) identified the prevention and treatment of pressure ulcers as a priority topic for the development of clinical practice guidelines.

AHCPR has defined the term **guideline** as "systematically developed statements to assist practitioner and patient decision making about appropriate health care for specific clinical circumstances." Clinical circumstances or conditions for which guidelines were to be developed were based on established priorities. These criteria included the following:

- A significant number of individuals are affected by the condition
- Significant variations occur in clinical practice
- Significant variations occur in the outcomes of care
- The condition is amenable to prevention
- An adequate scientific base of evidence exists to support the guideline.

An interdisciplinary non-Federal panel of experts and consumers was convened by the AHCPR's Office of the Forum for Quality and Effectiveness in Health Care to develop *Pressure Ulcers in Adults: Prediction and Prevention. Clinical Practice Guideline, No. 3.*

The panel considered the clinical benefits and harms of potential interventions as well as relevant health policy issues, such as cost constraints and feasibility. Specific to the guideline development is the fact that clinical practice must be based on empirical research.

The *Guidelines* make specific recommendations regarding at-risk adults as well as those with Stage I pressure ulcers. The guideline recommendations may not be appropriate for every at-risk adult, however, and should be adapted to the overall goals for the individual. Respecting individual preferences is especially important for older adults. The recommendations are not intended for infants and children; individuals with Stage II, III, or IV pressure ulcers; or individuals who are fully mobile.

Recommendations target four overall goals:

- Identify at-risk individuals who need prevention and the specific factors that place them at risk
- Maintain and improve tissue tolerance to pressure in order to prevent injury
- Protect against the adverse effects of external mechanical forces (pressure, friction, shear)
- Reduce the incidence of pressure ulcers through educational programs.

The guidelines are outlined below in italics; each recommendation is accompanied by a summary of the rationale behind it.

GUIDELINES FOR RISK ASSESSMENT TOOLS AND RISK FACTORS

Bed- and chairbound individuals or those with impaired ability to reposition should be assessed for additional factors that increase risk for developing pressure ulcers. These factors include immobility, incontinence, nutritional factors such as inadequate dietary intake and impaired nutritional status, and altered level of consciousness. Individuals should be assessed on admission to acute care and rehabilitation hospitals, nursing homes, home care programs, and other health care facilities. A systematic risk assessment can be accomplished by using a validated risk assessment tool such as the Braden Scale or Norton Scale. Pressure ulcer risk should be reassessed at periodic intervals. All assessments of risk should be documented.

Assessment is the first step in the identification and prevention of pressure ulcers. Assessment should occur on admission to a health care facility or at the initiation of a home care program.[2]

In addition to immobility and limited activity levels, other factors (eg, incontinence, altered levels of consciousness, and inadequate dietary intake or impaired nutritional status) should also be assessed.[2-5] Spector[6] found that cognitively impaired nursing home residents who were unable to feed themselves at all were at more risk than cognitively intact residents.

GUIDELINES FOR SKIN CARE AND EARLY TREATMENT

1. All individuals at risk should have a systematic skin inspection at least once a day, paying particular attention to the bony prominences. Results of skin inspection should be documented.

Routine skin inspection is customarily included in any skin care program. It provides essential information in formulating and evaluating skin care plans. A head-to-toe skin assessment with special attention to bony prominences should be performed at least once daily.

The nonblanchable erythema of a Stage I ulcer may be difficult to identify in individuals with darker skin and extra vigilance is required. Discoloration of the skin, warmth, edema, induration, or hardness may be useful indicators in these individuals.

2. Skin cleansing should occur at the time of soiling and at routine intervals. The frequency of skin cleansing should be individualized according to need and/or patient preference. Avoid hot water, and use a mild cleansing agent that minimizes irritation and dryness of the skin. During the cleansing process, care should be used to minimize the force and friction applied to the skin.

Metabolic wastes (including urine and feces) and environmental contaminants that result from daily activities are potential irritants and should be removed promptly and frequently. Use warm rather than hot water when bathing in order to minimize skin damage caused by excessive thermal energy. When the skin's "natural barrier" has been removed, the skin is drier and more susceptible to irritants. By using a mild cleansing agent, the removal of the skin's natural barrier is minimized. Frequency of cleansing should be based not only on the patient's skin condition, but also on the patient's preference.

3. Minimize environmental factors leading to skin drying, such as low humidity (less than 40%) and exposure to cold. Dry skin should be treated with moisturizers several times a day (in the a.m. following bathing and/or in the p.m.).

Decreased ambient air temperature and relative humidity are causes of clinically dry skin.[7] Preliminary research indicated a weak association between dry, flaky, or scaling skin and the development of pressure ulcers.[8]

Decreased skin hydration results in reduced pliability, and sometimes fissuring and cracking of the stratum corneum. The application of topical moisturizing agents improves skin hydration; however, the efficacy of a specific agent has not been established. In addition, although maintenance of relative temperature and humidity have not been linked directly to the prevention of pressure ulcers, adoption of these procedures appears to be prudent.

4. Avoid massage over bony prominences. Current evidence suggests that massage over bony prominences may be harmful as it may create a point of friction and may open an area of frayed skin.

Massage has been used for decades to stimulate circulation, contribute to a sense of patient comfort, and supposedly help prevent pressure ulcers. Preliminary evidence now suggests, however, not only that the purported benefits of such massage cannot be documented, but also that the practice may be harmful.[9,10] Back rubs are useful for promoting relaxation, but massaging areas over bony prominences should be avoided.

5. Minimize skin exposure to moisture due to incontinence, perspiration, or wound drainage. When these sources of moisture cannot be controlled, underpads or briefs can be used that are made of materials that absorb moisture and present a quick-drying surface to the skin.

Moisture alone can make the skin more susceptible to injury.[11-13] Urine, stool, perspiration, and wound drainage also may contain substances other than moisture that irritate the skin; therefore, it is important to keep skin exposure to these sources of moisture to a minimum.

The first line of attack should be management of incontinence.[14] Evidence indicates that underpads or briefs specifically designed to absorb moisture and present a quick-drying surface result in improvement of the skin condition.[15,16] The inclusion of the recommendation to use topical agents as moisture barriers is in accord with current clinical practice trends.[17,18]

For additional information about assessing and managing urinary incontinence, refer to *Urinary Incontinence in Adults: Clinical Practice Guideline* (available from AHCPR Publications Clearinghouse).

6. Skin injury due to friction and shear forces should be minimized through proper positioning, transferring, and turning techniques. In addition, friction injuries may be reduced by the use of lubricants (ie, cornstarch and creams), protective films (ie, transparent film dressings and skin sealants), protective dressings (ie, hydrocolloids), and protective padding.

Shear (when the skin remains stationary and the underlying tissue shifts) and friction (when the skin moves across a coarse surface, such as bed linens) predispose the skin to pressure-induced injuries. Most shear injuries can be eliminated with proper positioning. Cornstarch, emollient cream, barrier dressings, and heel and elbow pads also have been promoted as approaches to help reduce friction injuries, although none has been subjected to systematic research as it relates to preventing pressure ulcers.[12,19]

7. When apparently well-nourished individuals develop an inadequate dietary intake of protein or calories, caregivers should first attempt to discover the factors compromising intake and offer support with eating. Other nutritional supplements or support may be needed. If dietary intake remains inadequate and if consistent with overall goals of therapy, more aggressive nutritional intervention such as enteral or parenteral feedings should be considered. For nutritionally compromised individuals, a plan of nutritional support and/or supplementation should be implemented that meets individual needs and is consistent with the overall goals of therapy.

Pressure ulcer development has been found to be related to impaired dietary intake among chronic care patients. More specifically, Bergstrom[2] found that dietary intake below the recommended daily allowance for calories, protein, and zinc in elderly nursing home patients were predictors of pressure ulcer development.

To address the problem of impaired dietary intake, assistance with eating or nutritional supplements may be sufficient for the apparently well-nourished individual.[20-22] For the nutritionally compromised patient, a more aggressive nutritional intervention, such as parenteral feedings, should be instituted (if it is congruent with the patient's overall plan of carc).

8. If potential for improving mobility and activity status exists, rehabilitation efforts should be instituted if consistent with the overall goals of therapy. Maintaining current activity level, mobility, and range of motion is an appropriate goal for most individuals.

Immobility and inactivity are associated not only with the development of pressure ulcers, but also the development of larger ulcers.[23] Active and passive range of motion exercises reduce the deleterious effects of pressure on the tissues.[24,25] Encouraging ambulation, introducing physiotherapy, and supporting exercises that improve strength, flexibility, coordination, and range of motion are examples of other types of physical rehabilitation that may help prevent pressure ulcers.[26-28] Restraints (chemical or physical) impair mobility and should be avoided if possible.

9. Interventions and outcomes should be monitored and documented.

Detailed information regarding interventions including type, extent, and outcomes, should be individualized and readily available in written form. To ensure continuity of care, the plan of care should be periodically reevaluated by the multidisciplinary team.

GUIDELINES FOR MECHANICAL LOADING AND SUPPORT SURFACES

1. Any individual in bed who is assessed to be at risk for developing pressure ulcers should be repositioned at least every 2 hours if consistent with overall patient goals. A written schedule for systematically turning and repositioning the individual should be used.

The goal of repositioning is to allow tissue perfusion before the tissue becomes ischemic. Repositioning at least every 2 hours is usually sufficient for most bedridden patients. More frequent repositioning may be necessary for patients at extremely high risk, however, this can be very fatiguing for the very frail. In this case, individualize the plan of care to best meet the needs of the patient as well as minimize skin breakdown.

2. For individuals in bed, positioning devices such as pillows or foam wedges should be used to keep bony prominences (eg, knees or ankles) from direct contact with one another, according to a written plan.

Extremities should be supported in all positions.[29] An example of a positioning chart was developed by Abruzzese.[30]

3. Individuals in bed who are completely immobile should have a care plan that includes the use of devices that totally relieve pressure on the heels, most commonly by raising the heels off the bed. Do not use doughnut-type devices.

Because of the small surface area, it is difficult to redistribute pressure under the heels.[31] The use of pillows under the lower length of the leg (but not under the knee), suspending the heels, is one effective method. The pillow should raise the heels just enough so a piece of paper can be passed between the heels and the bed. Ring cushions (doughnuts), however, have been found more likely to cause than to prevent pressure ulcers and should not be used.[32]

4. When the side-lying position is used in bed, avoid positioning directly on the trochanter.

Studies have indicated that interface pressures are higher and transcutaneous oxygen tension is lower when individuals are positioned directly on their trochanter.[33,34] Patients should be positioned off the trochanter, ideally at a 30° angle.[34-36]

5. Maintain the head of the bed at the lowest degree of elevation consistent with medical conditions and other restrictions. Limit the amount of time the head of the bed is elevated.

When the head of the bed is elevated, the skin and superficial fascia remain fixed against the bed linens, while the deep fascia and skeleton slide down toward the foot of the bed (shear injury). This also is true when sitting individuals slide down in their chairs. Blood vessels in the sacral area are likely to twist and distort, and tissue may become ischemic and necrotic.[37] In order to prevent shear injury from semi-Fowler positioning, the head of the bed should not be elevated more than 30°. When this is not possible, positioning techniques and devices that help individuals maintain their position in the bed or chair should be used.

6. Use a lifting device, such as a trapeze or bed linen, to move (rather than drag) individuals in bed who cannot assist during transfers and position changes.

Although friction is most commonly associated with blisters and abrasions, it also can lead to more extensive injury. When transferring patients, care should be taken not to slide or drag the skin across the support surface.[38,39] The patient also may help to prevent friction injuries by taking an active role and using the trapeze in the turning and repositioning process.[39,40]

7. Any individual assessed to be at risk for developing pressure ulcers should be placed when lying in bed on a pressure-reducing device, such as foam, static air, alternating air, gel, or water mattresses.

Several studies have produced evidence that pressure-reducing devices can decrease the incidence of pressure ulcers when compared with standard hospital beds.[41,42] For many patients, foam overlays may be sufficient. In a study of 84 elderly patients, Kemp[43] found a significant relationship between the risk of developing a pressure ulcer and the type of mattress overlay used. The risk of pressure ulcer development was greater for patients on convoluted foam overlays than those on solid, sculptured, foam overlays. More research is required to determine the pressure-reducing device most appropriate given the patient's level of risk.

8. Any person at risk for developing a pressure ulcer should avoid uninterrupted sitting in a chair or wheelchair. The individual should be repositioned, shifting the points under pressure at least every hour or be put back to bed if consistent with overall patient management goals. Individuals who are able should be taught to shift weight every 15 minutes.

Relief of interface pressure during sitting is required at least every hour and preferably more frequently.

9. For chairbound individuals, the use of a pressure-reducing device, such as those made of foam, gel, air, or a combination, is indicated. Do not use doughnut-type devices.

Through the use of a pressure-reducing device, mechanical loading on tissue is reduced, and the risk of pressure ulcers is in turn diminished.[44-46] To ensure effectiveness, the device should be individually prescribed for the user so that it does not interfere with other aspects of mobility or personal autonomy.[47] King[38] suggested that patients shift their weight every 15 minutes for at least a 10-second duration.

10. Positioning of chair-bound individuals in chairs or wheelchairs should include consideration of postural alignment, distribution of weight, balance and stability, and pressure relief.

Proper postural alignment reduces the risk of deformities that could impair respiratory function and self-care activity. Distribution of weight influences the person's ability to transfer from the seat and defines the magnitude and location of maximum pressure. Balance and stability directly influence mobility, energy expenditure, and function performance. Use of pressure-reducing devices and positioning should be considered in conjunction with all these factors to ensure that the individual has maximum autonomy as well as protection from the possibility of pressure ulcers.

11. A written plan for the use of positioning devices and schedules may be helpful for chairbound individuals.

Written plans are important to document the use of positioning devices and ensure continuity of care for the patient confined to a chair. Consistency in the use of positioning devices is necessary in order to evaluate the nursing intervention. Individual comfort is a major consideration.

GUIDELINES FOR EDUCATION IN PRESSURE ULCER PREVENTION AND EARLY TREATMENT

1. Educational programs for the prevention of pressure ulcers should be structured, organized, comprehensive, and directed at all levels of health care providers, patients, and family or caregivers.

Effective pressure ulcer prevention depends on the coordinated effort of health care professionals in all health care settings and continued implementation of preventive interventions by family and the patient at home. A multidisciplinary approach that includes all caregivers is important and effective.[28,48] The multidisciplinary approach may be operationalized in the form of a pressure ulcer clinic, tissue management program, tissue team, skin care team/task force, or pressure ulcer committee. When appropriate and possible, the patient and family should be involved.[24]

2. The educational program for prevention of pressure ulcers should include information on the following items:

- *Etiology and risk factors for pressure ulcers*
- *Risk assessment tools and their application*
- *Skin assessment*
- *Selection and/or use of support surfaces*
- *Development and implementation of an individualized program of skin care*
- *Demonstration of positioning to decrease the risk of tissue breakdown*
- *Instruction on accurate documentation of pertinent data.*

Moody[49] has shown that educational programs decrease the incidence of pressure ulcers and are the basis of prevention programs in health care settings. A consensus exists that such programs should include the seven essential components noted in the guideline.[49-51]

3. The educational program should identify those responsible for pressure ulcer prevention, describe each person's role, and be appropriate to the audience in terms of level of information presented and expected participation. The educational program should be updated on a regular basis to incorporate new and existing techniques or technologies.

Continuity of care is assured when team approaches are documented and each member has identified his or her responsibilities.[25,52,53] The primary focus of the education program is to meet the needs of the learner. Written and illustrated guides are helpful for those who must position patients, including family members.[50,54-56] It is imperative to update the content of educational programs as new information becomes available.

4. Educational programs should be developed, implemented, and evaluated using principles of adult learning.

The primary purpose of pressure ulcer prevention programs is to reduce the occurrence of ulcers, and such programs must have a built-in evaluation mechanism that considers baseline data and compliance with quality assurance standards.

GERONTOLOGICAL NURSING IMPLICATIONS

Pressure ulcers are a serious but preventable problem for older adults. Elderly patients are usually at greater risk for pressure ulcers and suffer increased morbidity and mortality when they occur.

Gerontological nurses have a major responsibility to implement these guidelines through the use of:

- Identification of those at risk
- Assessment and reassessment through use of a clinically tested and reliable instrument
- Application of prevention measures that promote mobility
- Treatment and evaluation
- Documentation on a regular basis to determine treatment effectiveness
- Education of staff and family.

The true key to a successful program of prevention lies in good nursing care. Rudman[57] documented that more favorable staffing patterns and low staff turnover are significantly associated with a lower incidence of pressure ulcers. Although instituting this guideline may initially increase costs,[58] the cost of prevention is far less than the emotional and financial costs of treatment.[59]

If you would like more information or copies of the full guideline, contact AHCPR Publications Clearinghouse, PO Box 8547, Silver Spring, MD 20907; 800-358-9295.

REFERENCES

1. Bergstrom N, Bennett MA, Carlson CE, et al. *Treatment of Pressure Ulcers. Clinical Practice Guideline* (No. 15, AHCPR Publication No. 95-0652). Rockville MD: U.S. Department of Health and Human Services. Public Health Service, Agency for Health Care Policy and Research, December 1994.
2. Bergstrom N, Braden B. A prospective study of pressure sore risk among institutionalized elderly. *J Am Geriatr Soc.* 1992;40:747-758.
3. Allman RM. Pressure ulcers among bedridden hospitalized elderly. Unpublished data; 1991.
4. Berlowitz DR, Wilking SV. Risk factors for pressure sores. A comparison of cross-sectional and cohort-derived data. *J Am Geriatr Soc.* 1989;37(11):1043-1050.
5. Lowthian PT. Underpads in the prevention of decubiti. In: Kenedi RM, Cowden JM, Scales JT, eds. *Bed Sore Biomechanics. Proceedings of a Seminar on Tissue Viability and Clinical Applications.* London, England: Macmillan Press Ltd; 1976:141-145.
6. Spector WD. Correlates of pressure sores in nursing homes: evidence from the National Medical Expenditure Survey. *J Invest Dermatol.* 1994;102(6):42S-45S.
7. Dotz W, Berman B. The facts about treatment of dry skin. *Geriatrics.* 1983;38(9):93-95,99-100.
8. Guralnik JM, Harris TB, White LR, Cornoni-Huntley JC. Occurrence and predictors of pressure sores in the National Health and Nutrition Examination survey follow-up. *J Am Geriatr Soc.* 1988;36(9):807-812.
9. Dyson R. Bed sores—the injuries hospital staff inflict on patients. *Nurs Mirror.* 1978;146(24):30-32.
10. Ek AC, Gustavsson G, Lewis DH. The local skin blood flow in areas at risk for pressure sores treated with massage. *Scand J Rehabil Med.* 1985;17(2):81-86.
11. Leyden JJ, Katz S, Stewart R, Kligman AM. Urinary ammonia and ammonia-producing microorganisms in infants with and without diaper dermatitis. *Arch Dermatol.* 1977;113(12):1678-1680.
12. Leyden JJ. Corn starch, Candida albicans, and diaper rash. *Pediatr Dermatol.* 1984;1(4):322-325.
13. Zimmerer RE, Lawson KD, Calvert CJ. The effects of wearing diapers on skin. *Pediatr Dermatol.* 1986;3(2):95-101.
14. Urinary Incontinence Guideline Panel. *Urinary Incontinence in Adults: Clinical Practice Guideline* (AHCPR Publication No. 92-0038). Rockville, MD: Agency for Health Care Policy and Research, Public Health Service, U.S. Department of Health and Human Services, 1992.
15. Campbell RL, Seymour JL, Stone LC, Milligan MC. Clinical studies with disposable diapers containing absorbent gelling materials: evaluation of effects on infant skin condition. *J Am Acad Dermatol.* 1987;17(6):978-987.
16. Davis JA, Leyden JJ, Grove GL, Raynor WJ. Comparison of disposable diapers with fluff absorbent and fluff plus absorbent polymers: effects on skin hydration, skin pH, and diaper dermatitis. *Pediatr Dermatol.* 1989;6(2):102-108.
17. Hibbs P. Taking off the pressure. *Nurs Mirror.* 1985;160:3-6.
18. Kramer D, Honig PJ. Diaper dermatitis in the hospitalized child. *J Enterostomal Ther.* 1988;15(4):161-170.
19. Norton D, McLaren R, Exton-Smith AN. *An Investigation of Geriatric Nursing Problems in Hospitals.* London, England: Churchill Livingstone; 1975; 238.
20. Goode PS, Allman RM. The prevention and management of pressure ulcers. *Med Clin North Am.* 1989;73(6):1511-1524.
21. Kaminski MV Jr, Pinchcofsky-Devin G, Williams SD. Nutritional management of decubitus ulcers in the elderly. *Decubitus.* 1989;2(4):20-30.
22. Lidowski H. NAMP: a system for preventing and managing pressure ulcers. *Decubitus.* 1988;1(2):28-37.
23. Abildgaard AU, Daugaard K. Pressure sores. A study on prevalence. *Ugeskr Laeger.* 1979;141(46):3147-3151.
24. Colburn L. Pressure ulcer prevention for the hospice patient. Strategies for care to increase comfort. *Am J Hosp Care.* 1987;4(2):22-26.
25. Dimant J, Francis ME. Pressure sore prevention and management. *J Gerontol Nurs.* 1988;14(8):18-25.
26. Droessler D, Maibusch RM. Development of a nursing care plan for healing and preventing decubiti. *QRB Qual Rev Bull.* 1979;5(8):10-14.
27. Fugill GC. Pressure sores. *Physiotherapy.* 1980;66(2):46-47.
28. Levine JM, Simpson M, McDonald RJ. Pressure sores: a plan for primary care prevention. *Geriatrics.* 1989;44(4):75-76,83-87,90.
29. American Nurses Association. *Neuroscience Nursing Practice: Process and Outcome Criteria for Selected Diagnoses.* Kansas City, MO: Author; 1985.
30. Abruzzese RS. Early assessment and prevention of pressure sores. In: Lee BY, ed. *Chronic Ulcers of the Skin.* New York, NY: McGraw-Hill; 1985:1-19.
31. Parish LC, Witkowski LA. Clinitron therapy and decubitus ulcer: preliminary dermatologic studies. *Int J Dermatol.* 1980;19:517-518.
32. Crewe RA. Problems of rubber ring nursing cushions and a clinical survey of alternating cushions for ill patients. *Care Science Practice.* 1987;5(2):9-11.
33. Garber SL, Campion LJ, Krouskop TA. Trochanteric pressure in spinal cord injury. *Arch Phys Med Rehabil.* 1982;Nov;63(11):549-552.
34. Seiler WO, Allen S, Stahelin HB. Influence of the 30 degrees laterally inclined position and the "super-soft" 3-piece mattress on skin oxygen tension on areas of maximum pressure—implications for pressure sore prevention. *Gerontology.* 1986 May–Jun;32(3):158–166.
35. Braden BJ, Bryant R. Innovations to prevent and treat pressure ulcers. *Geriatr Nurs.* 1990;11(4):182-186.
36. Low AW. Prevention of pressure sores in patients with cancer. *Oncol Nurs Forum.* 1990;17:179-184.
37. Reichel SM. Shearing forces as a factor in decubitus ulcers in paraplegics. *JAMA.* 1958;15:762-763.
38. King RB, French ET. Procedures to maintain and restore tissue integrity. In: *Rehabilitation Nursing Procedures Manual.* Rockville, MD: Aspen; 1990:179-222.
39. Maklebust J. Pressure ulcers: etiology and prevention. *Nurs Clin North Am.* 1987;22(2):359-377.
40. Messner R. Infection control. The prevention of pressure sores. *J Pract Nurs.* 1987;37:16-17.
41. Andersen KE, Jensen O, Kvorning SA, Bach E. Decubitus prophylaxis: a prospective trial on the efficiency of alternating-pressure air-mattresses and water-mattresses. *Acta Derm Venereol.* 1982;63(3):227-230.
42. Goldstone LA, Norris M, O'Reilly M, White J. A clinical trial of a bead bed system for the prevention of pressure sores in elderly orthopaedic patients. *J Adv Nurs.* 1982;7(6):545-548.
43. Kemp MG, Kopanke D, Tordecilla L, et al. The role of support surfaces and patient attributes in preventing pressure ulcers in elderly patients. *Res Nurs Health.* 1993;16(2):89-96.
44. DeLateur BJ, Berni R, Hangladarom T, Giaconi R. Wheelchair cushions designed to prevent pressure sores: an evaluation. *Arch Phys Med Rehabil.* 1976;57(3):129-135.
45. Ferguson-Pell M, Cochran GV, Cardi M, Tractman LA. A knowledge-based program for pressure sore prevention. *Ann NY Acade Sci.* 1986;463:284-286.
46. Garber SL, Krouskop TA, Carter RE. A system for clinically evaluating wheelchair pressure-relief cushions. *Am J Occup Ther.* 1978;32:565-570.

47. Cooney TG, Reuler JB. Pressure sores. *West J Med.* 1984;140:622-624.
48. Hamilton L, Quek P, Lew N, Li K, Topp R. Pressure ulcers: an interdisciplinary protocol for prevention and treatment. *Perspectives.* 1989;13(1):9-15.
49. Moody BL, Fanale JE, Thompson M, Vaillancourt D, Symonds G, Bonasoro C. Impact of staff education on pressure sore development in elderly hospitalized patients. *Arch Intern Med.* 1988;148(10):2241-2243.
50. King RB, Boyink M, Keenan M, eds. *Rehabilitation Guide.* Chicago: The Rehabilitation Institute of Chicago; 1977:62-80.
51. Krouskop TA, Noble PC, Garber SL, Spencer WA. Effectiveness of preventative management in reducing the occurrence of pressure sores. *J Rehabil R D.* 1983;20(1):74-83.
52. Frye BA. A coat of many colors: a program to reduce the incidence of hospital-originated pressure sores. *Rehabil Nurs.* 1986;11(1):24-25.
53. Khun JK, Wygonoski C. A multidisciplinary team approach to decubitus ulcer care. *Nurs Homes.* 1984;33(1):29-33.
54. Di Domenico RL, Ziegler WZ. *Practical Rehabilitation Techniques for Geriatric Aides.* Rockville, MD: Aspen Publishers; 1989:147.
55. Lovett PA, Bridle MJ. *Your Skin: An Owner's Manual.* Charlottesville, VA: University of Virginia; 1986.
56. Morison MJ. Early assessment of pressure sore risk. *Professional Nurse.* 1989;4:428-431.
57. Rudman D, Slater EJ, Richardson TJ, Mattson DE. The occurrence of pressure ulcers in three nursing homes. *J Gen Intern Med.* 1993;8(12):653-658.
58. Hu TW, Stotts NA, Fogarty TE, Bergstrom N. Cost analysis for guideline implementation in prevention and early treatment of pressure ulcers. *Decubitus.* 1993;6(2):42-46.
59 Oot-Giromini B, Bidwell FC, Heller NB, et al. Pressure ulcer prevention versus treatment, comparative product cost study. *Decubitus.* 1989;2(3):52-54.

Chapter 14

Promoting Continence in the Elderly: Nursing Strategies for Behavioral Treatment

Deborah Lekan-Rutledge, MSN, RN, C, CCCN

OVERVIEW

Although urinary incontinence (UI) may not be viewed as a serious health problem, its high prevalence and significant impact among the elderly warrants recognition and intervention by professional nursing. Dissemination efforts by the federal government and professional nursing about the care and treatment of UI has addressed the importance of evaluation and treatment or management of UI. In particular, behavioral treatment is recognized as first-line intervention for the majority of individuals because of its low risk, its cost-effectiveness, and because it may be used as an adjunct to pharmacologic and surgical treatment. Behavioral treatment includes toileting regimens such as bladder training, pelvic muscle strengthening and rehabilitation, elimination of dietary bladder irritants, fluid management, and bladder urge suppression. Management techniques to control potential adverse sequela of UI include skin care regimens, absorbent products, and bowel training. While continence care has long been a nursing concern, new, state-of-the-art knowledge about assessment and targeted treatment strategies enhances nursing's effectiveness in promoting quality of care to incontinent individuals.

INTRODUCTION

UI is not usually viewed as a serious health problem among health professionals and the public. Urinary incontinence is not fatal, and, in many affected individuals, the magnitude of the problem may be categorized as mild or moderate. Nevertheless, among those who are affected, regardless of the magnitude of the problem, it is experienced as a socially distressing and disruptive problem with adverse psychosocial and financial consequences. The high prevalence of UI in older people is estimated at between 15% and 30%, with women being affected twice as often as men. As many as four out of 10 women older than 60 are affected with UI.[1]

UI is a significant public health issue since so many individuals are not properly diagnosed or treated. Recent developments at the national level have increased awareness of UI and stimulated changes in health services delivery related to UI. In 1988, the National Institutes of Health Consensus Conference on Adult Urinary Incontinence produced a consensus statement and recommendations on the state-of-the-art practice and research on UI. More recently, the Agency for Health Care Policy and Research published the *Clinical Practice Guideline on Urinary Incontinence in Adults*.[2] These documents provide vital information to health professionals about the research base for current practice regarding care of incontinent individuals. These documents have significant implication for nurses, since the care of the incontinent person has traditionally been a primary nursing concern and responsibility. It is significant that baseline evaluation and behavioral treatment methodologies for UI as recommended within these documents are within the role of the nurse.[3] The large population of underserved individuals with UI compels nurses to delve further into this clinical issue as a front-line provider.

UI has been defined as "the involuntary loss of urine sufficient to be a problem."[2] Urinary dysfunction is differentiated into two broad areas: failure to store urine and failure to empty urine. Problems with urine storage may be due to abnormalities such as poor bladder compliance, detrusor instability, impaired bladder contractility, and urethral sphincter incompetence. Problems with the emptying of urine may be due to obstruction of the urethra or bladder neck, sphincter hyperactivity, and impaired bladder contractility. In addition, sensory disorders may result in diminished sensation or pain as the bladder fills or during urination.

The lower urinary tract comprises the bladder, urethra, and pelvic floor muscles. The bladder is a hollow, muscular organ with the sole purpose of storing urine. As the bladder volume increases, the bladder wall relaxes to accommodate the urine. Simultaneously, urethral and pelvic floor muscles contract to increase bladder neck support and facilitate the storage of urine. In the adult, bladder capacity is approximately 350 mL to 600 mL.

As bladder capacity reaches about 150 mL, a sensation of bladder filling is perceived. This signal diminishes and passes, but will return as the bladder continues to fill, nearing its functional capacity or usual voiding volume. Bladder emptying occurs when the individual finds a socially acceptable toilet and initiates the micturition reflex in which the urethral sphincter and pelvic floor muscles relax. Detrusor muscles contract to expel urine. When voiding is complete, internal and external sphincter muscles contract and maintain resting tone to maintain urethral closure.

Normal Bladder Function

Continence is dependent upon a properly functioning urinary system, intact neurologic mechanisms between the bladder and pelvic floor muscles; spinal cord and brain; and competent urethral sphincter mechanisms. Alteration or dysfunction in any of these mechanisms may result in UI.[4]

NORMAL CHANGES IN THE AGING BLADDER

Gradual changes in the lower urinary tract occurring over a number of years may predispose the individual to maladaptive behavioral responses and increased risk for UI. Age-related lower urinary tract changes include diminished bladder capacity, decreased bladder compliance, decreased bladder contractility resulting in post-void residual urine, decreased "holding time," and increased number of unstable bladder contractions.[4,5]

TABLE 14-1

Types of Urinary Incontinence

TYPE	DEFINITION	SYMPTOMS
Urge	Leakage of urine associated with an unexpected sudden bladder urge that cannot be suppressed.	Loss of urine is sudden and unexpected, usually in moderate to large amounts. Associated symptoms include urgency, frequency, nocturia.
Stress	Leakage of urine associated with physical activity or an abrupt rise in intra-abdominal pressure such as coughing, sneezing, bending, laughing, walking, exercising.	Urine loss typically in small amounts, few drops to few teaspoons and in association with movement. Leakage may occur regardless of the fullness of bladder.
Overflow	Leakage of urine associated with a full bladder where small amounts of urine escape during movement or due to bladder overdistension.	Urine loss may be in dribbles. Obstructive voiding symptoms due to prostatic enlargement or stricture manifested in hesitancy, straining to void, intermittency, prolonged voiding, post-void dribbling, and sensation of full bladder.
Functional	Leakage of urine associated with the inability to appropriately toilet due to cognitive or physical impairments, restraints, environmental barriers, or medications.	Urine loss is spontaneous and without a pattern. Often UI is on way to toilet.

While normal voiding frequency is between four and nine times per day and once per night, some older people may report increased urinary urgency, frequency, and nocturia more than twice per night. Those symptoms combined are described as irritable voiding symptoms. In women, progressive muscle atrophy of the pelvic floor muscles (levator ani and other support structures), similar to the atrophy that occurs in lean body mass, contributes to pelvic muscle relaxation. These changes may be compounded by pudendal nerve denervation injury secondary to childbirth, a problem related to multiparity, vaginal delivery of large babies or prolonged Stage II labor. Estrogen decline in women contributes further to pelvic muscle atrophy and thinning and irritation of urethral mucosa. Maladaptive behavioral responses to these gradual changes include significant decreases in fluid intake, urinary frequency, nocturia, avoiding places without access to suitable toilets, and restricting leisure activities.[6-9] Psychological responses include increased anxiety, depression, social isolation, frustration, embarrassment, and preoccupation with one's voiding status.

TYPES OF UI

There are four types of UI: urge, stress, overflow, and functional.[2] Table 14-1 describes the definition and symptom profile for each UI type. Mixed incontinence refers to the coexistence of stress and urge UI, often documented in women. Functional incontinence may also occur with other UI types. Many conditions or medical problems outside the urinary tract influence the development of UI. Table 14-2 describes causes and contributing factors of UI.

TABLE 14-2

Causes and Contributing Factors to UI

Urologic: Carcinoma, bladder calculi, cystitis, prostatic obstruction, urethral stricture, bladder hypotonia or atonia, urethral sphincter incompetence, detrusor instability.

Gynecologic: Pelvic relaxation syndrome or pelvic muscle dennervation, multiparity, traumatic childbirth (heavy birthweight, lacerations, prolonged Stage II labor), previous pelvic surgery, obesity.

Metabolic: Paget's disease, diabetes mellitus, diabetes insipidus, pernicious anemia.

Neurologic: Multiple sclerosis, Parkinson's disease, CVA, dementia, spinal cord injury, or congenital abnormality.

Psychologic: Depression, delirium, regression, psychosis.

Pharmacologic: Diuretics, psychotropics, sedatives/hypnotics, narcotics, anticholinergics, alpha adrenergic agonists and antagonists, caffeine, alcohol, nicotine, post-anesthesia syndrome.

Functional: Acute illness affecting cognition or mobility, acute or chronic pain.

NURSING ASSESSMENT

Basic assessment of UI can be performed by nurses without specialized training, although knowledge of current practice guidelines for assessment and treatment is necessary.

Parameters for assessment include identifying acute or transient causes of reversible UI, a basic continence history, and using selected physical exam data, tests, and laboratory findings.[2,10] One example of a clinically useful assessment tool is illustrated in Figure 14-1. The basic assessment yields data to determine possible reversible and manageable/treatable causes of UI and factors that may be related to different types of UI. Table 14-3 lists the acute and potentially reversible causes of UI.

Rapid Assessment of Urinary Elimination

Instructions: Complete this form for patients who are incontinent. For each question, circle the appropriate response.

Patient Name: ____________ Date: ________ Date of birth/age: ________ Sex: ______

Diagnoses: ____________

Medications: ____________

HISTORY

1. Onset: a) recent onset within past 6 months, b) onset within past 3 yrs, c) persistent problem for >3 yrs
2. Frequency: a) once a day or less, b) at least once and up to twice a day, c) three times a day or more, d) nighttime only
3. Severity: a) small amounts of urine loss, b) moderate amount of urine loss, c) large amounts of urine loss
4. Risk factors: a) smoking, b) caffeine intake, c) alcohol, d) fluid intake inadequate, e) chronic constipation, f) obesity
5. Psychological impact: a) concerned about UI, b) not concerned about UI because it is well managed, c) unaware of denies UI, d) cost to manage UI burdensome, e) major change in lifestyle, f) social/family relationships adversely affected
6. Medical history: a) stroke, b) parkinson's disease, c) dementia, d) CHF, e) diabetes mellitus, f) diabetes insipidus, g) multiple or difficult childbirth, h) pelvic surgery, i) pernicious anemia, j) multiple sclerosis, k) kidney disease, stones, recurrent infection, l) back injury or surgery
7. Current management: a) pads/diapers, b) toileting regime, c) catheters or devices, d) medication, e) skin care
8. Incontinence Symptom Profile

STRESS UI	URGE UI
a. Leakage with cough, sneeze, physical activity b. UI in small amounts (drops, spurts) c. No nocturia or UI at night d. UI without sensation of urine loss	a. Strong, uncontrolled urge prior to UI b. Mod./large volume of urine loss (gush) c. Frequency of urination d. Nocturia > 2 times e. Enuresis
OVERFLOW UI	**FUNCTIONAL UI**
a. Difficulty starting urine stream b. Weak or intermittent stream (dribbles) c. Post-void dribbling d. Prolonged voiding e. Feeling of fullness after voiding f. Voiding small amounts often or dribbling with changes in position	a. Mobility or manual dexterity impairments b. Lack of toilet or toilet substitute c. Restraints d. Sedative, hypnotic, CNS depressant, diuretic, anticholinergic, alpha-adrenergic antagonist e. Depression, delirium, dementia f. Pain

PHYSICAL EXAM

1. Abdominal exam: a) normal b) palpable bladder c) abdominal masses d) bowel distended e) poor peristalsis
2. Genitalia: a) normal b) reddened, irritated tissue c) discharge d) infection e) odor f) lesions
3. Pelvic exam:
   Vaginal inspection: a) normal b) tissue pale, thin, dry c) pelvic organ descent with valsalva d) lesions
   Pelvic muscle assessment: a) palpable, voluntary contraction, rating 0-5:___ b) pt. unable to elicit voluntary contraction
4. Rectal exam: a) snug anal sphincter tone and good sensation b) lax or absent anal sphincter tone c) fecal impaction
5. Diagnostics:
   Post-void residual urine measurement:
   Urine dipstick: nitrite _____ WBC _____ sp. gravity _____ pH ___ RBC ___ protein _____ glucose _____
   Urine culture if ordered: date: _________ positive for bacterial growth ___ negative for growth ___
   Voiding diary: # voids/day ___ #UI episodes/day ___ # pads used/day ___ type of pad _______________
   approx. volume of UI ____ cc, maximal bladder capacity ____cc, functional capacity ____cc

FUNCTIONAL ASSESSMENT

1. Mobility: a) can toilet self without assistance b) needs physical assistance or verbal prompting to toilet c) unable
2. Manual dexterity: a) independent b) needs assistance c) unable
3. Voiding functions: a) able to voluntarily start urine stream b) often unable to voluntarily start urine stream c) refuses to toilet when prompted or offered assistance
4. Cognitive function: a) intact b) impaired - Mini Mental State Exam Score: _____ (<24 abnormal)

Clinical Impression:

Nurse:

Figure 14-1. Form for rapid assessment of urinary elimination. Copyright © 1995 Deborah Lekan-Rutledge, MSN, RN, C, CCCN.

Bladder Diary: To better understand your bladder problem, it is helpful to record a Bladder Diary. A Bladder Diary can create a day-to-day picture of your incontinence and bladder symptoms. A Bladder Diary is a dialy tracking of your voids, liquid intake, urges to urinate, and symptoms. Many people may overestimate or underestimate the severity of their bladder problem. While keeping the Bladder Diary, go about your daily life and avoid making any chages in your bathroom habits so it will be an accurate account of your situation.

	DAY 1					DAY 2				
Time	Void (s/m/l)	Leak (s/m/l)	Urge	Liquid Intake	Activity	Void (s/m/l)	Leak (s/m/l)	Urge	Liquid Intake	Activity
6 am										
7 am										
8 am										
9 am										
10 am										
11 am										
12 N										
1 pm										
2 pm										
3 pm										
4 pm										
5 pm										
6 pm										
7 pm										
8 pm										
9 pm										
10 pm										
11 pm										
12 M										
1 am										
2 am										
3 am										
4 am										
5 am										
Number of pads used:			Type:			Number of pads:			Type:	
Comments:						Comments:				

Figure 14-2. Bladder diary.

History taking for UI includes determining onset, frequency, and severity of UI, medical problems that may possibly affect continence, psychological impact, and current management. Patient interview ascertains the incontinence symptom profile describing the circumstances of urine loss. The voiding diary is a vital data collection tool that reveals the older person's natural pattern of voiding and incontinence. The voiding diary is recorded for at least 3 consecutive days. The voiding diary (Figure 14-2) is an important reference for determining the individual's daily and nocturnal urine volume, fluid intake patterns, bowel habits, behavioral and environmental circumstances associated with UI, and functional and maximal bladder capacity. The voiding diary also documents the number and types of absorbent products used.

TABLE 14-3

Acute or Transient Causes of Potentially Reversible UI

- Psychological: delirium, depression
- Infection: urinary tract
- Inflammation: atrophic vaginitis or urethritis
- Dehydration
- Polyuric states: diabetes mellitus or insipidus, congestive heart failure, low albumin states, hypocalcemia
- Stool impaction
- Restricted mobility: mobility impairments, progressive weakness, post-surgery
- Medications

The physical exam is targeted toward identifying objective data on findings related to UI and contributing factors, including stool impaction, inflammation or infection of external genitalia or vaginal tissues, and urinary tract infection and dehydration (via the urine esterase dipstick test for nitrite, leukocyte/WBC, specific gravity, glycosuria). In certain instances, measuring post-void residual urine volume is helpful to rule out a bladder emptying dysfunction that may require further medical or urologic evaluation. Patients with neurological problems (Parkinson's disease, multiple sclerosis, cerebral vascular accident (CVA), spinal cord injury, brain tumor), diabetes mellitus, or urethral obstruction may require further evaluation. In the absence of documented neurological or urological problems, incomplete bladder emptying has been documented in some older people with urge UI. This clinical finding has been termed detrusor hyperactivity with impaired contractility (DHIC).[11] These patients may experience recurrent urinary tract infection due to urine stasis and are at risk for acute urinary retention secondary to anticholinergic drugs. To obtain the post-voiding residual (PVR), the patient's voiding volume is recorded, and a post-void urine measurement is obtained using straight catheterization. The use of a portable ultrasound instrument provides indirect measurement of urine volume. Post-void measurements of >100 mL suggests poor bladder emptying. In the elderly, measurements <100 mL are considered normal. Patients with PVRs >100 mL should be carefully monitored as urologic evaluation may be indicated. Post-void residual measurements exceeding 200 mL (on at least two occasions) warrant urologic referral.[10]

Assessment of pelvic muscle contraction is necessary if pelvic muscle exercises are an appropriate and feasible treatment option. This is accomplished by performing a digital vaginal exam with a lubricated, gloved finger and asking the patient to contract the muscles around the finger. The strength of the contraction is rated as absent (0), flicker (1), weak (2), moderate (3), good (4), or strong (5).[12] The ability to voluntarily contract pelvic muscles can also be ascertained indirectly by observing the anal sphincter when the patient is asked to contract the sphincter "as if you are holding back gas." The anal sphincter should visibly close and draw inward. The ability to voluntarily contract pelvic muscles is a condition for initiating a pelvic muscle exercise program.

Functional assessment determines the older person's abilities to manage toileting independently or with assistance. Manual dexterity problems may prolong the time needed to undress prior to voiding, long enough to exceed the person's "holding time." Physical limitations that are identified and assessed may be corrected with physical therapy or assistive devices. The ability to initiate the urine stream is an important marker of bladder function, wherein the lack of voluntary voiding suggests a bladder emptying problem that may require further evaluation. In addition, if the person is cognitively impaired, assessment of mental status using the Mini-Mental Status Exam is helpful to determine the extent to which the person may be able to independently carry out self-managment strategies versus the need for caregiver-assisted strategies.[13]

Assessment of the physical and social environment should not be overlooked. Environmental conditions that may contribute to UI include lack of an available toilet (too far away, unable to climb stairs), a toilet that is too low or lacks grab bars, bathroom that does not accommodate a wheelchair, poor lighting, or cluttered walkway.[10] Within the social environment, the availability and willingness of a caregiver to remind or directly assist the older person to toilet can be a vital link to continence.

BEHAVIORAL TREATMENT

Behavioral treatment is an approach that involves self-monitoring and self-regulation to influence symptoms or maladaptive behaviors. Behavioral interventions are recommended as first-line treatment for UI in contrast to pharmacologic or surgical intervention because they are cost-effective, noninvasive, and are readily learned and implemented by the patient.[2,14] Additionally, behavioral interventions may be used in conjunction with pharmacologic treatment, or prior to or after surgery. Patients with overflow UI are not candidates for behavioral treatments.[2]

Behavioral interventions include toileting regimens (scheduled toileting, prompted voiding, habit training, bladder training), dietary modifications, bowel management, urge suppression, pelvic muscle exercises, and adjuvant technologies including biofeedback, weighted vaginal cones, and electrical stimulation. Behavioral interventions are tailored to the patient's underlying problems and require a high degree of patient participation over 6 to 12 weeks. The type of intervention is highly contingent upon the patient's cognitive status, motivation, and willingness to engage in self-management strategies. Behavioral interventions may be categorized into two groups: general approaches, which are oriented toward health promotion and problem prevention; and targeted interventions, which are directed at treating the underlying type of UI in cognitively intact or impaired individuals. Cognitively impaired individuals can achieve continence goals with the assistance of caregivers; however, certain interventions such as pelvic muscle rehabilitation, may not be achievable. Behavioral interventions for continence promotion are illustrated in Table 14-4.

TABLE 14-4

Behavioral Interventions for Continence Promotion

GENERAL APPROACHES

- Toileting regimens
- Dietary modifications: fluid management, bladder irritants
- Bowel management
- Skin care
- Continence aides: absorbent products, equipment, devices

TARGETED APPROACHES

Cognitively Intact	Cognitively Impaired
• Bladder training	• Prompted voiding
• Pelvic muscle exercises	• Habit training
• Biofeedback	
• Vaginal cones	
• Urge suppression	
• Electrical stimulation	

GENERAL APPROACHES

Toileting regimens can reduce UI through consistent bladder emptying. Four types of toileting regimens and their indications are described in Table 14-5. Adhering to a toileting regimen helps increase awareness of bladder function and reinforce the role of the bladder as a receptacle to hold urine. Toileting regimens are often the foundation of any continence care program in the elderly.

Dietary modifications including fluid management and elimination of bladder irritants can reduce bladder urgency, frequency, nocturia, and urge UI. Caffeine is a strong bladder irritant found in coffee, tea, chocolate, soft drinks, and some cold and allergy medications and should be restricted. Self-imposed fluid restriction is very common among individuals with UI. Inadequate fluid intake contributes to bladder urgency due to concentrated urine and decreased bladder capacity due to deconditioning of the bladder muscle and subsequent muscle atrophy. Odor, skin problems, and increased risk for urinary tract infection also result from concentrated urine. Daily fluid goals may be individualized by taking the patient's body weight in pounds and dividing by two to calculate the number of ounces of liquids needed per day.[15] Fluid intake should be increased beyond the minimum goal in individuals with febrile states, respiratory disorders, diarrhea, and during exercise. Under-hydration is addressed with a fluid hydration protocol, which gradually increases the daily ingestion of fluid in small amounts, for example, 2 to 4 ounces twice a day. One helpful strategy is for the person to measure out the extra fluid needed to reach his or her daily fluid goal into a large tumbler or sport bottle, to be sipped during the morning and afternoon until it is consumed. This approach allows for gradual bladder filling that is unlikely to increase UI episodes.

TABLE 14-5

Acute or Transient Causes of Potentially Reversible UI

TYPE	DESCRIPTION	INDICATIONS
Scheduling Toileting	Fixed pattern of voiding (ie, every 2 hours).	Voiding pattern infrequent. Stress or urge UI.
Prompted Voiding	Voiding schedule, either fixed or variable, with a communication protocol for caregiver to increase patient's expectations for continence, and provide reinforcement and praise for toileting and staying dry.	Patient is cognitively impaired and has a caregiver to assist to toilet. Used in nursing home and home health. Stress and urge UI.
Habit Training	Voiding schedule is individualized according to patient's baseline UI and voiding pattern.	Voiding record indicates variable pattern of urine volume and UI (ie, diuretic use in a.m. creating polyuria). Stress and urge UI.
Bladder Training	Voiding schedule incorporates progressively longer intervals between voids.	Stress and urge UI, irritable bladder symptoms, nocturia, small bladder capacity. Requires motivated patient with ability to learn urge suppression.

Bowel management is an important part of continence care. Chronic constipation increases the older person's risk for fecal impaction in which hard stools obstruct the bowels. Distended bowel and rectum compress the bladder neck, which may decrease bladder capacity, encourage urine retention, and cause reflex bladder contraction and UI.[16] Constipation also increases the local fecal flora that may migrate upward through the urethra into the bladder, increasing risk for infection. Chronic constipation may also be associated with repeated straining during bowel evacuation, thus weakening pelvic floor muscles. Good bowel action is dependent upon adequate fluid, fiber, and physical activity. A fiber supplementation program can aide the individual with constipation to restore regular bowel action. Daily requirements for fiber are between 20 grams and 30 grams. In addition to increasing fruits and vegetables, adding high-fiber cereal or unprocessed wheat bran to the daily diet can be very effective.

A skin care regimen is imperative in those incontinent individuals prone to contact dermatitis from urine and fungal infections. When urine is in prolonged contact with skin, maceration and inflammation occurs. Local irritation also contributes to urinary urgency and frequency. Special skin care products are widely available for cleansing, moisturizing, and protection.[17] A variety of absorbent products are also available to accommodate individual needs related to absorbancy, pad design and sizing, skin protection, and comfort. Absorbent product designs include pad inserts with adhesive backing, belted undergarments, a coordinated pad and pant system, and full undergarments.[17] Appropriate product selection matches the individual's unique needs related to amount of wetness, comfort, cost, and availability[18] (see Chapter 13, *Clinical Practice Guideline: Prediction and Prevention of Pressure Ulcers*).

TARGETED INTERVENTIONS

Bladder training is a toileting schedule with progressively increased intervals between voids, which gradually allows the bladder to hold greater urine volumes. The patient learns self-management strategies for urge suppression by monitoring his or her behavior and identifying triggers associated with the onset of bladder urges, and practicing urge suppression techniques when bladder urges occur. Voiding occurs on a strict schedule, and urge suppression allows the patient to maintain the schedule to facilitate bladder stretching to hold increasing volumes of urine. The voiding interval may initially be hourly, with 15- to 30-minute adjustments made on a weekly or biweekly basis until a 3 to 4 hour voiding interval is attained. Bladder training is appropriate for stress or urge UI.[19]

Urge suppression uses pelvic muscle exercises and self-monitoring techniques to reverse the crescendo of a bladder urge and delay voiding until a convenient time. At the onset of the urge, the patient should stand still or sit down, repeatedly contract pelvic muscles, inhale and exhale in a slow relaxed manner, and concentrate on suppressing the urge with "self-talk." Phrases for self talk include "I can make this urge go away—I am in control of my bladder"; or "My bladder is not full, and it is able to hold much more urine than it is now." Urge suppression is necessary for bladder training, to prevent urge UI, and for irritable bladder symptoms.

Pelvic muscle exercises, also known as Kegel exercises, improve UI by increasing urethral resistance by contraction of pelvic muscles, primarily via the levator ani complex. An individualized exercise program is designed based on the patient's ability to perform an effective contraction and the degree of muscle weakness, atrophy, and fatigueability. A pelvic muscle exercise program typically consists of endurance contractions (hold contraction for count of 3, 5, or 10 seconds, and relax for 10 to 15 seconds) and strength contractions (exert maximal contraction, then release). At least 3 months is needed for muscle rehabilitation, and improvements can still be attained at 6 months with continued exercise.

Vaginal cones are tampon-shaped devices weighing 20 grams to 70 grams designed for pelvic muscle weight training. The cone is placed in the vagina, and in the standing position, the patient actively contracts the pelvic muscles in order to retain the cone. Proper muscle isolation is achieved via the proprioceptive sensations (pelvic muscle pressure with reciprocal pelvic muscle contraction) yeilded with the retained cone. This procedure is done twice per day, progressively increasing to 15 minutes in each session. Progression from standing, walking, to coughing and jumping with the lightest cone is then followed in the same sequence with the next weighted cone.[20] Patients with stress UI can benefit from vaginal cone therapy.[21]

Another targeted intervention is electromyographic (EMG) biofeedback-assisted pelvic muscle retraining. This is used for muscle assessment and ongoing evaluation of muscle performance. Biofeedback translates muscle activity into an understandable event using visual displays and auditory signals. This technology helps the patient recognize and control physiologic processes. Immediate information displayed from the biofeedback instrument allows the patient to better control muscle strength, endurance, and coordination.[20] Physiologic signals are transmitted via skin electrodes placed on either side of the anus, rectal, or vaginal probes.[22-24]

GERONTOLOGICAL NURSING IMPLICATIONS

Elderly people often experience problems with continence. Nurses can introduce behavioral interventions that offer a range of approaches to better treat and manage UI. When working with the older person, it is often recognized that significant lifestyle modifications may be required to gain improvements in continence status. For many older people, "a little change goes a long way," and even modest changes should be considered within the context of the person's belief system, preferences, values, and priorities. Modest changes may be difficult for some individuals to undertake. Nurses need to identify meaningful, realistic continence goals, plan the intervention so that small changes lead to success, and monitor progress toward therapeutic results. This will lead to an effective nurse-patient relationship. The nurse assists the older person in finding workable solutions to achieve continence goals, provides ongoing reinforcement and praise for successful implementation, and validates clinical progress.

Nurses also play a critical role in health education and promotion, early identification and basic assessment, and in the design and implementation of behavioral treatment programs. They often underestimate their unique preparedness as health educators and clinicians. A number of reports concerning why incontinent individuals do not seek treatment document that UI is viewed as a normal part of aging and that little can be done for the problem.[25-27] One survey found that more than half of the respondents had sought help about their UI, reporting that their visit to the doctor or nurse was "no help at all," that some providers did not seem knowledgeable about UI, and some were embarrassed or unsympathetic.[28] This area is fast becoming a specialty within gerontological nursing. UI requires a commitment on the part of the nurse and patient to work together for effective results. Public misconceptions combined with lack of preparedness of physicians and nurses to properly address the problem hampers the provision of appropriate treatment. Fortunately, many cases of UI can be improved or cured with appropriate assessment and treatment. In any care setting—

community, home, nursing home, corporate, or hospital—nurses hold responsibility for early identification and intervention for UI and thus contribute to improved quality of life for many incontinent individuals.

REFERENCES

1. Herzog AR, Fultz NH. Prevalence and incidence of urinary incontinence in community dwelling population. *J Am Geriatrics Society.* 1990;38(3):273-81.
2. Urinary Incontinence (UI) Guideline Panel. *Urinary Incontinence in Adults: Clinical Practice Guideline.* AHCPR Publication No. 92-0038. Rockville, MD: Agency for Health Care Policy and Research, Public Health Service, U.S. Department of Health and Human Services. March 1992.
3. Colling J. An update on the AHCPR Guideline implementation. *Nurs Pract Forum.* 1994;5(3):134-137.
4. Staskin DR. Age-related physiologic and pathologic changes affecting lower urinary tract function. *Clin Geriatr Med.* 1986;2( ):701-710.
5. Wozniak-Petrofsky J. Urinary incontinence in the elderly: Not a normal part of aging. *Urol Nurs.* 1993;13:12-16.
6. Hunskaar S, Vinsnes A. The quality of life in women with urinary incontinence as measured by the sickness impact profile. *J Am Geriatr Soc.* 1991;39(4):378-382.
7. Wyman JF, Harkins SW, Fantl JA. Psychosocial impact of urinary incontinence in the community-dwelling population. *J Am Geriatric Society.* 1990;38(3):282-288.
8. Dowd TT. Discovering older women's experience of urinary incontinence. *Res Nurs Health.* 1991;14:179-186.
9. Mitteness LS. The management of urinary incontinence by community-dwelling elderly. *Gerontologist.* 1987;27:185-193.
10. McDowell BJ. Care of urinary incontinence in the home. *Nurs Pract Forum.* 1994;5(3):138-145.
11. Resnick NM, Yalla SV. Detrusor hyperactivity with impaired contractile function: an unrecognized but common cause of incontinence in elderly patients. *JAMA.* 1987;257:3076-3081.
12. Wyman JF. Level 3: Comprehensive assessment and management of urinary incontinence by continence nurse specialists. *Nurs Pract Form.* 1994;5(3):177-185.
13. Folstein MF, Folstein S, McHugh PR. Mini-mental state: a practical method for grading the cognitive status of patients for the clinician. *J Psychiatr Res.* 1987;12:189-198.
14. Colling J, Newman DK, McCormick KA, Pearson BD. Behavioral management strategies for urinary incontinence. *J ET Nurs.* 1993;20(1):9-13.
15. Pearson BD, Larson JM. Urine control by elders: Noninvasive strategies. In: Funk SG, Tournquist EM, Champagne MT, Wiese RA, eds. *Key Aspects of Elder Care: Managing Falls, Incontinence, and Cognitive Impairment.* New York: Springer Publishing Co.; 1992:154-168.
16. Rousseau P, Fuentevilla-Clifton A. Urinary incontinence in the aged, Part 1 and 2. *Geriatrics.* 1992;47(6):22-26,33-34,37-40,45,48.
17. H.I.P. *Resource Guide: Products and Services for Incontinence.* (6th ed.). 1994. Help for Incontinent People, Inc., PO Box 544, Union, S.C. 29379. 1-800-BLADDER.
18. Bierwirth W. Which pad is for you? *Urol Nurs.* 1992;12(2):75-77.
19. Fantl JA, Wyman JF, McClish DK, Harkins SW, Elswick RK, Taylor JR, Hadley EC. Efficacy of bladder training in older women with urinary incontinence. *JAMA.* 1991;265(5):609-13.
20. Laycock J. Pelvic muscle exercises: physiotherapy for the pelvic floor. *Urol Nurs.* 1994;14(3):136-140.
21. Moore K, Metcalfe JB. Effectiveness of vaginal cones in treatment of urinary incontinence. *Urol Nurs.* 1992;12(2):69-72.
22. Burns PA, Parnikoff K, Nochajski T, Hadley EC, Levy KJ, Ory MG. A comparison of effectiveness of biofeedback and pelvic muscle exercise treatment of stress incontinence in older community-dwelling women. *J Gerontol.* 1993;48(4):M167-M174.
23. Wall LL, Norton PA, DeLancey JO. *Practical Urogynecology.* Baltimore: Williams and Wilkins Publishing, 1993.
24. Sand PK, Richardson DA, Staskin DR, Swift SE, Appell RA, Whitmore KE, Ostergard DR. Pelvic floor electrical stimulation in the treatment of genuine stress incontinence: a multicenter, placebo-controlled trial. *Am J Obstet Gynecol.* 1995;173(1):72-79.
25. Goldstein M, Hawthorne ME, Engeberg S, McDowell BJ, Burgio KL. Urinary incontinence: why people do not seek help? *J Gerontol Nurs.* 1992;18(4):15-20.
26. Simons J. Does incontinence affect your client's self-concept? *J Gerontol Nurs.* 1985;11(6):37-40,42.
27. Mitteness LS. Knowledge and beliefs about urinary incontinence in adulthood and old age. *J Am Geriatr Soc.* 1990;38:374-378.
28. Jeter KF, Wagner DB. Incontinence in the American home: a survey of 36,500 people. *J Am Geriatr Soc.* 1990;38:379-383.

Chapter 15

Geriatric Depression

Carla Groh, PhD, RN, CS, and Ann L. Whall, PhD, RN, FAAN

OVERVIEW

Depression in older adults is a major health problem. Although the great majority of older adults negotiate late life changes with grace, good humor, and equanimity, there is a minority of older adults who don't. This chapter deals with the minority—either those who have a life history of clinical depression, which often increases in frequency and severity with age, or those for whom stresses associated with aging have triggered their first episode of a major clinical depression[1] as identified in the fourth edition of *Diagnostic and Statistical Manual of Mental Disorders* (DSM-IV).[2]

Several topics are covered: the demographics of geriatric depression; the prevalence of suicide and known risk factors; the predictive factors that influence relapse rate; the factors that contribute to the etiology of geriatric depression; the symptoms of depression in older adults; and the major components of a comprehensive nursing assessment. A brief review of the traditional treatment modalities (eg, medications, ECT, psychotherapy) is presented. The concept of restorative environments is introduced as a viable option for nursing research, which might result in the development of nursing interventions that could improve nurses effectiveness in caring for older adults who are depressed. The significance of geriatric depression to the profession of nursing and nursing implications are discussed throughout the chapter.

INTRODUCTION

Most human beings experience ups and downs in their lives without succumbing to a prolonged, unhealthy state of depression. The process of aging represents a special challenge in this respect, with increased potential for sudden, often irreversible, declines in physical health or for slow progressions of chronic illness, which is compounded by the loss of friends, family, and autonomy. Even among older adults, the great majority negotiate these life changes with only minor disruptions in their lives.

It is important for nurses to remember that many older adults diagnose themselves as being "blue," "in the dumps," or "feeling down." They may not, however, be experiencing a major clinical depression. Nurses can effectively intervene with older adults suffering from major clinical depression. Nurses in a variety of settings (eg, long-term care, community health, primary care, psychiatric facilities) are in critical positions to identify and treat depression in the elderly. The nurse who understands the complex interrelationships among physical health, mental health, and the consequences of drugs commonly prescribed to treat illness in older adults is in a unique position to assist in the differential diagnosis of depression and to assist older adults to improve their mood states.[3]

DEMOGRAPHICS

Depression is the most prevalent and troublesome mental health problem among older adults.[4,5] Even though the Epidemiologic Catchment Area (ECA) study showed that only 1% to 2% of people 65 years and older living in the community meet criteria for major depression as identified in the DSM-IV; 27% of this population experience depressive symptoms that do not meet DSM-IV criteria.[5]

The prevalence of depression is even higher in institutions. A major depressive disorder is diagnosed in 12% of patients in institutions providing long-term or short-term care; 23% to 31% of these populations have significant depressive symptoms that do not meet DSM-IV criteria.[5]

The elderly comprise the age group most at risk for suicide, and the rate of suicide among the elderly is 50% higher than the rate for young people. Suicide rates peak for men between the ages of 80 and 90 and for women between the ages of 50 and 65. Compared to younger people, older adults communicate their suicidal intent less frequently, use more violent and lethal methods, and less often attempt suicide as a means of manipulation.[6] The elderly account for 25% of suicides, yet they make up only 10% of the total population.[7]

Relapses and chronicity are important issues in geriatric depression. Studies of geriatric depression covering 1 to 6 years of follow-up have shown that chronicity occurs in 7% to 30% of all cases. The chronicity figures are higher and range from 40% to 42% if partially improved people are included. The chronicity of a depressive episode may be predicted by the presence of a coexisting medical illness, the long duration of previous episodes, and poor social supports. About one third of those who recover will relapse within 1 year. Several factors are predictive of early relapse: if there is a history of three or more depressive episodes, late onset of the first depressive episode, concurrent medical illness, and concurrent traumatic life events.[5]

ETIOLOGY OF GERIATRIC DEPRESSION

Nurses need to view geriatric depression as a heterogeneous condition that can result from a variety of factors. Three factors will be discussed: medical/physical, psychosocial, and gender (Table 15-1).

TABLE 15-1

Related Factors in Onset of Depression in Older Adults

ILLNESSES

- Hypothyroidism
- Hyperthyroidism
- Cushing's disease
- Infections
- Lymphoma
- Cancer: pancreatic, breast, prostate
- Other malignancies

MEDICATIONS

- Reserpine (Serpasil)
- α-methyldopa (Aldomet)
- Clonidine (Catapres)
- Hydralazine (Apresoline)
- Propranolol (Inderal)
- Digitalis
- Cimetidine (Tagamet)
- Steroids
- Estrogens
- Progestational agents
- Indomethacin (Indocin)
- Propoxyphene (Darvon)
- Codeine
- Antibacterials
- Levodopa (Larodopa)
- Tamoxifen (Nolvadex)
- Vincristine (Oncovin)
- Vinblastine (Velban)
- Benzodiazepines
- Barbiturates

NUTRITIONAL DEFICITS

- Lack of B vitamins
- Tooth loss
- Malfitting dentures
- Loss of interest in eating alone

NEUROLOGIC CHANGES

- Reduction in norepinephrine
- Reduction in dopamine
- Reduction in serotonin brain concentrations
- Increase in monoamine catabolic enzyme monoamine oxidase

PSYCHOSOCIAL STRESSORS

- Restricted social contacts
- Reduced vocational, social, and recreational activities
- Financial impoverishment with poor living conditions
- Widowhood
- Separation from children and others
- Lack of adequate social supports
- Loss of "beauty" in western world
- Loss of status in western world
- Loss of employment and "self-worth" in western world
- Lack of stimulating environment

PHYSIOLOGIC CHANGES

- Sleep disturbances
- Slowed gait
- Decreased eye sight
- Decrease in hearing
- Chronic illnesses as loss (eg, benign prostatic hypertrophy and surgery leading to loss of potency)

Medical/Physical Factors

Physiological changes of aging, medical illnesses, and medications may all contribute to geriatric depression. Normal physiological changes associated with aging can predispose the older adult to geriatric depression. In addition to normal physiological changes, medical illnesses can also increase an older adult's risk for depression. People with neurological disease experience a high rate of depression; about 15% to 20% of people with Alzheimer's disease experience major depressive symptoms while up to 50% have less intense depressive symptoms.[5] Multi-infarct dementia is associated with depression even more frequently than is Alzheimer's disease. In addition, a cerebrovascular disease is often accompanied by depression as are about 50% of people with Parkinson's disease.

Many drugs prescribed for common physical problems have psychoactive properties that can precipitate symptoms of depression, major psychosis, anxiety disorder, and dementia. In addition, drugs prescribed to alleviate mental symptoms have side effects that can mimic other mental conditions such as mood disorder and/or dementia.[8]

Psychosocial Factors

There are several psychosocial factors that predispose an older adult to geriatric depression: restricted social contacts, financial difficulties, feelings of loneliness and hopelessness, lack of social supports, death of significant others, and change in living arrangements.

Gender

Gender has long been considered a risk factor for depression. Community surveys show that adult women are twice as likely as men to be treated for depression. Longitudinal research suggests that depressed women have longer episodes of depression than men and a lower rate of spontaneous remission. For women, there is a peak in first onset during the childbearing years and a decrease in onset after age 45. There is no evidence for an increase of depression during the menopausal years.[9]

After the age of 65 years, however, the frequency of depression in men increases so that the rates tend to approach each other or even reverse.[7] Among men and women who have a lifetime history of depression, there is no gender difference in risk of recurrence.[7] Although frequency of depression in men and women approach each other after age 65, older women are at greater risk for iatrogenic drug abuse involving psychoactive drugs than any other age-by-gender group. A study of the prevalence and correlates of long-term regular use of anxiolytics reports regular users to be older people, predominantly women, with high levels of emotional distress and chronic somatic health problems.[10]

Many gaps remain in our understanding of the differential rates of depression in men and women. We lack a coherent explanation of why the rates of major depression are higher in women than in men during the childbearing/child-rearing years and also why the rates begin to equal each other after age 65. One could speculate that biologic factors, such as endocrinologic and genetic influences, as well as social factors (eg, role-related stress) contribute to the relative excess of depression in women during the childbearing/child-rearing years.[9] However, much remains to be learned about the basic pathogenesis of depression in men and women after age 65.

RECOGNIZING GERIATRIC DEPRESSION

Depressed people live in varying degrees of pain and desperation, often undiagnosed or misdiagnosed. Even the sufferer may not be aware of having the disorder, which can be masked by body aches and pains. It is atypical to be depressed in late life. Depression is a serious illness that needs to be identified and treated. In order for nurses to actively participate in the identification and differential diagnosis of clinical depression in older adults, it is essential that they become familiar with mood disorders; delirium, dementia, amnesia, and other cognitive disorders, as well as mental disorders attributed to a general medical condition in the DSM-IV.

The clinical features of geriatric depression are similar to those of depression in young adults. People who are depressed look sad, tired, and forlorn. Reassurance by others gives little comfort. They usually move slowly (psychomotor retardation), although in some situations they will appear anxious and restless (agitation). The disturbance is prominent, persistent, and associated with impaired functioning. Often, attention to grooming and hygiene are neglected due to lack of motivation and energy. The feelings most often reported by depressed people include guilt, feelings of worthlessness, disinterest in life, isolation, loneliness, lack of pleasure in usually pleasurable activities, feelings of failure, and thoughts of death and suicide. Neurovegative symptoms include anorexia and weight loss, sleep pattern disturbances, constipation, tachycardia, and somatization.

Although geriatric depression is similar to depressive symptoms found in the young, there are some key differences. Older adults who are depressed are more likely to have numerous somatic complaints even in the absence of physical disease. They are more likely to express somatic anxiety (eg, panic attacks), which may be severe, leading to agitation.[11] These people tend to be highly irritable and hostile.

Feelings of sadness are not necessarily experienced or expressed. Older depressed adults tend to have blunted emotions or only mild expressions of sadness. In addition, they do not blame themselves for their current situation[11] nor do they admit to feelings of inappropriate guilt.[5] Elderly depressed people may be malnourished and agitated for weeks to months before being diagnosed. Depression left untreated or undertreated can lead to an increased risk for cardiac disease,[12] memory loss, and decreased attention,[13] with a three-fold increase in mortality.[14]

ASSESSMENT

The interview is the initial step in the assessment of an older adult and the most important procedure in differentiating depression from other psychiatric disorders.[15] Many older adults are aware of only some symptoms and may minimize their disability. Many factors may inhibit older adults from expressing their feelings: sensory loss, confusion, communication problems, cultural influences, shame, and fear of stigmatization.[3] Interviewing someone who knows the individual well (eg, spouse, close friend, relative) can be extremely valuable in obtaining an accurate picture of the older adult's symptoms, degree of disability, and course of illness. It is also important that the nurse make the person comfortable, conveying a sense of empathy, respect, and caring.

The interview should include the following:

- Physiologic status, including recent illnesses and operations, nutritional status, chronic diseases
- Alcohol intake, including amount and type of alcohol (see Chapter 20, *Elderly and Alcohol: A Deadly Combination*), duration of alcohol intake
- Cognitive functioning, including a mental status exam, changes in cognition over time, educational level
- Current living arrangements, including social supports, recent deaths
- Financial situation, including any recent loss of income
- Past psychiatric history, including prior manic, psychotic, or depressive episodes
- Family history of major depression or bipolar disorder, including family history of suicide attempt(s)
- Current medications, including over-the-counter and prescription (see Chapter 19, *Screening for Polypharmacy in a Nursing Home Care Unit*)
- Suicidal ideations, including a current plan or past attempts.

SUICIDE RISK ASSESSMENT

The potential for suicide should never be minimized. There are four important points that nurses need to be aware of when assessing suicide risk. The most at-risk individual is the elderly white man who is widowed and living alone.[4] There is a strong association between alcohol intake and suicide, especially among the elderly.[16] Older adults who are considering suicide tend not to contact crisis intervention and hotlines, but may make contact with physicians or other health care providers. A study conducted by Foster[17] found that 75% of older adults who committed suicide had seen a physician shortly before the act. Since nurses are often the first health care provider seen by patients, it is critical that nurses be knowledgeable of the clues and warning signs of suicide (Table 15-2). And finally, if you suspect the person might be thinking of suicide but does not share that information with you, ask the question directly. If you believe the person poses a serious risk for suicide or if a person is in a high-risk category, he or she should be hospitalized for protection and further evaluation.[4] Nurses need to be aware of their legal responsibility when they believe that an older adult poses a harm to himself or herself. Since suicidal people often resist psychiatric hospitalization, nurses need to know that there is a court process for involuntary commitment as delineated in each state's mental health code. A copy of your state's mental health code can be obtained by contacting the Department of Mental Health or the local community mental health board in the area you work.

TREATMENT

The nursing goals for treatment should include reducing symptoms, risk of relapse, and recurrence; increasing quality of life; improving general and medical health status; and decreasing mortality.[18] Thus, treatment of geriatric depression must be multi-faceted for the most effective results.

TABLE 15-2

Warning Signs of Suicide Risk in the Depressed Elderly

VERBAL CLUES

- I'm going to kill myself.
- I'm going to commit suicide.
- Life just isn't worth living anymore.
- You would be better off without me.
- I just want out.
- I can't stand this anymore.

BEHAVIORAL CLUES

- Purchasing a gun
- Stockpiling pills
- Making or changing a will
- Making funeral plans
- Giving away money or possessions
- Changes in behavior (eg, episodes of screaming or hitting, throwing things)
- Suspicious of noncharacteristic behavior (eg, going out at odd times, kissing or waving goodbye)
- Loss of physical skills, general confusion or loss of understanding, judgment, memory
- Scheduling of appointment with doctor for no apparent physical cause or shortly after the last visit to the doctor
- Increase in amount of alcohol intake
- Drinking in spite of medical advice against alcohol use
- Sudden change in mood from depressed to happy, cheerful

SYMPTOMS OF DEPRESSION

- Change in sleep patterns
- Change in eating patterns (eg, loss of appetite, weight loss)
- Extreme fatigue
- Increased concern with bodily function (eg, frequent complaints of constipation, loose bowels, aches and pains, increased heart rate)
- Change in mood (eg, listless, apathetic, angry, hostile, nervous, irritable, sad)
- Feelings of worthlessness

SITUATIONAL CLUES

- Recent move
- Death of a spouse or significant other
- Diagnosis of terminal illness
- Argument with relative or close friend
- Isolating self from relatives or friends
- Financial problems
- White man, living alone

Adapted from Osgood NJ. Suicide in the elderly. *Carrier Foundation Letter.* April 1988;133.

There are currently three major treatment options for geriatric depression: medications, ECT, and psychotherapy. In addition to these three traditional treatment modalities, restorative environments are an adjunct to treatment. Research findings by Kaplan[19] support the hypothesis that restorative environments are effective in people who are mentally fatigued. This might be an important area for nurses to explore since it has been hypothesized that mental fatigue may be prodromal to depression.[20] Many excellent articles and chapters are available on medications,[4,8,21] ECT,[22,23] and psychotherapy[24]; therefore, this will be briefly discussed.

TABLE 15-3

Common Side Effects of the Major Antidepressants

HETEROCYCLIC	MAOIs	SSRIs
Amitriptyline Amoxapine (Asendin) Bupropion Clomipramine (Anafranil) Desipramine (Norpramin) Doxepin (Sinequan) Imipramine (Tofranil) Nortriptyline (Pamelor) Trazodone (Desyrel) Trimipramine (Surmontil)	Isocarboxazid (Marplan) Phenelzine (Nardil) Tranylcypromine (Parnate)	Fluoxetine (Prozac) Paroxetine (Paxil) Sertraline (Zoloft) Venlafaxine (Effexor)
SIDE EFFECTS	**SIDE EFFECTS**	**SIDE EFFECTS**
Orthostatic hypotension Sedation Cardiac toxicity effects: • AV block • Prolonged PR, QRS and QT intervals Anticholingeric effects: • Constipation • Dry mouth • Urinary retention • Increased anxiety • Agitation • Confusion • Restlessness • Disorientation • Assaultiveness • Paranoia	Orthostatic hypotension Weight gain Dry mucous membranes Insomnia Overstimulation Sexual dysfunction Hypertensive crisis ** Peripheral neuropathy (eg, weakness of legs, paresthesias memory loss, and confusion in demented persons) ** People on MAOIs need to avoid foods with tyramine (eg, all cheese [except cottage cheese and cream cheese], yeast extract, caviar, sausage, herring, liver, avocado, chocolate, caffeine, red wine, beer)	Dizziness Anxiety and nervousness Insomnia Drowsiness Fatigue Tremors Anorexia and weight loss Sexual dysfunction Dry mouth Headaches Sweating

MEDICATION

Many older adults with clinical depression have a robust response to antidepressant medication. The drug of choice should be based on previous responses to treatment and anticipation of which side effects might pose the greatest problems or produce the greatest therapeutic benefits for that person. Three important points are critical to remember when working with older adults who are taking antidepressants. Older adults metabolize and excrete drugs more slowly than younger people, so they may require a lower dose of the medication. Older adults respond more slowly to an antidepressant—maximum effect is usually not achieved before 2 to 6 weeks. Older adults tend to be more responsive to the toxic effects of antidepressants; thus, the nurse must be knowledgeable regarding the common side effects of the three major antidepressant groups: heterocyclic, MAOIs, and SSRIs antidepressants (Table 15-3).

Electroconvulsive treatment is one of the most effective and safest available treatments for depression in all age groups.[22] This is especially true for the elderly depressed patient whose depression is accompanied by self-destructive behavior (eg, suicidal ideations and refusal to eat); in patients who become catatonic from severe depression;[4] in patients who have medical illnesses where the use of antidepressants may be dangerous;[23] in patients who cannot tolerate the medication and/or the side effects of the antidepressants; and/or in patients who are non-responders to antidepressants.[4]

Although ECT is considered an effective alternative for the high-risk elderly patient with depression,[23,25] it has been suggested that the aging brain might be more vulnerable to ECT's adverse effects, particularly those affecting memory.[26] Memory deficits consist of three types: anterograde amnesia (loss of ability to accomplish new learning); retrograde amnesia (loss of memory for events that occurred before ECT); and, memory complaints.

The memory impairments that occur with ECT and the expected recovery patterns have not been well established. Many patients continue to report persistent memory problems for several months after treatment. Freeman[27] found that 75% of their patients reported that memory loss was the worst side effect of ECT with 30% stating that their memories have never returned to normal. Others have suggested that by 6 months after ECT treatment, new learning ability and remote memory return to baseline.[28] However, the results of numerous studies have still not provided a definitive answer to the question of whether and, if so, to what degree ECT is associated with persistent memory loss.[25]

Since the care of the depressed elderly patient following ECT is often the responsibility of nurses, it is important that nurses develop intervention strategies that acknowledge these memory deficits. For example, nurses might want to avoid having the patient perform tasks that require new learning; provide the patient memory cues about recent events; support and reassure the patient and family that the confusion and memory loss is probably temporary; and not expect more of the patient than he or she is able to do.

Psychotherapy can help older adults better understand the anxieties, conflicts, and pain involved with depression and to develop coping skills to manage their stressful situations. There are four major types of psychotherapy used to treat depressive disorders that nursing has traditionally been involved with: cognitive therapy, behavioral therapy, interpersonal therapy, and group therapy. Cognitive therapy can be used to help older adults change negative thinking patterns, whereas behavioral therapy emphasizes the importance of daily experiences and behavior. Interpersonal therapy focuses on relationship problems and role conflicts that might contribute to depression. Group therapy is also an important treatment modality that provides older adults an opportunity to connect with others in similar type situations. Nurses, especially advanced practitioners, need to continue to assume an active role in psychotherapy, both inpatient and outpatient.

RESTORATIVE ENVIRONMENTS

Researchers have begun to explore the relationship between the restorative qualities of the natural environment and psychological well-being. Kaplan[19] has developed a theory of attentional restoration, which focuses on the relationship between mental fatigue, directed attention, and restorative environments. They postulate that mental fatigue is a state of reduced effectiveness and increased discomfort following overuse of directed attention. Mental fatigue manifests in decreased attentional capacity resulting in distractibility, increased errors, declining ability to focus, to achieve clarity, to problem-solve, and to make or carry out plans. Directed attention is the capacity to inhibit distractions and focus on needed information. Thus, Kaplan suggests that mental fatigue is reduced in restorative environments because these environments allow for the recovery of directed attention. The types of environments that help to restore humans most often include natural elements, such as plants, animals, flowing water, and fresh air. In addition, walking, touching, smelling, inhaling, savoring the sights, listening to the sounds, and tasting as appropriate are all factors that help restore mental and physical health and allow the person to take full advantage of his or her restorative experience.[29]

Kaplan's theory of restoration has the potential to be important in the nursing care of older depressed adults for several reasons. It has been suggested that older adults may demonstrate increased susceptibility to mental fatigue and distractibility.[19,20] Symptoms labeled as depression in older adults such as concentration and attention difficulties, indecisiveness, disorientation, easy distractibility, irritability, and memory impairment resemble the manifestations of mental fatigue. Having noted that, Yankou[20] speculates that attentional fatigue may have at times been labeled as depression, dementia, or "old age." Furthermore, the etiology of depressive symptoms in some older adults may be chronic mental fatigue. Restorative environments may have positive effects on depression related to mental fatigue in older adults. Yankou,[20] in a study with older women (n=57), found an association between women who reported participating in restorative activities and decreased depression.

Although the concept of restorative environments is relatively new, nurses have been concerned about the effects of the environment on health since Nightingale. Nightingale[30] wrote extensively about the importance of the environment in the promotion of health, suggesting ways for providing relief from pain such as needlework, plants, pets, flowers, and a window with a view. In recent years, nurse researchers have begun to look at incorporating the concepts related to restorative environments in the nursing care of patients.[20,31] It is an exciting area of research with multiple potentials for nursing interventions.

The following case study provides an example of how restorative environments could be used in the care of an older adult who is depressed. It is important to note that while there is much potential for the use of restorative environments, many of the findings are tentative and there are no current nursing studies that support a direct relationship between depression and restorative environments. Thus, restorative environments must be viewed as adjunct to the more traditional therapies discussed earlier.

CASE STUDY

The geriatrician was sincere and quite frustrated. He and his colleagues had tried everything. Nevertheless, the elderly woman remained depressed. In his view, asking the question, "What can nursing do to help this woman?" was a logical next step.

The situation for the 78-year-old woman appeared gloomy. Her husband of many years had died the previous year. Because she was unable to manage her home and personal care, she moved in with her daughter, son-in-law, and two grandsons. Although the daughter's home was in the same city, the connections with her and her husband's past were severed.

She began complaining of lower back pain—the situation that had brought her to the geriatrician. She was "worked up" at an excellent health center; minor arthritis was found in her lumbar spine, but nothing that would account for the degree of pain that she reported. The usual treatment for back strain did not work; as time progressed, the pain worsened.

The patient was sent for a second opinion to an equally qualified health center. The health care workers there confirmed the first diagnosis and suggested that depression was most likely making the problem seem worse to the elderly woman. The geriatrician started the patient on an antidepressant, which initially seemed to help but later seemed only to maintain the same level of depression. This situation prompted the geriatrician to ask for nursing assistance.

The nurse and her colleagues assessed the situation, answering in part the following questions: What is there in the patient's life that began about the time of the depression that is distressing her? How might this depression be related to grief and loss? Why is the antidepressant not working? and What could be done to put the patient in the best possible position for nature to heal her? The patient's symptoms seemed to be clues to the situation.

Some of the topics the nurses discussed included the pain of "working through" grief in isolation and the pain caused by her sudden losses of neighborhood, home, and familiar people and activities. Finally, the nurses realized that these elements were likely the reasons why the drugs were not effective.

The nurses knew that when a situation seems hopeless, changing one major element would change the nature and magnitude of all elements/problems. They also knew that the environment seemed wrong for this woman. Viewing the environment from a holistic bio-psychosocial perspective, the nurses saw many things that needed to be addressed. For example, in the psychosocial realm, several needs of the patient had to be addressed (see Chapter 6, *Gerontology, Spirituality, and Nursing*).

This woman did not venture outside of her daughter's home because she was unfamiliar with the area and was concerned about her low back pain and falling. Since her daughter and son-in-law worked and the grandsons were in and out, the woman was home alone most of the day with no outside contacts. At night when the family was home, the woman retired to her room shortly after dinner. She often felt like she was "in the way," and the amount of activity and noise at night made her nervous. Thus, many of the elements that contribute to health and life satisfaction, eg, the opportunity to move about and to be active in the environment, the opportunity to get fresh air, to have meaningful social interactions, and to feel "normal," were missing from this woman's life. Staff felt that there was good reason for the nonefficacy of the antidepressant, as too many other elements mitigated against their effect.

It was felt that this woman lived in a depleted and nonhealthy environment, and it was decided to approach her depression from a slightly different perspective with a modified environment so that the patient was in the best position for nature to heal the depression. Several interventions were implemented. A geripsychiatric consultation was initiated to assess the patient's medications and to check for any drug interactions that might be implicated. The patient was asked to identify the one or two most important elements to change in order to help heal her mind, body, and spirit. The patient reported that she missed feeding the birds in the backyard of the home she and her husband had lived in. While it was not possible for her to feed the birds at her old home, the daughter was willing to put a birdfeeder in her backyard, and it became the woman's responsibility to feed the birds every day. Since she was still concerned about going outside with her low back pain and feared falling, arrangements were made with the daughter's neighbors to be available on a rotating schedule. As the woman became more confident in her abilities, she began to spend longer periods of time outside doing a little gardening and listening to the birds. After a while, the neighbors were no longer needed. The nurses discussed recent losses, such as the death of her husband, the change in her living arrangements, and loss of close contact with her friends. She expressed a great deal of sadness and longing for the past. Looking at pictures of her husband and friends, she began to share her stories with us and was able to begin appropriate grieving of these many losses.

Over the next 6 months, the woman reported that she felt "a little better," and her behavior and willingness to get more involved was significantly improved. Her complaints of back pain lessened, and she did not require as frequent visits to the doctor. Modifying the environment was healthful for this woman, and that improvement was noted.

GERONTOLOGICAL NURSING IMPLICATIONS

It is imperative that nurses in all realms of the heath care system be able to recognize geriatric depression and how to treat it. There are multiple implications for nurses working with older adults in all phases of illness. Depression is often overlooked and may play an important part in the care provided. If overlooked, the patient may not experience better health.

There is a danger in nursing and other disciplines of believing that because depression in older adults is "understandable," it need not be explored further and that treatment is not necessary. Depression in older adults cannot be dismissed as unimportant to function, and new methods of treatment must be sought and encouraged.[32] Nurses are in powerful positions to conduct research studies that examine cutting edge theories about depression and new treatment strategies.

Geriatric depression is a heterogeneous condition that can result from a variety of factors. Nurses need to be aware of these factors and actively participate in the assessment and treatment of older adults who are diagnosed as clinically depressed. Nurses will always be involved with older adults who are prescribed antidepressants, receive ECT and/or psychotherapy. A substantial body of new research on geriatric depression is now available. Implementing these findings in clinical practice and measuring their outcomes can vastly improve nurses' effectiveness as caregivers.

Nightingale had a vision that the actions taken by nurses to promote health would be focused on control of the environment. Nurses need to recapture this vision today if our health care system itself is not to be "toxic" to older adults.[33] We must help nature heal depression by putting the patient in the best environment possible. Nurses in institutional settings can promote/advocate for plant, pet, and music therapy, providing their patients a sunny or brightly lit setting and use of touching to not only reach their depressed patients, but also to prevent exacerbations of depressive episodes. Nurses in the community/home care setting can also access the environment for clues that can promote restoration: proximity to a radio, plants, and windows. Gerontological nurses, as consultants to corporations, have the expertise to discuss and develop appropriate environments where restorative modalities are a major consideration. Working with families is important as many older adults live with spouses or children. Referrals will be needed to promote continuity of care and to assist families in understanding behavior changes and reactions to medication.

Inherent in any discussion of depression is an in-depth awareness of older patients, in addition to their past medical history. Who they are in relation to a family/community, what experiences/skills have brought them to older age and allowed them to achieve success or failure are important. Positive coping skills, behavior modification, and appropriate medication can be provided to older patients to promote resiliency in the twilight of their lives.

REFERENCES

1. Gaylord S, Zung W. Affective disorders among the aging. In: Carstensen L, Edelstein B, eds.. *Handbook of Clinical Gerontology*. New York: Pergamon Press; 1987:76-95.
2. American Psychiatric Association. *Diagnostic and Statistical Manual of Mental Disorders* (4th ed). Washington, D.C.: American Psychiatric Association; 1994.
3. Love C, Buckwalter K. Reactive depression. In: Maas M, Buckwalter K, Hardy M, eds. *Nursing Diagnoses and Interventions for the Elderly*. Menlo Park: Addison-Wesley Nursing; 1991:419-432.
4. Jenike MA. Affective disorders in the elderly. In: Jenike MA, ed. *Geriatric Psychiatry and Psychopharmacology*. St. Louis: Mosby Year Book, Inc.; 1989:33-126.
5. Alexopoulos G. Mood disorders. In: Kaplan H, Sadock B. *Comprehensive Textbook of Psychiatry/VI*. Baltimore: Williams & Wilkins; 1995:2566-2568.
6. Osgood NJ. Suicide in the elderly. *Carrier Foundation Letter*. April 1988;133.
7. Roy A. Suicide. In: Kaplan H, Sadock B, eds. *Comprehensive Textbook of Psychiatry/VI* (Vol. 2). Baltimore: Williams & Wilkins; 1995: 1739-1752.
8. Whall AL. Geropsychiatry: the psychoactive properties of commonly prescribed drugs. *J Gerontol Nurs*. 1988; 14(11):31-32.
9. Weissman MM, Olfson M. Depression in women: implications for health care research. *Science*. August 1995; 269:799-801.
10. Mellinger GD, Balter MB, Uhlenhuth EH. Prevalence and correlates of the long-term regular use or anxiolytics. *JAMA*. 1984:251:375-379.
11. Monfort J. The difficult elderly patient: curable hostile depression or personality disorder? *International Psychogeriatrics*. 1995; 7:95-111.
12. Tsuang MT, Woolson RF, Fleming JA. Premature deaths in schizophrenia and affective disorders. *Arch Gen Psychiatry*. 1980; 37:979-983.

13. Sweeney JA, Wetzler S, Stokes P, Locsis J. Cognitive functioning in depression. *J Clin Psychology*. 1989; 6: 836-842.
14. Ashby D, Ames D, West CR, et al. Psychiatric morbidity as prediction of mortality for residents of local authority homes for the elderly. *International J Geriatric Psychiatry*. 1991; 6:567-575.
15. Lazarus LW, Davis JM, Dysken MW. Geriatric depression: a guide to successful therapy. *Geriatrics*. 1985; 40:43-53.
16. Blazer D. *Depression in Late Life*. St. Louis: CV Mosby, 1982.
17. Foster BG, Burke WJ. Assessing and treating the suicidal elderly. *Fam Pract Recertification*. November 1985; 7:33-45.
18. Schneider LS, Olin JT. Efficacy of acute treatment for geriatric depression. *International Psychogeriatrics*. 1995; 7: 7-25.
19. Kaplan R, Kaplan S. *The Experience of Nature: A Psychological Perspective*. Cambridge: Cambridge Press; 1989.
20. Yankou DJ. *Depression and directed attentional fatigue in older women*. Unpublished doctoral dissertation, University of Michigan; 1996.
21. Salzman C. *Clinical geriatric psychopharmacology* (2nd ed). Baltimore: Williams & Wilkins; 1992.
22. Dubovsky SL. Electroconvulsive therapy. In: Kaplan H, Sadock B, eds. *Comprehensive Textbook of Psychiatry/VI* (Vol. 2). Baltimore: Williams & Wilkins; 1995; 2129-2140.
23. Karlinsky H, Shulman K. The clinical use of electroconvulsive therapy in old age. *J of Nervous and Mental Disease*. March 1984; 32:183-186.
24. Alonso A, Swiller H. *Group Therapy in Clinical Practice*. Washington, D.C.: American Psychiatric Press; 1993.
25. Weiner R. The role of electroconvulsive therapy in the treatment of depression in the elderly. *J American Geriatrics Society*. November 1982;30:710-712.
26. Fraser R, Glass I. Recovery from ECT in elderly patients. *Br J Psychiatry*. 1978; 133:524-528.
27. Freeman C, Kendell R. Patients' experience of and attitudes to electroconvulsive therapy. *Annals New York Academy of Science*. 1986; 341-345.
28. Squire L, Slater P. Electroconvulsive therapy and complaints of memory dysfunction: a perspective three-year follow-up study. *Br J Psychiatry*. 1983; 142:1-8.
29. Whall AL. Geropsychiatry: what is the nursing treatment for depression? *J Gerontol Nurs*. 1994; 20(1):42-45.
30. Nightingale F. *On Nursing: What it is and What it is Not*. New York: Dover (originally published 1859).
31. Cimprich B. Development of an intervention to restore attention in cancer patients. *Cancer Nursing*. 1993; 16(2):83-92.
32. Lichtenberg PA, Ross T, Millis SR, Manning CA. The relationship between depression and cognition in older adults: a cross-validation study. *J Gerontology*. January 1995; 50B:25-32.
33. Whall AL. Using the environment to improve the mental health of the elderly. *J Gerontol Nurs*. 1991;17(7):39.

Chapter 16

Cerumen Impaction and Hearing Impairment Among Nursing Home Residents: Nursing Implications

Diane Feeney Mahoney, PhD, RN, CS, GNP

OVERVIEW

Impacted cerumen (earwax) is a reversible cause of conductive hearing loss. Interpretive difficulties arise from impaired hearing, which negatively affect older adults' quality of life. One hundred four randomly selected nursing home residents from nine facilities were examined to determine the prevalence of cerumen impaction and hearing impairment. A prevalence rate of 24.8% for cerumen impaction and 55% for moderate to profound hearing impairment were found. Notably, the only facility that employed a gerontological nurse specialist had no cases of cerumen impaction. Without this unique facility, the cerumen rate would have been identical to the 34% reported in community and hospital settings. Cerumen impaction and hearing impairment are common problems among older adults and warrant attention.

RATIONALE FOR THE STUDY

Cerumen impaction is a reversible, frequently overlooked cause of a conductive hearing loss.[1] Many nursing home residents are not aware that their hearing is reduced and consequently do not request hearing evaluations.[2] Impacted cerumen occludes 100% of the canal, darkens in color, and hardens with the passage of time. The person with this condition may notice nothing or complain of a sensation of itchiness, fullness, decreased hearing, and/or an achy feeling in the affected ear(s). Rubin[3] recommends evaluating every patient presenting with hearing loss for cerumen impaction. In a convenience sample of 123 community-residing older adults, 34% had cerumen impaction.[4] Similar results (35%) were found among a randomized sample of hospitalized elderly.[5] Unknown at present is the prevalence of cerumen impaction in the institutionalized elderly population.

The underlying theoretical basis for this study lies within the philosophy of gerontological nursing. There is a unifying belief among gerontological nurses, and it is applied within the American Nurses Association (ANA) standards of gerontological nursing practice, that nurses should strive to maximize older adults' achievable independence in everyday living.[6]

Treatable disorders in nursing home residents are important to discover in order to improve residents' quality of life by optimizing their present functional status and reducing excess disability. The purpose of the present study was to determine the prevalence of impacted cerumen in a population of elderly nursing home residents, evaluate the difference in hearing perception after the removal of impacted cerumen, and identify the factors in the nursing home setting that impede or promote the detection and treatment of cerumen impaction.

HEARING LOSS AS A MAJOR GERIATRIC PROBLEM

In contrast to the numerous hearing research studies conducted in primary care settings, few studies have occurred in nursing homes. Estimates indicate that 70% to 90% of nursing home residents exhibit a hearing impairment.[7-9] Humphrey[10] suggests that many people, including health care professionals, believe that hearing loss is a normal part of aging and that little can be done to improve older adults' hearing. If the staff and physicians believe that hearing loss among nursing home residents is expected due to advanced age, then the likelihood of further evaluation of hearing impairments is minimal. There are, however, three hearing disorders common in the older population:

- Presbycusis, the progressive irreversible bilateral loss of high tone perception often associated with aging
- Central deafness (sensorineural hearing loss), which occurs from nerve damage within the brain
- Conduction deafness (conductive hearing loss) that results from blockage or impairment of the mechanical movement in the outer or middle ear.[11]

The first two disorders usually result in permanent hearing loss. Conduction deafness, however, can be reversed if it is due to a treatable disorder such as cerumen impaction.

Hearing loss is a serious health problem among the elderly. Social isolation, depression, acting out inappropriately, and paranoia have been related to impaired hearing.[12,13] Older adults with hearing loss may feel that people around them are mumbling or deliberately excluding them from the conversation.[14] If ignored, a hearing impairment can cause older adults to become inappropriately labeled as "confused" or "uncooperative" when they misinterpret communication and respond improperly.[2,9] In a study of 153 non-institutionalized elderly, Bess[15] found that poor hearing was associated with functional—as well as psychosocial—impairment. One of the key health status objectives for older adults in *Healthy People 2000* is to reduce the prevalence of significant hearing impairment.[16] Thus, it is important that treatable causes of hearing loss such as cerumen impaction are identified and treated. Four questions guided this research:

1. What is the prevalence of cerumen impaction among a random sample of elderly nursing home residents?
2. Is there a significant difference in demographic and health care characteristics between residents with and without cerumen impaction?
3. Is there a measurable difference in hearing perception after the removal of impacted cerumen?

4. What factors in the nursing home setting impede or promote the detection and treatment of cerumen impaction?

METHODS

SUBJECTS

The study sample consisted of 104 residents randomly chosen from eight Massachusetts nursing homes. The nursing homes were randomly chosen from the Massachusetts State listing of adult long-term care facilities for 1990. Facilities were excluded if they had fewer than 50 residents since small homes are less likely to have an adequate pool of eligible residents and tend to have unique characteristics that limit generalizability. Residents were ineligible if they were not able to understand and follow audiological testing directions, were acutely ill, or younger than 62. Five residents were ineligible according to these criteria. Of the 107 residents eligible for the study, 104 (97%) agreed to participate.

The study occurred in two phases. Initially, all the subjects were examined to determine the prevalence rate for cerumen impaction in the nursing home population. Then, to assess if a measurable difference occurs when impacted cerumen is removed, a pretest/post-test two-group comparison design was chosen. The subjects with impacted cerumen comprised the study group, and the subjects without impacted cerumen were the comparison control group. Subjects in both groups received the initial hearing test and would be scheduled for a second test after the impacted cerumen was removed from the study group.

DATA COLLECTION AND INSTRUMENTS

Subjects were interviewed and examined by a specially trained nurse research assistant to determine their eligibility to participate, their level of cerumen impaction, and their hearing perception. Participants with hearing aids wore them during the interview. The individual's medical record was reviewed to ascertain eligibility, demographic, behavioral, medication, and treatment data. Cerumen impaction was determined through otoscopic examination and defined as 100% occlusion of the tympanic membrane due to wax obstruction. Descriptive features concerning the level of impaction were coded according to pre-established categories.[4] Mental status was assessed using the 10 item Mental Status Questionnaire[17] and the number of errors were recorded. Speech discrimination, a test for conversational hearing ability, was determined by the percentage of correct responses to a standard list of 10 phonetically balanced monosyllabic words.[18] The data collection measures were chosen to balance obtaining the most relevant information while limiting the burden on the resident.

The audiometry was conducted according to a standardized protocol using a Beltone Model D portable pure-tone audiometer. This particular model has been tested and used as the "gold standard" in research conducted in field settings. It permits objective, numerical calibrations of hearing ability to be recorded for comparative purposes.[19,20] The audiometer was calibrated to American National Standards Institute specifications immediately prior to use in the field.

The audiometer produces and measures tones of varying frequency and intensity. The frequency is measured in Hertz (Hz) or cycles per second and is perceived as pitch. Human hearing ranges from approximately 20 to 20,000 Hz. Intensity is measured in decibels (dB) and is perceived as loudness. Measurements are made by air conduction where the sound is introduced through a headset into the ear. Threshold is the faintest sound that an average listener can just hear in the quiet. Pure tone thresholds (PTT) were measured at the frequencies found in the speech range of 500, 1000, 2000, and 4000 Hz using the standard 10-down 5-up bracketing technique. The participants' thresholds were recorded for each frequency and ear. Thresholds were interpreted as normal (0 to 25 dB), mild hearing loss (26 to 40 dB), moderate (41 to 55 dB), moderately severe (56 to 70 dB), or profound (>70 dB).[21] Duplicate assessments were incorporated in the testing as a reliability check on the residents' responses. Also, the mean three-frequency pure-tone average (500, 1000, and 2000 Hz) in the participants better ear was calculated. People with pure-tone averages in excess of 40 dB are considered to be hearing impaired.

A charge nurse in each facility was interviewed using a semi-structured questionnaire to obtain information about the factors that promote or impede the detection and treatment of cerumen impaction in the nursing home. An administrative representative shared data on the characteristics of the nursing home, which were validated by state data.[22]

RESULTS

Prevalence of Cerumen Impaction

Impacted cerumen was observed in 26 out of the 104 nursing home residents for a prevalence rate of 25%. Of the 104 residents, 21 had cerumen unilaterally (20%), and five had both ears occluded (4.8%). Moreover, an additional 18 (23%) of the 78 people without impaction had a strong potential to develop the condition; that is, at the time of the study the cerumen in the canals was greater than 75% but less than the criteria of 100% necessary to be categorized as impaction. Taken together, 42% of the residents had severe to complete cerumen impaction.

Characteristics

Personal characteristics mentioned in the literature as being associated with impacted cerumen were compared between those with and without cerumen impaction. Characteristics are reported using mean values (+/- SD) or percentages where applicable (Table 16-1). The only notable difference between the two groups occurred with speech discrimination in which those with impacted cerumen scored significantly worse (t test, p=.05, t=2.0).

Prevalence of Hearing Impairment

The majority of the nursing home residents were hearing impaired. Only a minority (4%) had hearing levels within normal limits while the majority (55%) were moderately to profoundly hearing impaired. If those with mild hearing loss are included, the overall prevalence rate of residents with any hearing loss was 96%.

The level of hearing ability was compared among the residents with and without impacted cerumen. The mean three frequency pure-tone average in the better ear was 44.2 dB with a range of 18 dB to 77 dB (SD 12). Although the mean level at 47 dB was higher in impacted residents than the 43 dB level in non-impacted residents, the difference was not statistically significant.

TABLE 16-1

Characteristics of Cerumen Impacted and Non-Impacted Residents

	RESIDENTS					
	Total		**Impacted**		**Non-impacted**	
Characteristics	N	(%)	N	(%)	N	(%)
Female	83	(80)	21	(81)	62	(79)
Wore hearing aid	16	(15)	5	(19)	11	(14)
	N	(SD)	N	(SD)	N	(SD)
Mean age	84	(7.6)	85.3	(6.9)	83.4	(7.9)
Mean number of diagnoses	4.8	(2.4)	5.3	(2.5)	4.7	(2.3)
Mean number of drugs	5	(2.6)	5.7	(3.1)	4.6	(2.4)
Mean length of stay in months	28	(3.5)	28.1	(5.3)	28.5	(4.2)
Speech discrimination	72	(26)	63	(28)	75	(25)*

Total number of residents=104; total number impacted=26, total number nonimpacted=78.
*Independent sample t-test, p=.05; t(2.0), F-ratio(1.34).

POST-TEST

The second hearing evaluation scheduled to be performed after the cerumen removal was unable to be conducted because of two major problems:

- There was difficulty in obtaining the necessary physicians' orders that would permit nursing home nurses to administer cerumenolytic ear drops.
- Of those who did receive treatment, the vast majority of residents' ears remained impacted.

Obtaining an order for cerumen removal and or locating the physician was difficult at times. This difficulty frequently meant that the patient's condition continued. Of the 17 residents who received treatment for cerumen impaction, 12 remained 100% impacted, four were greater than 75% impacted, and one was greater than 50% impacted.

CERUMEN IMPACTION FACTORS

The key charge nurse in each nursing home was interviewed using a combination of structured questions, probes, and open-ended opportunities to discern the factors affecting the assessment and treatment of cerumen impaction. The nurses (N=8) were all female, employed full-time, primarily were LPNs (62%), and were on average 40 years old. They had worked 14 years in long-term care, and none had any additional educational preparation in gerontological nursing. They primarily were supervisors (100%), with the majority administering medications (75%) and only a minority providing direct care (25%). The major obstacles to detecting cerumen impaction that they reported are listed in Table 16-2; the factors that facilitate detection are outlined in Table 16-3.

TABLE 16-2

Nurse Impressions of Impediments to Detecting Cerumen Impaction*

RESPONSE	*N*	(%)
Must obtain physician order	6	(75)
Low priority, competing demands	5	(63)
Knowledge deficit about detection	4	(50)
Lack of awareness about impaction	4	(50)
Unfamiliar with use of otoscope	4	(50)
Difficult and time-consuming to remove	3	(38)
Residents not competent to inform staff	1	(13)

**N*=8; nurses could have more than one response.

The typical nursing home in this study was for-profit (75%), part of a chain (62%), had 99 licensed beds, a 99% occupancy rate, and was in operation for 43 years. The nursing homes represented all traditional levels of skilled care and the majority of their residents (73%) were on Medicaid. None of the homes employed or contracted the services of a gerontological nurse practitioner. They all were served by private physicians (100%) and had their own medical director (100%). One home had both a gerontological clinical nurse specialist and a RN certified by the ANA in gerontological nursing. This home had no problems with cerumen impaction. Compared to the other nursing homes in the sample, the facility with the gerontological nurses was the newest (5 years old). It was of private non-profit ownership, fully occupied (100%), slightly smaller (82 beds), but with more level II (100%) and Medicaid residents (90%) than the other homes.

Discussion

Although one quarter of the nursing home residents were found to have impacted cerumen, this may be a conservative finding. One of the nursing homes uniquely differed from the others because no residents had cerumen impaction. This was the only home that employed two nurses who had specialty preparation in gerontological nursing. Interestingly, if that home had been excluded, the impaction rate would have been 34%, supporting prior findings in the community[4] and hospital setting.[5]

Surprisingly, many of the characteristics alluded to in the literature as being associated with greater potential for cerumen impaction were not statistically significant in this study. In particular, it is frequently reported that being older, male, wearing a hearing aid, and in frail health predisposes an elder to increased cerumen production. These variables did not emerge as important features perhaps due to the small number of residents in this sample who wore hearing aids (15%) or were men (20%). Of interest would be a replication study in a predominantly male institutionalized population.

In order to gain entry into multiple nursing homes and reduce concerns about liability, it was necessary to rely on the nursing home staff to coordinate the residents' treatment for cerumen impaction. Initially, 3 months were allowed for this process; however, treatment could not be effectively rendered within a 6-month period even with weekly telephone contacts with the nursing homes.

TABLE 16-3

Nurse Impressions of Factors that Promote the Detection/Treatment of Cerumen Impaction*

RESPONSE	*N*	(%)
Train charge nurse in methods	8	(100)
Institute an ear check reminder schedule	8	(100)
Conduct monthly ear checks	7	(88)
Develop a standardized treatment protocol	6	(75)
Document impaction in the record	5	(63)
Document impaction in the care plan	5	(63)
Make ear checks part of the charge or treatment nurse's role	3	(38)
Increased physician responsiveness	3	(38)
Encourage residents to inform staff	1	(13)

**N*=8; nurses could have more than one response.

It is apparent that practice and policy conflicts exist in long-term care. Physicians are reluctant to personally perform ear irrigations, and the nurses reported that they were unable to independently administer cerumenolytic ear drops, use an otoscope, or perform ear irrigations. Otologic examination and treatment for cerumen impaction has become part of professional nursing practice.[23] The continued use of licensed practical nurses, untrained in gerontological nursing, adds to the difficulty of being unskilled in treatment protocols.

FINDINGS

The findings from this study portray a striking difference in clinical practice between the nursing home with gerontological nurses and the other facilities. Unintentionally, this study documented objective evidence that access to physician services for cerumen impaction is a problem. Otoscopic inspection for cerumen impaction and audiometric testing for presbycusis are two of the 10 screening programs recommended for the elderly based upon the research literature, findings of the U.S. Preventive Services Task Force, and the consensus of experts in geriatrics.[24] Cerumen impaction did not exist in the home where the gerontological clinical nurse specialist performed otoscopic examinations and ear irrigations. In the other homes, residents who received treatment remained impacted, even after cerumenolytic ear drops were administered. One possible explanation for this phenomenon may be that the four or five ear drops typically administered daily for 2 to 4 days was inadequate to dissolve hard, impacted cerumen. More intensive treatment with the ear drops or an ear irrigation to complement the ear drops probably would have been effective.

TABLE 16-4

Practice Recommendations Related to Cerumen Impaction

- Use a gerontological clinical nurse specialist/practitioner in the nursing home.
- Conduct staff development programs on hearing impairment and cerumen impaction.
- Sensitize staff to the following:
  - Ambient room noise
  - Hearing aid use
  - Speech discrimination problems vs. confusion
- Check for cerumen impaction on admission and then monthly.
- Obtain an otoscope and train charge/treatment nurse in its use.
- Evaluate present treatment practices.
- Develop a standard protocol for cerumen impaction prevention and treatment.

Additional findings document that physician and professional nursing services to treat cerumen impaction are lacking. Nursing home residents with impaired hearing experience a reduced quality of life from missed opportunities for socialization and nutrition when announcements are not heard.[2] Nursing homes come under the Americans with Disabilities Act[25] and are required to provide reasonable accommodations for those with impaired hearing. Training the staff to detect and treat cerumen impaction and to be more aware of measures to improve communication with hearing impaired residents is a reasonable expectation.

GERONTOLOGICAL NURSING IMPLICATIONS

This study revealed that the foremost need is to teach nursing home nurses the methods of cerumen detection and treatment. Hiring a geriatric clinical nurse specialist or nurse practitioner as a consultant to teach, demonstrate, and establish the relevant policies and treatment protocol is one possibility. Another possibility is to use the services of an audiologist since cerumen detection and removal is within the audiologist's scope of practice.[26,27]

The advocacy role of the registered nurse becomes apparent in this clinical situation. The client becomes the victim of negligence; the nurse becomes the observer of a situation that demands/needs an immediate professional response. As an advocate, the nurse has the opportunity to enlighten/discuss this with the administrator(s), the client, and the client's family. In-service educational programs will assist the staff to better understand conductive hearing loss, its reversible condition, and the positive results when appropriate intervention is effective.

On admission, the nurse should elicit a detailed history of any damage or surgery to the internal ear and refer those with a likelihood of non-intact eardrum(s) to a health care provider experienced in dry removal techniques. When treating cerumen impaction, the nurse should avoid procedures that infuse solutions using high pressure techniques because that could rupture an eardrum and lead to infection.[28] Aural irrigating syringes should be used at an angle pointing above or below the eardrum, not directly at it.

Given the high rate of hearing impairment among nursing home residents, staff should generally treat everyone as having an impairment. Measures to improve communication within nursing homes have been published.[2,29,30] Consultant geriatric nurse specialists and/or audiologists could conduct staff education programs to help the nursing homes create more sensitive environments for the hearing impaired. Practice recommendations (Table 16-4) are made considering these constraints.

Although it was disappointing that a post-cerumen hearing evaluation could not be conducted,[31] an institutional study started after this research did find that almost 50% of the 40 hearing impaired patients with cerumen impaction had their hearing restored after removal of the cerumen. This supports prior findings in which removing cerumen impaction from a hospitalized elderly sample resulted in improved hearing scores for 75% of the ears.[5] These two studies lend credence to the contention that removing impacted cerumen can improve older adults' hearing. Given the prevalence of hearing loss and cerumen impaction among the elderly, greater attention to the detection and removal of impacted cerumen is warranted.

REFERENCES

1. Flugrath J, Lutz D, Hamdy R. Hearing impairment and cerumen impaction in older patients. *J Tenn Med Assoc.* 1993;86(7):301-302.
2. Mahoney D. Hearing loss among nursing home residents: perceptions and realities. *Clin Nurs Res.* 1992;1(4):317-332.
3. Rubin I, Dwyer F. Management of the geriatric population. In Rubin I, Crocker A eds. *Developmental Disabilities.* Philadelphia, PA: Lea and Febiger; 1989:128-139.
4. Mahoney D. One simple solution to hearing impairment. *Geriatr Nurs.* 1987;8(5):242-245.
5. Lewis-Cullinan C, Janken J. Effect of cerumen removal on the hearing ability of geriatric patients. *J Adv Nurs.* 1990;15:594-600.
6. American Nurses Association. *Scope and Standards of Gerontological Nursing Practice.* Washington, D.C.: American Nurses Foundation Publishing; 1995.
7. Ciurlia-Guy E, Cashman M, Lewsen B. Identifying hearing loss and hearing handicap among chronic care elderly people. *Gerontologist.* 1993;33(5):644-649.
8. Glass L. Rehabilitation for deaf and hearing impaired elderly. In Brody S, Ruff G eds. *Aging and Rehabilitation.* New York: Springer; 1986.
9. Weinstein B, Amstel L. Hearing loss and senile dementia in the institutionalized elderly. *Clin Gerontol.* 1986;4(3):3-15.
10. Humphrey C. Some characteristics of the hearing impaired elderly who do not present themselves for rehabilitation. *British Journal of Audiology.* 1981;15(25):3-6.
11. National Institute on Aging. *Hearing and the Elderly.* (Publication No. 1983-416-520). Washington, D.C.: U.S. Government Printing Office; 1983.
12. Ebersole P, Hess P. *Toward Healthy Aging* (4th ed.) St. Louis: C.V. Mosby; 1994.
13. Ham R. *Primary Care Geriatrics.* Boston: John Wright; 1983.
14. Sanders D. *Aural Rehabilitation.* Englewood Cliffs, N.J.: Prentice-Hall; 1971.
15. Bess F, Lichtenstein M, Logan S, Burger C, Nelson E. Hearing impairment as a determinant of function in the elderly. *J Am Geriatr Soc.* 1989;37:123-128.
16. Public Health Service. *Healthy People 2000: National Health Promotion and Disease Prevention Objectives. DHHS (PHS) 91-50212.* Washington, D.C.: U.S. Department of Health and Human Services; 1991.
17. Kahn R, Goldfarb A, Pollack M, Peck A. Brief objective measures for the determination of mental status in the aged. *Am J Psychiatry.* 1960;117:326-328.
18. Butler PM. Physical appraisal of the ear and hearing. In: Sana J, Judge R eds. *Physical Appraisal Methods in Nursing Practice.* Boston: Little, Brown, and Co; 1975.
19. Corbin S, Reed M, Nobbs H, Eastwood K, Eastwood M. Hearing assessment in homes for the aged: a comparison of audiometric and self-report methods. *J Am Geriatr Soc.* 1984;32(5):396-400.

20. Ohta R, Carlin M, Harmon B. Auditory acuity and performance on the mental status questionnaire in the elderly. *J Am Geriatr Soc.* 1981;29(10):476-478.
21. Weinstein B. Validity of a screening protocol for identifying elderly people with hearing problems. *American Speech-Language Hearing Association (ASHA).* 1986;28(5):41-45.
22. Goldman D, Veisbergs B, eds. *Guide to nursing and rest homes in Massachusetts, 1990/91* (13th ed.). Boston: Women's Educational and Industrial Union and Massachusetts Department of Public Health; 1990.
23. Burke M, Walsh M. *Gerontologic Nursing: Care of the Frail Elderly.* St. Louis: Mosby-Year Book; 1992.
24. Beers M. Screening recommendations for the elderly. *Am J Public Health.* 1991;81(9):1131-1140.
25. Americans with Disabilities Act. ADA 28 Code of Federal Regulations. *Federal Register.* 1991; part 36:35544.
26. American Speech-Language-Hearing Association. External auditory canal examination and cerumen management. *ASHA.* 1992; Supplement (7):22-24.
27. Ballachanda B, Peers C. Cerumen management: instruments and procedures. *ASHA.* 1992;34(2):43-46.
28. Zikk D, Rapoport Y, Himelfarb M. Invasive external otitis after removal of impacted cerumen by irrigation. *N Engl J Med.* 1991;325(13):969-970.
29. Brunner M. Managing hearing loss in the nursing home. *SHHH (Self-help for the hard of hearing).* 1988;9(5):12-15.
30. Voeks S, Gallagher C, Langer E, Drinka P. Hearing loss in the nursing home: an institutional issue. *J Am Geriatr Soc.* 1990;38:141-145.
31. Morley JE, Kahl MJ, Peak M. Hearing impairment in the nursing home. *Gerontologist.* 1990;30:296A.

Chapter 17

Tuberculosis Comeback: Impact on the Elderly

Evelyn Lancaster, RN, BSN, PHN

OVERVIEW

Most of today's elderly are at risk for having been infected with tuberculosis (TB) in childhood or as young adults and are a large reservoir for active disease in the future. This article reviews the basic TB epidemiology, transmission, pathogenesis, infectiousness, and treatment of infection and disease. The implications of TB in the elderly are discussed in terms of management and follow-up of elderly who are infected with TB or have active TB disease.

INTRODUCTION

Tuberculosis (TB) in the United States had been declining by approximately 5% per year until 1985. From 1985 to 1991, the number of TB cases increased by 18%.[1] In 1993, the TB case rate per 100,000 population in the United States was 9.8; however, the case rate that year for those older than 65 years of age was 17.8.[2] A 1987 study revealed that the elderly accounted for 27% of the cases reported in the United States that year, which represented 12% of the total population.[3] What meaning does this have for health care providers who serve the elderly? It means the likelihood of one of your patients having TB is increasing. Most of the cases reported annually arise from people who were infected many years ago, and alarmingly TB case fatality rates increase with increasing age.[1]

To properly screen and treat elderly patients for TB, one needs to understand the epidemiology, transmission, pathogenesis, infectiousness, and treatment of TB. These topics and current recommendations for the prevention, control, and surveillance for TB will be discussed.

EPIDEMIOLOGY: GROUPS WITH A HIGH INCIDENCE OF TUBERCULOSIS

TB crosses all levels of our society, but is not evenly distributed. Each region of the country may have a slightly different profile of its local TB patient caseload. Nationally, however, the groups that have a high prevalence of TB[4] include the following:

- Close contacts to an infectious case
- Foreign born people from areas where TB is common (eg, Asia, Africa, Latin America)
- Medically underserved, low-income populations
- The elderly
- Residents of long-term care facilities, such as correctional institutions and nursing homes
- Injecting drug users
- Locally identified high-prevalence groups (migrant workers, homeless, workers with occupational exposure).

TRANSMISSION AND PATHOGENESIS

TB is generally spread via airborne routes. The TB organisms are carried in particles suspended in the air and are referred to as "droplet nuclei." These droplet nuclei are produced when a person coughs, sneezes, laughs, speaks, or sings. Large particles that are produced fall out of air circulation and do not cause infection. It is the small particles (droplet nuclei), 1 to 5 μm in size, which stay suspended in the air that can cause infection. These droplet nuclei can become distributed throughout a room or building by normal air currents. A susceptible person who inhales the droplet nuclei containing TB organisms may become infected.

TB organisms that land on the mucociliary blanket of the respiratory tree or intact mucosa rarely invade tissue to result in infection. If droplet nuclei contaminated with TB organisms are inhaled and reach the alveoli, infection can occur. The organisms are engulfed by macrophages. A systemic infection occurs when the organisms, engulfed by macrophages, are spread via the lymph and blood streams. This systemic infection is usually silent; that is, the person is not ill or symptomatic. It takes the body 2 to 10 weeks to mount an immune response to limit further spread of the TB organisms and control the infection.[5] Most people (90%) who are infected with TB never progress from infection to active disease.[6] However, 10% of people infected with TB will progress to active disease sometime later in their life. The risk of progressing to active disease is much greater for those individuals who are also infected with the HIV virus.[7] Additionally, as a person ages, his or her immune system becomes less effective; therefore the elderly, who were infected in childhood, may break down with active TB as their immune systems become suppressed. Many elderly were infected in childhood when TB was prevalent in the United States and worldwide.

There are two stages in the TB process. The first stage is TB infection, the second stage is TB disease. Table 17-1 compares these two stages. The similarities are that in both stages the person has the TB organisms in his or her body, is considered infected, and usually has a positive tuberculin skin test. The differences are that a person who is infected only usually has a normal chest X-ray, sputum smears and/or cultures for TB are negative, has no symptoms, is not infectious, and is not considered a "case" of TB but rather infected (a tuberculin reactor). A person who has active pulmonary TB disease usually has an abnormal chest X-ray; sputum or bronchoscopy specimens are usually positive for AFB (acid fast bacillus) smear and/or culture; have pulmonary symptoms of cough, sputum production, and occasionally hemoptysis or chest pain; has generalized symptoms of fever, night sweats, and weight loss; is frequently considered infectious before the patient starts responding to treatment; and is considered a case of TB disease.

TABLE 17-1

Usual Features Distinguishing Tuberculosis Infection from Pulmonary Tuberculosis Disease

FEATURES	INFECTION	DISEASE
Similarities		
Tuberculosis organisms present in the body	Yes	Yes
Infected with tuberculosis	Yes	Yes
Tuberculin skin test usually positive	Yes	Yes
Differences		
Chest x-ray	Usually normal	Usually abnormal
Specimens for acid fast bacilli (AFB) smears and/or cultures	Negative	Usually positive
Symptoms	None	Cough, sputum, night sweats, weight loss, fever
Infectious	No	Often, before treatment
A "case" of tuberculosis	No	Yes

Adapted from table printed in CDC. *Tuberculosis Medical Orientation Course*. 3rd ed. September 1989.

The questions exist: who is infectious, and how infectious are they? A person is considered infectious if he or she is capable of transmitting TB germs. Generally, only people with active pulmonary or laryngeal TB present the possibility of being infectious around the time of diagnosis. Many providers confuse TB infection and TB disease when assessing infectiousness and deciding on treatment regimens.

INFECTION

People with a positive tuberculin skin test but who do not have active disease are not considered infectious.[5] They are diagnosed with TB infection. However, if their TB infection has not been adequately treated, they are at risk for the rest of their lives to become ill with active disease.

DISEASE

People who do have active disease may or may not be infectious. There are many factors that determine whether a person may be infectious or not.

Non-pulmonary TB. Patients with non-pulmonary TB are usually not considered infectious. This form of TB may or may not be treated.

Pulmonary TB. There are many factors that influence infectiousness of pulmonary and laryngeal TB. These factors can be grouped into three basic categories:

1. Clinical features of the case
2. Environment
3. Contact's exposure information.

Each case must be looked at individually and all factors assessed to evaluate how infectious they may have been and the likelihood of transmission for each setting. This information helps to determine the extent of contact (exposure) investigation that is pursued after diagnosis.[3]

TREATMENT OF TB: INFECTION AND DISEASE

The recommendations for treatment of infection and of disease are usually simple and straightforward. The guidelines discussed below are for the usual simple situations. If drug resistance or drug intolerance is encountered, consult with your local Health Department TB Program.

INFECTION

Treatment for TB infection is usually referred to as preventive therapy or chemoprophylaxis. The recommendation is for isoniazid (INH) to be given for 6 to 12 months. The usual adult dose is 300 mg daily. If the person is 35 years of age or older, preventive therapy is usually only offered if the person has medical conditions that increase his or her risk of breaking down with disease; however, all people with a positive Mantoux tuberculin skin test should be evaluated carefully to see if they are candidates for preventive therapy.[8]

DISEASE

There are two main treatment regimens (Table 17-2) recommended in conjunction with some basic guidelines:

- Two or more anti-TB drugs, to which the organism is susceptible, are given to treat active disease (note: only one drug, INH, is used for infection).
- In general, regimens adequate to treat pulmonary TB in adults are adequate to treat children and non-pulmonary TB.
- Be aware of drug resistance trends in your area, and when initiating treatment, include additional TB drugs to the treatment regimen selected to cover for drug resistance.

Both the 6-month and the 9-month regimens have two phases: the initial and the continuation. The 6-month regimen includes INH, rifampin (RIF), pyrazinamide (PZA), and ethambutol or streptomycin (to cover for drug resistance) for at least 2 months, followed by another 4 months of just INH and RIF. Ethambutol or streptomycin should be continued until drug susceptibility results are known. If drug resistance is found, it takes longer than 3 months for the patient to convert his or her sputum to culture negative, or patient noncompliance develops, the regimen needs to be re-evaluated and lengthened or changed appropriately. The 9-month regimen is the same as the 6-month except that PZA is not included among the drugs used so the continuation phase is lengthened from 4 months to 7 months.

Outbreaks of multidrug-resistant TB have been reported in recent years.[1,9] The outbreaks identified nosocomial transmission not only to HIV-infected patients, but also to the health care workers. There were many factors that contributed to the nosocomial and community outbreaks. These factors delayed recognition of active TB disease inadequate infection control and non-recognition of drug resistance. Patients infected with HIV and TB may not present for care with symptoms typically associated with pulmonary TB. Failure to suspect and cover for drug resistance (pending sensitivity results) can result in additional problems:

- Inducing further drug resistance for the patient.
- Increasing transmission of the resistant organism due to prolonged periods of infectiousness. Management of infected contacts is problematic because INH is usually one of the drugs to which the organism is resistant.

TABLE 17-2

Disease Treatment: Basic Drug Regimens*

6-Month Protocol*

Initial Phase: INH+RIF+PZA+EMB** for 2 months***
Continuation Phase: INH+RIF for 4 months

9-Month Protocol*

Initial Phase: INH+RIF+EMB** pending sensitivities
Continuation Phase: INH+RIF to complete 9 months

INH=isoniazid, RIF=rifampin, PZA=pyrazinamide, EMB=ethambutol.
* Regimens may need to be changed as a result of:
1. Sputum did not convert to culture negative within 3 months of starting treatment
2. Patient noncompliance
3. Drug resistance
4. Drug intolerance.

** Ethambutol (EMB) or Streptomycin to cover for drug resistance until susceptibility results are known.
*** For the 6-month protocol: INH, RIF, and PZA must be given for at least the first 2 months of therapy. Most clinicians will keep patients on all four drugs until susceptibility results are known, even if it is longer than 2 months. If the initial phase is longer than 2 months, the continuation phase may be shortened so that the total length of therapy is 6 months.

Health care providers should consult with their local Public Health TB Control Program when patients have drug-resistant TB, do not adhere to treatment protocols, or develop intolerance to the drugs. Additionally, the Centers for Disease Control and Prevention (CDC) recommends the following centers for expert consultation on the management of drug-resistant TB:

- National Jewish Center for Immunology and Respiratory Medicine
- Infectious Disease Consultation Service, 303-389-1279
- Model TB Centers funded by CDC:

New Jersey, 201-982-3270
New York, 212-491-8403
San Francisco, 415-502-4700

General information on TB and its management may be obtained by calling the National TB Center (funded by CDC), New Jersey Medical School at 1-800-4TB-DOCS (482-3627) Monday through Friday 9 am-5 pm EST. You may call CDC for information on current TB policies at 404-639-3311.

The elderly may have an atypical presentation of symptoms because the immune system weakens with increased age and some of the clinical symptoms, such as fever, may be slow to appear. Additionally, because of immune suppression, elderly who are infected may have a false negative Mantoux TB skin test due to anergy or waned sensitivity. Many elderly have other pulmonary problems, and because TB symptoms are not unique, patients are not screened for TB or have been improperly screened.[10] A TB test should be performed on initial examination. Unnecessary delays in diagnosis can result in death.[11] TB should be considered in any patient who has a persistent cough or other general symptoms of weight loss, fever, anorexia, and night sweats.[3,8]

NON-INSTITUTIONALIZED ELDERLY

An initial history and physical should include questions about past exposure to TB as well as a Mantoux tuberculin skin test, using the "two-step" method if indicated, to establish a baseline.[5] Having a TB history and skin test data will help identify which patients have a "high index of suspicion for active TB" in case the patient develops symptoms consistent with active TB in the future. Patients known to be infected with TB must have this documented on their care plan. In the event they progress to active disease, it can be diagnosed early.

The elderly were raised in a time when there was no cure for TB; those diagnosed with TB were ostracized, others were sent away to TB Sanitoria, and most died from their illness. Today's elderly may feel TB is a death sentence, and the provider should carefully explain TB is now treatable and curable provided medication is taken as directed.

Advise the patient that TB is a reportable disease, and that there is a need to report the diagnosis to the Health Department. Alert the patient that a Public Health Nurse may be contacting him or her and will be a part of the medical team during treatment for TB. Many areas have Public Health Nurses who contact patients to assess their understanding of TB, conduct a follow-up of exposed people, and assist in monitoring the TB care. Providers may call the local Public Health TB Control Program to familiarize themselves with the services offered by the program. Directly observed therapy (DOT) is a service many programs offer. DOT means a health care worker watches the patient ingest each dose of TB medication. Candidates for DOT are patients who have difficulty remembering to take their medication, who have drug-resistant TB, who have alcohol or other drug use problems, or who have displayed non-adherence patterns to medical recommendations in the past. Every dose of medication is important to achieve a cure.

ELDERLY IN LONG-TERM CARE SETTINGS

Elderly who live in nursing homes are at greater risk for TB than elderly people who live at home in the community. A CDC-sponsored study from 29 states indicated that the incidence of TB among nursing home residents was 39.2 cases of active TB per 100,000 population compared to 21.5 cases per 100,000 among elderly who lived in the community. This fact is not surprising, as many of our elderly were infected in childhood and are placed in nursing homes at a time when their immunity is compromised due to their failing health. Preliminary TB data indicate that 6% of cases reported in 1994 resided in long-term care facilities at the time of diagnosis.[12] The CDC provides guidelines for control of TB in long-term care facilities.[3] The guidelines are divided into *four* categories: surveillance, containment, assessment, and education, which are summarized below.

SURVEILLANCE

The facility should have a policy and procedure for screening all residents and staff for TB infection. Residents should be screened on admission, as well as when any exposure to TB occurs. Staff should be screened on hire and periodically thereafter (check with your local TB control program for recommendations in your area). The Mantoux (intradermal) tuberculin skin test should be used to identify infected people. The "two-step" method should be used when indicated. The multiple puncture devices are not recommended. Because false-negative skin test reactions can occur, staff or residents who have symptoms of active TB should have a complete work up to rule out active TB regardless of the skin test reaction size.

The local or state health department should be notified when TB is suspected or confirmed among residents or staff. Reporting requirements vary by state law and local requirements. The TB program receiving reports should be able to assist with recommendations regarding appropriate follow-up.

CONTAINMENT

People with suspected or confirmed infectious TB should be placed under appropriate isolation until they have become non-infectious to prevent the spread of infection. If the following conditions are met, the suspected case may remain in his or her usual environment:

- Treatment with adequate chemotherapy is initiated promptly.
- Recent and current contacts are evaluated and placed on appropriate therapy.
- New contacts can be prevented until the patient has become non-infectious.

Treatment recommendations published by the American Thoracic Society and the CDC should be followed. Staff should not only dispense but also observe that the TB medication is in fact ingested by the patient.

An exposure usually occurs when a resident or staff member develops active disease. All too often the disease is not diagnosed until after the person has become infectious, requiring contact follow-up to be initiated. When an exposure occurs, consult the CDC guidelines and your local health department TB program for consultation regarding which contacts should be examined.

Recommendations for administration of preventive therapy should be followed. People who refuse or are unable to complete a recommended course of preventive therapy should be reminded of the symptoms of active TB and be advised to seek medical attention promptly should those symptoms develop.

Assessment

Each facility should keep records of their TB surveillance data, compliance with preventive therapy, and results of contact follow-up activities. The guidelines published by CDC have a sample record-keeping system in the Appendix.[3]

Education

Education is an integral part of the whole program. Staff need to be knowledgeable in order to be alert to the signs and symptoms of TB. They also need knowledge about TB transmission and pathogenesis to understand the importance of following appropriate infection control procedures and to cooperate with surveillance activities. Residents and patients need to understand current TB treatment recommendations and how successful they are today if patients are compliant. As health care providers, we need to remember that each of us has our own knowledge base about TB and those beliefs are going to influence our behavior. The education of both staff and patients should begin with an assessment of their knowledge about TB so that old, erroneous beliefs can be corrected and current knowledge imparted. Only then will we be able to improve understanding and cooperation to ensure success in our TB control efforts.

GERONTOLOGICAL NURSING IMPLICATIONS

The epidemic proportions surrounding TB and the potential risk of immunocompromise with the elderly clearly indicate the importance of remembering that of the 80% of the elderly who become infected with TB, 95% live in the community.[13]

Gerontological nurses have a challenge to make certain that their patients discharged from acute care facilities have access to the resources needed in the community and that appropriate follow-up will be undertaken by home health nurses as well as the health department. In addition to what has been discussed previously, nurses working in the home have an additional opportunity to work with families. The family may be experiencing fear and emotional discomfort associated with hearsay, myth, and misinformation. Alleviating fears about the spread of infection, death and dying, and the course of treatment and follow-up is easily accomplished by the gerontological nurse. Inviting questions each visit will not only promote trust but also positively impact upon treatment. Assessment of contacts and follow through with preventive therapy, as well as developing an individualized educational plan for each person or family member, will assure that continuity of care is maintained.

The resurgence of TB in the United States and the current health care focus on prevention of disease and promotion of health requires a priority effort to once again eliminate this life-threatening disease. TB, once considered eliminated, is a challenge for all health care providers. Elderly people are at high risk for this disease. They must be screened and preventive therapy initiated so that they can be restored to optimal health.

REFERENCES

1. American Thoracic Society, CDC. Control of tuberculosis in the United States. *Am Rev Respir Dis.* 1992;146(6):1623-1633.
2. CDC. *Reported TB in the United States.* 1993.
3. CDC. Prevention and control of tuberculosis in facilities providing long-term care to the elderly. *MMWR* 1990;39/No.RR-10.
4. CDC. *TB Care Guide: Highlights from Core Curriculum on TB.* 1994.
5. American Thoracic Society, CDC. Diagnostic standards and classification of TB. *Am Rev Respir Dis.* 1990;142:725-735.
6. American Thoracic Society, CDC. Diagnostic standards and classification of TB and other mycobacterial diseases. *Am Rev Respir Dis.* 1981;123:343-355.
7. CDC. TB and human immunodeficiency virus infection: recommendations of the Advisory Committee for the Elimination of TB (ACET). *MMWR.* 1989; 38:236-238,243-250.
8. American Thoracic Society, CDC. Treatment of TB and TB infection in adults and children. *Am Rev Respir Dis.* 1994;149:1359-1374.
9. CDC. Guidelines for preventing the transmission of tuberculosis in health-case settings, with special focus on HIV-related issues. *MMWR.* 1990;39(no.RR-17):1-26.
10. Price L, Rutala W. Tuberculosis screening in the long-term care setting. *Infection Control.* 1987;8(9):353-356.
11. Grennen C, Muder R, Muraca P. Occult endemic tuberculosis in a chronic care facility. *Infection Control Hosp Epidemiol.* 1988;9(12):548-552.
12. CDC. Tuberculosis morbidity—United States, 1994. *MMWR.* 1995;44/No.20.
13. Walsh K. Guidelines for the prevention and control of tuberculosis in the elderly. *Nurse Practitioner.* 1994;19(11):79-84.

Chapter 18

Immunizing Older Adults

Diane M. Holt, RN, MS, CS, GNP

OVERVIEW

Of the 19 national health objectives for the year 2000 that target vaccination and infectious diseases, 10 are related to vaccination of adults (Table 18-1). Although similar goals were set in the previous decade, immunization levels remain very low and substantial morbidity and mortality from preventable diseases persist in our nation's older adult population. As the proportion of those at greatest risk for adverse complications from influenza and pneumococcal disease increases with our aging population, and with rising concerns about health care financing, major changes in clinical practice are required. Increasing provider and patient awareness about the safety and effectiveness of vaccines is important, but is not sufficient to boost vaccine usage to recommended levels. Recommendation by a health care provider significantly affects whether a person will be immunized, and creative organizational strategies may help remove barriers to immunization. This chapter discusses vaccine recommendations, side effects, and efficacy; in addition, strategies and nursing implications for improving immunization levels in older people are examined.

INTRODUCTION

Nursing's active role in immunization programs in the United States has helped to dramatically reduce the occurrence of many childhood infectious diseases and to achieve the 90% objective for children's immunizations targeted by *Healthy People 2000*. In contrast, and in spite of the much heavier financial and social burden of disease, vaccines recommended for older adults are not widely used by health care providers. Experience with children's immunization programs and current research, however, suggest that nurses may be instrumental in reversing current trends of vaccine underutilization in the older adult population.

In their recent update on adult immunizations, the Advisory Committee on Immunization Practice (ACIP) strongly advised that all adults 65 years of age or older receive a single vaccination against pneumococcal pneumonia, an annual influenza vaccination, and a combined tetanus-diphtheria toxoid booster every 10 years after completion of a primary series.[1] Yet only about 20% of the older adult population are adequately immunized against pneumonia and influenza disease,[2] and 49% to 66% of older adults lack protective antitoxin levels against tetanus.[1] As a result, significant morbidity and mortality attributed to these vaccine-preventable diseases persist in the older adult population.

TABLE 18-1

Healthy People 2000 Objectives Related to Immunizing Older Adults

- Provide influenza and pneumococcal vaccines to at least 60% of the non-institutionalized chronically ill or older people.
- Reduce epidemic-related pneumococcal and influenza deaths and pneumonia-related days of restricted activity.
- Increase to 90% the proportion of primary care providers and public health departments that provide adult vaccines for tetanus and for influenza and pneumococcal disease.
- Increase to at least 85% the proportion of tertiary care hospital labs and to at least 50% the proportion of secondary care hospital and health maintenance organization labs possessing technologies for rapid viral diagnosis of influenza.
- Improve financing and delivery of adult immunizations so that virtually no individual has a financial barrier to receiving recommended vaccines.

Adapted from U.S. Public Health Service. *Healthy People 2000: National Health Promotion and Disease Prevention Objectives.* Washington, D.C.: U.S. Department of Health and Human Services, Public Health Service; 1991.

Although there are no accurate estimates of overall disease incidence, a conservative estimate is that 172,000 excess hospital admissions have occurred in moderate influenza outbreaks.[3] Additionally, nosocomial influenza contributes to prolonged hospital stays for the elderly. Pneumococcal pneumonia occurs more frequently as people age, with a two-fold increase among those older than 60.[3] Hospital admission rates for pneumococcal pneumonia and bacteremia are estimated at 40,000 to 120,000 per year.[1] Mortality from the two diseases is substantial and results not only from these specific disease states but also from exacerbations of underlying chronic illnesses. Influenza epidemics can account for 10,000 to 40,000 excess deaths per year, and an estimated 40,000 deaths occur annually from pneumococcal disease.[3] More than 90% of deaths attributed to influenza and pneumonia occur in people older than 65 years of age.

VACCINE RECOMMENDATIONS, SIDE EFFECTS, AND EFFICACY

TETANUS-DIPHTHERIA VACCINE

Tetanus-diphtheria (Td) vaccine is recommended every 10 years to maintain immunity in the older adult. If a primary series against diphtheria and tetanus was not completed in childhood, an adult should receive a series of three intramuscular doses of combined Td. Two doses should be at least 4 weeks apart, with the third dose administered 6 to 12 months after the second. Because 40% to 84% of those older than 60 lack protective levels of circulating antitoxin against diphtheria,[1] the combined Td preparation is preferred to tetanus toxoid.

In wound management, a Td booster within 10 years is adequate for clean or minor wounds; for all other wounds, a booster within the previous 5 years is recommended. In cases where immunization status is unknown or incomplete, tetanus immunoglobulin may be given concurrently with Td. The only contraindication to the use of Td is previous severe hypersensitivity or neurologic reaction following a dose. Mild local reactions of erythema and induration, with or without tenderness, are common. Following these guidelines, Td immunization is 95% to 100% effective against these two diseases.[1] Although the economic efficiency of increased efforts to improve tetanus vaccination levels has been challenged as a "questionable use of health care resources,"[4] private-sector payment and strategies that optimize Td vaccination at the time of routine medical appointments and through existing public health programs may provide for cost-effective Td vaccination.

Pneumococcal Vaccine

Pneumococcal vaccine consists of purified capsular polysaccharide antigens from 23 of the most prevalent or invasive pneumococcal types, responsible for 85% to 90% of bacteremic pneumococcal disease in the United States. Replacing a 14-valent vaccine in 1983, a 0.5-mL intramuscular dose of this 23-valent vaccine is given as a single, lifetime vaccination. Revaccination is generally not recommended except for those groups at highest risk of serious or fatal pneumococcal infection who have received the 23-valent vaccine at least 6 years previously or for those who have only received the 14-valent vaccine.

Vaccination is recommended for all adults older than 65 who are healthy or for immunocompetent adults with chronic illness, such as cardiovascular disease, pulmonary disease, diabetes mellitus, cirrhosis, alcoholism, or cerebrospinal fluid leaks. Immunocompromised adults who require immunization due to increased risk for pneumococcal disease or its complications include those with splenic dysfunction or anatomic asplenia, Hodgkin's disease, chronic renal failure, multiple myeloma, or conditions associated with immunosuppression such as organ transplants or HIV infection. About half of those vaccinated report mild local reactions of erythema and pain; fever and myalgia are reported by less than 1%. Pneumococcal vaccine can be administered at the same time as influenza vaccine, provided each is given at a separate site.

Assessing the clinical efficacy of pneumococcal vaccine, studies of young, healthy populations in South Africa and New Guinea with high prevalence for pneumococcal infection demonstrated an 80% to 90% reduction in disease rates.[5] Studies in older adult populations have been less consistent in demonstrating vaccine efficacy. Three case-control studies in the United States and a large, ongoing, prospective study in France have shown an overall protective efficacy of 60% to 70% in the immunocompetent elderly.[5-10] Two Veterans Administration case-control studies, however, demonstrated no protection against pneumococcal disease.[10,11] A relatively low incidence of pneumococcal infection and the inclusion of older, more immunocompromised patients in the groups studied may account for these findings. Cost-analysis studies by the U.S. Office of Technology indicate that pneumococcal vaccine, which is reimbursed by Medicare, improves the health of older adults at a reasonable cost.[9] Administering vaccines through public programs may in fact make them cost-effective.

Influenza Vaccine

Based on antigenic characteristics of disease-causing virus strains from the previous season, influenza vaccine is typically a trivalent preparation of three strains—generally two type A and one type B—expected to cause outbreaks during the upcoming influenza season. Administered annually via intramuscular injection, influenza vaccine is composed of inactivated or killed virus, which cannot cause disease. Local reactions of pain, erythema, and induration are common in about one-third of recipients. Fever, myalgia, and malaise occur infrequently for 1 to 2 days. Serious systemic reactions are rare; increased risk of Guillain-Barre syndrome has not been associated with the vaccine since the 1976 swine influenza vaccine.[1] The only contraindication to the vaccine is severe anaphylactic sensitivity to eggs, since vaccines contain a small amount of egg protein.

Influenza activity in the United States typically peaks in late December and early March, so the optimal time for immunizing those at risk is usually the period from mid-October through mid-November. Typical influenza illness is characterized by an abrupt onset of fever, myalgia, sore throat, and nonproductive cough and may be accompanied by severe malaise. Primary influenza pneumonia and secondary bacterial pneumonia may cause more severe illness, especially among older adults. Older adults considered to be at risk for influenza-related complications and who should receive influenza vaccine are healthy adults older than 65 years; adults with chronic cardiovascular or pulmonary disease; adults who have required regular medical follow-up or hospitalization in the previous year for chronic metabolic disease such as diabetes mellitus, renal dysfunction, hemoglobinopathies, or immunosuppression; and residents of nursing homes and other chronic care facilities. Also, those who have extensive contact with high-risk patients; for example, health care workers and family members should also be immunized to minimize the risk of nosocomial influenza.

Influenza vaccine appears to be effective and cost-saving. Eighty to 90% of immunocompetent adults achieve protective antibody levels with a decline in titers after about 6 months.[12] Protection also depends on how closely the vaccine strains resemble the circulating strains of influenza. The elderly and the immunocompromised may develop lower or less-sustained antibody levels. Although these patients may remain susceptible to upper-respiratory tract infection, they are often protected against lower-respiratory tract involvement and other complications, thus reducing the risk of hospitalization and death.[3] Studies have shown that influenza vaccination can cause a 37% reduction in illness, a 72% reduction in hospitalization, and a 79% to 87% reduction in mortality rates among the elderly during influenza outbreaks.[3,13] With cost estimates of influenza epidemics between $3 billion and $12 billion annually,[14,15] the economic impact of such reductions in morbidity and mortality rates is substantial.

STRATEGIES FOR IMPROVING IMMUNIZATION LEVELS

Discussion of how to improve immunization levels of older adults must include examining provider and patient knowledge, behavior, and attitudes about immunization. Although vaccines recommended for the older adult appear safe and effective, misconceptions about vaccine efficacy and adverse side effects, inadequate knowledge of indications, and failure to consider vaccination during patient appointments contribute to low usage of both pneumococcal and influenza vaccines.

Centers for Disease Control and Prevention (CDC) surveys conducted in the 1980s demonstrated that 81% to 98% of internists and general practitioners believed that pneumococcal and influenza vaccines were indicated for older adults, but most failed to translate their knowledge into practice.[14] Similarly, in a study of 45,000 patients at the Minneapolis and Pittsburgh Veterans Affairs Medical Centers, more than 90% of high-risk vaccine recipients and nonrecipients acknowledged that influenza is a serious disease in the elderly that can result in death.[16] Yet, this study revealed that patient behavior was largely influenced by attitudes, rather than knowledge, about vaccination. Factors positively associated with vaccination behavior were intention to follow physician or nurse recommendations for "flu shots" and previous vaccination behavior. Factors negatively associated with vaccination behavior were difficulty in getting to the medical center and concern about vaccine side effects. Reasons for non-vaccination identified in other studies include lack of a physician's recommendation and a feeling of general "good health" and, therefore, that vaccination was unnecessary.[17,18]

Educational programs to improve immunization practices of providers and consumers may prove helpful. Although providers and patients appear aware of the serious nature of these diseases, greater emphasis should be placed on implementing prevention practices, such as immunizations, in health provider education. The public should also be better informed not only of the recommendations for, but the benefit and safety of, current vaccines. Public-awareness programs are promoted by the American Lung Association and other organized groups, such as the National Foundation for Infectious Disease, which raise money for immunization programs and promote alternative sources of vaccine funding. Increasing public- and private-sector collaboration for adult immunization programs is a primary focus of the National Coalition for Adult Immunization. In addition to these resources, information about current immunization practice is available for providers through the recommendations of the ACIP, the American College of Physicians' *Guide for Adult Immunization*, and CDC's publication, *Morbidity and Mortality Weekly Report* (ie, MMWR), an excellent resource for disease surveillance and immunization policy updates.

Relying on individual providers to achieve the nation's immunization goals may not be enough. Organizational and administrative interventions may help to boost immunization usage to more acceptable levels. Clinic-based strategies include mailed reminders, which have been shown to improve vaccination rates by 20% to 28%, especially when baseline immunization levels are less than 35%.[19-21] Adding physician reminders and performance feedback may improve levels to 40% to 60%.[21] Medical record checklists, which included immunization status, improved vaccination rates from 40% to almost 60% in several studies, especially when nurses played an active role.[22,23] Combining several organizational strategies, which include non-physician provider support, may prove most successful. A Minneapolis VA program, for example, utilized several interventions—an informational mailing to patients, a standing order policy allowing nurses to administer vaccines, a vaccine reminder on daily appointment lists, and the availability of walk-in visits for vaccines—and sustained influenza vaccination rates of 60% to high-risk outpatients for several years; the program was successfully generalized from the teaching hospital to a community outpatient setting as well.[16] Only one study demonstrated as high as a 95% vaccination rate.[24]

Interventions were physician reminders and completion of a questionnaire where patients' reasons for vaccine refusal were documented. Patient education about vaccine side effects and efficacy likely reduced refusal rates and may represent a significant focus for nursing.

In addition to clinic-based strategies, hospital-based strategies may prove helpful. Fifty to 60% of non-immunized elderly accepted pneumococcal and influenza vaccines as part of their care in the emergency department setting.[25] Also, since 20% to 30% of those who die from pneumonia and influenza are hospitalized within the last year of life,[26,27] older adults hospitalized any time between September and March could receive needed vaccinations before discharge.

Removing administrative and financial barriers may also be helpful. Increasing the availability of immunizations at sites where older adults congregate or reside should be considered. Possible sites include institutional settings, such as long-term care facilities; outpatient facilities providing care to high-risk patients, for example, hemodialysis centers and urgent care facilities; home health agencies; and retirement communities and senior centers.[12] Although reducing vaccine cost through Medicare financing has not improved vaccine usage as expected, simplifying the reimbursement process to providers may be a key factor in removing financial barriers.[28]

GERONTOLOGICAL NURSING IMPLICATIONS

Gerontological nurses are in an optimal position to facilitate decisive change in reaching the national objectives for adult immunization policy through interventions both within their own clinical practices and collectively with other health care providers within the communities and clinical settings where they live and provide health care. Nursing has taken a strong leadership role in the past in promoting and realizing national objectives for childhood immunization levels during the past decade. With these goals met, nurses will need to direct their attention and activity to the adult immunization arena as well. Current research strongly supports an active role for gerontological nurses in all aspects of promoting adult immunization policy: that is, in educational, organizational, and research-based approaches.

As patient educators and advocates with increasing autonomy, nurses can significantly impact present program limitations by promoting current vaccine guidelines and by developing new strategies to improve vaccine delivery to older adults in their clinical settings and communities. In any practice setting, gerontological nurses can assess not only immunization status, but also knowledge and attitudes about immunizations of older adult patients, provide appropriate immunizations, and impart information to promote vaccine acceptance. On a broader scale, nurses' involvement in community education programs, often with support of consumer-based awareness groups or public health programs, will help promote a stronger educational message to patients about the importance and safety of vaccination. Educating peers and other health disciplines about clinical practice and public policy regarding adult immunizations is also paramount.

Another focus where nurses may actively impact immunization levels within their practice setting is in designing improved, research-based interventions and evaluating outcomes of strategies implemented in immunization program policy. Increasing understanding of patient and provider vaccination behavior and attitudes through clinical research may be instrumental in developing more effective immunization programs. Developing studies to identify barriers to immunization and success of program strategies will be of continued importance. Ongoing outcome evaluation of immunization programs may elucidate key factors that positively predict and promote optimal immunization behavior. Initiating mailed reminders and provider feedback, educating patients about vaccine safety and efficacy, and implementing physician standing orders are just a few of the possible directions for program development.

Gerontological nurses have taken a leadership role in identifying and responding to the unique needs of the geriatric patient. Immunizing the older adult is another forum for discussion and intervention. Only by their active participation and contribution in this important preventive health practice will national health objectives for adult immunization be met.

REFERENCES

1. U.S. Department of Health and Human Services. Update on adult immunization: recommendations of the Immunization Practices Advisory Committee. *MMWR.* 1991;40(RR-12):5-7,33-42.
2. U.S. Public Health Service. *Healthy People 2000: National Health Promotion and Disease Prevention Objectives.* Washington, D.C.: U.S. Department of Health and Human Services, Public Health Service; 1991.
3. Le C, Chang RS. Tetanus; diphtheria; influenza; pneumococcal diseases. In: Hudson TW, et al. *Clinical Preventive Medicine: Health Promotion and Disease Prevention.* Boston: Little, Brown & Co.; 1988:595-599,615-619.
4. Hutchison BG, Stoddart GL. Cost-effectiveness of primary tetanus vaccination among elderly Canadians. *Can Med Assoc J.* 1988;139:1143-1151.
5. Fedson DS. Adult immunization. In: Becker DM, Gardner LB, eds. *Prevention in Clinical Practice.* New York: Plenum Medical Book Co.;1988:39-48.
6. Williams WW, Hicksom MA, Kane MA, et al. Immunization policies and vaccine coverage among adults. *Ann Intern Med.* 1988;108(4):616-625.
7. Spika JS, Fedson DS, Facklam RR. Pneumococcal vaccination: controversies and opportunities. *Infect Dis Clin N Amer.* 1990;4(1):11-27.
8. Sims RV, Steinmann WC, McConville JH, et al. The clinical effectiveness of pneumococcal vaccine in the elderly. *Ann Intern Med.* 1988;108(5):653-57.
9. Riegelman RK. Pneumococcal vaccine. In: Riegelman RK, Povar GL, eds. *Putting Prevention into Practice: Problem Solving in Clinical Prevention.* Boston: Little, Brown & Co.; 1988:145-55.
10. LaForce FM, Eickhoff TC. Pneumococcal vaccine: an emerging consensus. *Ann Intern Med.* 1988;108(5):757-59.
11. Simberkoff MS, Cross AP, Al-Ibrahim M, et al. Efficacy of pneumococcal vaccine in high-risk patients. *N Engl J Med.* 1986; 315(21):1318-27.
12. Centers for Disease Control and Prevention. Prevention and control of influenza. *MMWR.* April 21, 1995;44(RR-3):1-22.
13. Shann F. Modern vaccines: pneumococcus and influenza. *Lancet.* 1990;335(8694):898-901.
14. Fedson DS. Influenza and pneumococcal strategies for physicians. *Chest.* 1987;91(3):436-43.
15. Schoenbaum, S. Economic impact of influenza. *Am J Med.* 82(6A):26-30.
16. Margoli KL, Nichol KL, Wuorenma J, Von Sternberg TL. Exporting a successful influenza vaccination program from a teaching hospital to a community outpatient setting. *J Am Geriatr Soc.* 1992;40:1021-23.
17. Centers for Disease Control and Prevention Update: influenza—United States, 1989-90. *MMWR.* March 16, 1990;39(10):157-67.
18. Centers for Disease Control and Prevention. Adult immunization: knowledge, attitudes, and practices—DeKalb and Fulton counties, Georgia, 1988. *MMWR.* November 4, 1988;37(43)657-61.
19. Mullooly JP. Increasing influenza vaccination among high-risk elderly: a randomized controlled trial of a mail cue in an HMO setting. *Am J Public Health.* 1987;77(5):626-7.
20. Barnas GP, McKinney WP. Postcard reminders and influenza vaccination. *J Am Geriatr Soc.* 1989;37(2):195.
21. Barton MB, Schoenbaum SC. Improving influenza vaccination performance in an HMO setting: the use of computer-generated reminders and peer comparison feedback. *Am J Public Health.* 1990;80(5):534-36.
22. Cheney C, Ramsdell JW. Effect of medical records checklists on implementation of periodic health measures. *JAMA.* 1987;83:129-36.
23. Davidson RA, Fletcher SW, Retchin S, Duh S. A nurse-initiated reminder system for the periodic health exam. *Arch Intern Med.* 1984;144:2167-70.
24. Walker CL, Patterson R, Wu A, Bennett E. Influenza vaccination: a successful outpatient program. *Allergy Proc.* 1992;13(6):317-19.
25. Rodriques RM, Baraff LJ. Emergency department immunization of the elderly with pneumococcal and influenza vaccines. *Ann Emerg Med.* 1993;22(11):1729-1731.
26. Fedson DS. Influenza and pneumococcal vaccine through a strategy of hospital-based immunization: a review of its rationale and implications. *J Am Geriatr Soc.* 1985;33(2):142-49.
27. Fedson DS, Kessler HA. A hospital-based influenza immunization program, 1977-78. *Am J Public Health.* 1983;73(4):442-45.
28. Centers for Disease Control and Prevention. Implementation of the Medicare influenza vaccination benefit—United States, 1993. *MMWR.* 1994;43(42):771-73.

Chapter 19

Screening for Polypharmacy in a Nursing Home Care Unit

Judith S. Schainen, RN, CS, PhD, and Virginia Burggraf, RN, C, MSN

OVERVIEW

Polypharmacy is defined as the concurrent use of several drugs.[1] This condition occurs when a person receives too many medications for an extended period of time or in exceedingly high doses. The older person is impacted not only by alterations in pharmacokinetics and pharmacodynamics, but also by concomitant illnesses requiring medication administration. It is important for all health care providers of the elderly to assess for polypharmacy and develop interventions to prevent additional health risks from occurring. This chapter addresses a screening program for polypharmacy currently being conducted in a nursing home care unit (NHCU) at a VA medical center.

INTRODUCTION

Elderly patients comprise only 12% of our population, yet they consume nearly one-third of all prescription medications.[2] Almost 30% of nursing home patients receive as many as 12 medications daily.[3] It has been reported that the potential for an adverse drug reaction is only 6% when two drugs are taken, while the risk rises to 50% when five drugs are taken and to 100% when eight drugs are taken.[4] Adverse reactions are a significant cause of morbidity and may account for 20% of hospital admissions of the elderly, as well as complicate the treatment of many elderly patients.[5-8] As the number of somatic complaints and diseases increase over time, the need arises for more medications to be administered and hence increases the risk of polypharmacy.[9] This chapter will describe the following:

- A screening program to minimize the incidence of polypharmacy
- The roles of the screening team: physician, pharmacist, and nurse
- Ways in which the team works to prevent polypharmacy in older patients.

THE NURSING HOME CARE UNIT (NHCU)

The NHCU, a 56-bed unit, is subdivided into three categories determined by the resident's length of stay (LOS). The categories are:

- Actual nursing home beds: 44. LOS is from 1 month to 2½ years. These residents require continuous care. Their discharge to the community is dependent on their restorative potential.
- Geriatric Evaluation Management (GEM) 10 beds. LOS is from 10 to 30 days. These residents are housed in the NHCU and followed by a multidisciplinary team of professionals from the VA Medical Center and not necessarily from the NHCU. These residents undergo an intensive rehabilitation program of care prior to their return to the community.
- Respite care: two beds. LOS is 1 to 2 weeks, after which time residents usually return to their home. This is a period of time that the family can rest from the burdens associated with caregiving. These patients are frequently boarders, however, they do receive care if needed.

The mean age of the residents on the unit at the time of this study was 77; this places them within the age range that many elderly experience the adverse effects of polypharmacy.[9-11] The average number of medical diagnoses was seven compared to five diagnoses described in a similar setting.[12] An average of 12 medications per resident supported current research.[3,13] Table 19-1 lists the medical problems encountered by the residents. The medications prescribed also supported the treatment of these disease entities.

The NHCU physician serves the unit part-time. Medical coverage on off tours of duty is provided by the staff of the emergency walk-in-clinic at the medical center. The nursing staff consists of 10 RNs, seven LPNs, 13 NAs, a nurse practitioner, and a clinical nurse specialist. The nursing staff covers all tours of duty. The pharmacist rotates through the unit on a monthly basis. Pharmacy service provides 24-hour coverage.

THE POLYPHARMACY SCREENING TEAM

The team meets once a week for 30 to 60 minutes to review the computerized medication profiles of up to 20 residents. Data include the start date and time of all medications. They consider altered pharmacokinetics and pharmacodynamics and any change that may be occurring since the last review. Suggestions are made about changing drugs, alterations in dosage, and possibly discontinuing certain drugs. Certain criteria have been designated by the team in order to be consistent with their review process. These criteria include the following:

- Medications are periodically reviewed for each resident, in light of his or her medical problems.
- Dosage levels are set at the minimum therapeutic concentration level.
- Potential drug interactions are monitored and regimens altered to minimize any harmful side effects.
- The optimal dosage form (liquid, tablet, or capsule) is determined on an individual basis.

The individual roles of the team members have been defined in terms of their functions. The NHCU physician (MD) and nurse practitioner (NP) discuss potential medication changes with the other members of the team. During the following week, the MD and NP take the team's recommendations and review each resident's physical examination, laboratory results, and other medications.

TABLE 19-1

Medical Problems in NHCU Residents

CATEGORY	EXAMPLES	INCIDENCE
Gastrointestinal	Peptic ulcer, hiatal hernia, constipation	68
Dermatological	Xerosis, candidiasis, seborrheic dermatitis	41
Pain Management	Headache, muscle and bone pain	36
Neurological	TIA, CVA, seizures, Parkinson's, MS	33
Psychosocial	Depression, anxiety, agitation, insomnia, dementia	28
Renal	Incontinence, UTI, renal failure, BPH	20
Endocrine	NIDDM, IDDM, hypothyroid, malnutrition	18
Respiratory	COPD, asthma, URI, pneumonia	15
Cardiovascular	HTN, CAD, MI, angina, PVD, arrhythmias	11
Musculoskeletal	Osteoporosis, RA, gout, fractures/falls	4
Hematological	Iron deficiency, Vitamin B_{12}, Folic Acid	3
Glaucoma	Wide and narrow angle glaucoma	3
Gynecological	Estrogen replacement therapy to treat osteoporosis	1

The pharmacist plays a major role as educator and participates with the physician in a national drug utilization review (DUR) program for all Medicaid patients. Access to computer technology enhances the pharmacist's role to monitor medication regimens and drug-drug and drug-food interactions. The physician also reviews all medications prescribed and addresses the efficacy of those drugs taken for a long period of time. The pharmacist brings the Unit Dose Medication Profile (Figure 19-1), a computerized printout, which lists the resident's current medication regimen. This profile also serves as a medication order form that can be used by the MD or the NP for changing or reordering medications. When possible, alternatives to drug therapy are instituted.

The nurse not only administers medication but also has the major responsibility to immediately monitor the resident for any side effects that may occur. He or she attends each meeting of the screening team and functions as team leader. The nurse has additional responsibility to assess residents' charts in need of review and provide any anecdotal reports or documentation concerning medications. Often a patient is an ad hoc member of the team and is frequently asked to participate at a meeting. This patient presence helps to focus the team on their ultimate charge to identify and, if necessary, reduce the incidence and effects of polypharmacy in elderly residents.

Unit Dose Medication Profile				
A new order must be written for any new medication or to make any changes in dosage or directions on an existing order.				
Name of Patient:	Ward:		Team#:	
Social Security:	Weight (kg):		Admit Date:	
Date of Birth:	Sex:		Room/Bed:	
Diagnosis: NKDA				
Reactions:				
NUMBER OF DRUG	**NAME**	**START**	**STOP**	**STATUS INFO**
O Take No Action	O Discontinue	O Renew	O Cost Unit	
O Take No Action	O Discontinue	O Renew	O Cost Unit	
Physician's Signature:			Date:	

Figure 19-1. The Unit Dose Medication Profile lists a patient's current medication regimen and serves as a medication order form for the physician or nurse practitioner.

The establishment of a polypharmacy screening program is a positive and valuable service. It creates a team spirit among the professionals caring for the elderly as well as maximizes the health potential of the residents. It is an ongoing method of assessment that promotes the quality of care provided to the residents. The professional exchange of information among the three disciplines promotes a respect for holistic care of the older adult.

GERONTOLOGICAL NURSING IMPLICATIONS

Nurses play a key role in facilitating drug treatment efficacy and reducing drug side effects, interactions, and adverse reactions in the elderly. There is a defined need for nursing research on the pharmacologic effects of drugs in the elderly. Replicated studies are needed to examine the effect of nutritional status, smoking, concomitant disease, and the effects of immobility on medications in aging adults. If pharmacologic studies were undertaken in middle-aged individuals and comparisons made on these adults when older, a physiological basis for drug efficacy could be established.

Gerontological nurses are in the nursing home unit on a continuous basis and serve as advocates for their patients. This advocacy role takes on a significant challenge when monitoring medications, their side effects, as well as efficacy. The challenge lies in their ability to suggest alternatives to drug therapy. Exercise sometime in the early evening can eliminate a sleeping medication. The idea of warm milk should not be dismissed, and the time it takes for this to be prepared is well worth the sleep that it imposes minus the effect of a drug. Using laxatives needs to be discouraged and increasing fluids and fiber in the diet encouraged. Creating a team atmosphere where all disciplines play a role can enhance the wellness of the resident. The creation of a polypharmacy screening team is only one step in addressing polypharmacy. There is a need for staff continuing education. The nurse practitioner and/or clinical nurse specialist have a responsibility to provide this on an ongoing basis in the form of in-service programs and resource information when new drugs are introduced. Family members can be a part of this educational experience in order to minimize any anxiety in the event new medications are introduced. Many families visit the nursing home on a daily basis and need to be reassured that their friend or loved one is being cared for in a positive way.

In 1990, the American Nurses Association (ANA) introduced a position statement on Polypharmacy and the Older Adult. In this statement, ANA makes reference to the need for a drug profile being initiated on older adults upon admission to any health care facility; the evaluating/monitoring of this drug profile for unnecessary and excessive drugs by appropriate professionals; supporting nurses in their actions to communicate, document, and refuse to give medications that in their judgment may adversely affect their older patients; conducting research in pharmacodynamics; and promoting safe medications self-administration in the older population.[1] The development of a polypharmacy screening team is one way to assure that older patients in nursing homes will receive quality care.

REFERENCES

1. Council on Gerontological Nursing. Position statement: polypharmacy and the older adult. *American Nurses Association.* 1990.
2. Santo-Novak D, Moore-Edwards R. Rx: take caution with drugs. *Geriatric Nurs.* March/April 1989;72-75.
3. Clark BE, Vestal RE. Adverse drug reactions in the elderly: case studies. *Geriatrics.* 1984;39:53-63.
4. Shaughnessy AF. Common drug interactions in the elderly. *Emergency Medicine.* 1992;24:21-31.
5. Mitchell GW, Stanazek WT, Nichols NB. Documenting drug-drug interactions in ambulatory patients. *Am J Hosp Pharm.* 1979;36:653-657.
6. Carasanos GJ, Stewart RB, Cluff LE. Drug-induced illness leading to hospitalization. *JAMA.* 1974;228:713-717.
7. Ives TJ, Bentz EJ, Gwyther RE. Drug related admission to a family medicine inpatient service. *Arch Intern Med.* 1987;147:1117-1120.
8. Hutchinson TA, Fiegel KM, Kramer MS, LeDuc DG, Kong HH. Frequency, severity, and risk factors for adverse drug reactions in adult outpatients: a retrospective study. *J Chronic Disease.* 1986;39:533-542.
9. Colley CA, Lucas LM. Polypharmacy: the cure becomes the disease. *J Gen Intern Med.* May 1993;8:278-283.
10. Rosenbloom AA. Essential factors in the care of elderly patients. *J Am Optometry Assoc.* 1988;59(10):774-779.
11. Potempa KM, Folta A. Drug use and effects in older adults in the United States. *Internat J Nurs Studies.* 1992;29(1):17-26.
12. Shimp LA, Ascione FJ, Glazer HM, Arwood BF. Potential medication-related problems in non-institutionalized elderly. *Drug Intell Clin Pharmacy.* 1985;19:766-772.
13. Montamat SC, Cusak B. Overcoming problems with polypharmacy and drug misuse in the elderly. *Clin Geriatr Med.* 1992;8(1):143-158.

Chapter 20

Elderly and Alcohol: A Deadly Combination

Richard Barry, MDiv, MLS, and Virginia Burggraf, RN, C, MSN

OVERVIEW

It is estimated that 3 million elderly older than 60 have problems with alcohol.[1] Health care providers' lack of knowledge and awareness of problems with alcohol among the elderly is as pervasive as the problem itself. Knowledge is the key to assessing this very treatable problem, which has a very high success rate among the elderly. Gerontological nurses in trusting and therapeutic patient relationships can provide the opportunity to increase quality of life among elderly having problems with alcohol.

INTRODUCTION

Alcohol, alcoholism, and alcoholic—a substance, a condition, and a label—all part of an issue that affects every family. The use and abuse of alcohol are pervasive in our society. Alcohol (ethanol) is the most widely personally prescribed over-the-counter drug in use today. Older people, just as others in our society, use and abuse alcohol. Americans tend to disbelieve that the elderly can have alcohol problems, and some hold the view that one of the few remaining pleasures should not be taken away at this time of life.[2] The awareness of alcohol's specific impact upon the elderly, its diagnosis, use, and dependence are under-reported in this population.

Alcohol is a legalized part of our society that can have deleterious effects upon anyone, especially the elderly. Regarding the notion of not wanting to confront an elder's alcohol problem, it is important to note that alcohol dulls any pleasure an older person may have. Not addressing an alcohol problem actually helps to damage the individual's quality of life. For alcoholics of any age, drinking is never pleasure; it is connected instead with pain. And if they can become and remain sober, the quality of the rest of their lives improves dramatically, whether it's 20, 10, 5, or just 1 year.[3] The importance of recognizing alcohol's impact upon health cannot be ignored. Successful treatment of the whole person involves knowledge and awareness of all the factors that contribute to or detract from a state of optimal health.

Primary care providers frequently do not screen for alcohol use. Studies and research indicate 60.7% use alcohol in the general public.[4] Alcohol is part of the culture, yet not part of health assessment. Alcohol of and by itself has a diverse judgment associated with it with laws regulating its use (minimum age requirements by state) and laws indicating its misuse (blood alcohol content percentage and operation of a motor vehicle). On the other hand, it also is indicated therapeutically in some limited medical situations.

The religious and moral judgments surrounding alcohol are as diverse as the population who voice an opinion. Health care providers often have personal opinions about alcohol use and abuse as well as opinions and judgments about alcohol use and abuse by others. As a result, there is such a maze of opinion, judgment, value, standards, and bias about alcohol that a clear understanding is not easily obtained. Compounding the issue is the Diagnostic and Statistical Manual of Mental Disorders (DSM-IV) that categorizes alcoholism as a mental illness. Although true, it must be remembered that the physical effects on the person are profound whether it is one drink or 20.

Assessing for alcohol intake is similar to taking a sexual history. Providers must override their discomforts and incorporate screening questions into everyday practice. Relying on cues to trigger an evaluation of alcohol and drug use is not effective.[5] While interacting with patients during a sexual history, providers "suspend" personal values and focus upon the person, the individual needing care at the time. The same behavior and compassionate care are requisites in taking a history for substance abuse.

The major drawback with alcohol use is that it is a self-reported activity based upon a memory that alcohol affects. Alcohol distorts physical perceptions (drinking and driving don't mix). Alcohol also distorts other perceptions such as how long and how much drinking has occurred, the emotional level of interactions, and remembering or recalling duties and tasks to be performed. This is compounded by the fact that many elderly were raised during a time when the prohibition movement's effects were felt or remembered. To question a person about his or her use of alcohol is to immediately put him or her on the defensive. Acknowledging that they drink alone or have more than "a couple" drinks tends to generate defensiveness and guilt, the major activity of denial. Denial associated with alcohol is the self-protective mechanism for rationalizing the use of alcohol. Not until objective demonstration of the consequences of alcohol use or abuse can be shown (missed appointments, lack of self-care, withdrawal) will there be any behavioral change in the use of alcohol.

ALCOHOL AND THE ELDERLY

Individuals older than 65 who claim to drink alcohol are currently 43.3% of the population. Of this group, 11% consider themselves to be heavy drinkers.[3] These statistics do not distinguish between individuals who have been drinking for the better part of their life, (early-onset, EO) and those who have recently begun to drink (late-onset, LO). LO drinkers are those who begin drinking in their 40s or early 50s. The EO drinkers have a life-long pattern of alcohol use or abuse.

It is important to make some distinctions that are not applicable to hard-and-fast definitions. Alcohol affects everyone differently. Some individuals can have an occasional drink for years and never experience any adverse side effects. Other individuals need only one experience with alcohol, and it becomes a life-long struggle to break free of its influence. There are those people who drink socially. There are those individuals who occasionally use alcohol to cope with stress or as a sleeping aid. There are those people who depend on alcohol to get them through each and every day; they are unable to be without alcohol in their system for very long. There are those people who abuse alcohol, who continually drink an amount of alcohol that alters their normal thinking and behavioral patterns. The range is very wide—from the occasional social drink to the life-threatening abuse. The ambiguity of attempting to define alcohol abuse, of exactly when a particular "threshold" is crossed, focuses upon the frequency and quantity of alcohol consumed. The quantity yardstick fails to take into account how alcohol is affecting patients dynamically, socially, or physiologically.[6] It needs to be remembered that any and every drink of alcohol has its effect upon the individual's health. Some have tried to show the "medicinal" effect of alcohol related to cardiovascular function, but findings are inconclusive. Alcohol is a drug, and every drug taken has an effect on the body. This situation is only compounded in the elderly.

The National Institute on Alcohol Abuse and Alcoholism definition for a drink is considered 0.5 ounces of alcohol. This is equal to 1.5 ounces of distilled spirits, 12 ounces of beer, or 5 ounces of wine. The impact of 0.5 ounces of alcohol on the body of a 45-year-old is very different from that of a 70-year-old. Between the ages 25 and 60, the proportion of total body weight represented by fat almost doubles in men and increases by 50% in women. As lean body mass diminishes and adipose tissue increases, the volume of total body water decreases. Because ethanol is a water-soluble compound, it is distributed in total body water. The volume of distribution is smaller in elderly individuals; a drink of alcohol to an older and a younger individual of similar size and of the same gender produces a higher blood alcohol concentration in the older individual.[7]

Abuse of alcohol is a serious health problem and needs to be dealt with appropriately in all populations; however one drink of alcohol, whatever form that may take, compromises the health of the elderly. It is important to separate the medical consequences of drinking from the problem of alcohol dependence.[4] Alcohol being absorbed into the blood stream so quickly influences each and every organ of the body. The effects, though immediate, do not manifest themselves in terms of impaired organ function for a long time. As a drug, its function in the body needs to be taken into account. As a drug interacting with other drugs, its presence needs to be calculated for potential negative effect.

LITERATURE REVIEW

The use of alcohol in cultures and societies is a centuries-old custom. The pleasurable sensations associated with alcohol have caused it to become a topic of questionable moral and social acceptability. Studies of alcohol use and abuse have predominantly focused upon the "younger" person and most frequently upon the alcoholic or abuser of alcohol. Using the term "alcohol problem" helps to move away from all the subjective relative markers and denial. To say an individual has an alcohol problem is to acknowledge that alcohol has had a negative influence upon interpersonal, financial, legal, and medical dimensions of life.[8] This is understandable when we realize that the consequences of alcohol abuse are more apparent among younger people. When an individual fails to show up for work, neglects preparing meals for his or her children, has a police record due to erratic driving or antisocial behavior, and fails to properly groom himself or herself, then attention is afforded this behavior. These types of behavior are not part of normal social activities.

Remove many of these indicators for the elderly and retired: absence of the workplace; the children are grown and on their own, with no one directly dependent upon a parental role function; limited income; and a diminished social life, no one will notice a drink or three during prime-time television. The elderly have a diminished responsibility in our society, so that little or no attention has been given to the use or abuse of alcohol in this population.[9] Another barrier to alcohol detection in the elderly is pervasive stereotypes. Health care providers can miss the opportunity to help an elderly person if the stereotype exists that older people do not have alcohol problems. We can easily think that they have had all of these years to work through every problem, and now it is just a matter of dealing with the physical "shell." Part of the stereotype about the alcoholic is that years of alcohol abuse have eliminated them from the elderly population. Alcoholics just don't live that long is not true. Older people with alcohol problems are unique and do not fit into media portrayals or those of the younger population. Older alcoholics were less likely to be diagnosed if they were white, female, or had completed high school. Older alcoholics were also less likely to be referred for and receive treatment.[7]

At any age, the most frequently cited reason for drinking is to relieve stress. This is no different for the elderly, yet there are additional issues. Alcohol problems increase after retirement, with the loss of a loved one, due to loneliness, and social isolation. Older women are at risk for alcohol problems particularly when drinking increases following retirement of a spouse. Survivors of these relationships are not identified as having an alcohol problem until after the death of the spouse. Even without a history of drinking with their spouses, widowhood causes an increase in alcohol consumption among some women.[10] Other influences on drinking could be changes in or the loss of role function, which has given identity and purpose for many years, that now translates into feelings of uselessness. Release from a structured daily schedule, not knowing how to use time well, and having not developed hobbies or leisure time activities create boredom for which alcohol is the easiest solution. Chronic illness is another factor that often becomes a "cause" for drinking. This is of major concern, since it compromises all other treatment regimens.

Alcohol, itself a drug, is often harmful if mixed with other drugs, including those sold by prescription and those bought over-the-counter. People older than 65 run the greatest risk of bad drug interaction since they make up 12% of the population and take 25% of all medications. Also, older Americans are heavy users of over-the-counter drugs.[11] The potential for drug interactions and death should not be minimized.

Elderly often have adverse reactions from multiple medication regimens that result in emergency hospitalization. Without a knowledge of patterns of alcohol abuse, these situations could wrongly be interpreted as iatrogenic illness.[12] Polypharmacy (see Chapter 19) has a certain "X" factor if the use of alcohol is not considered. There are numerous prescription drugs that interact with alcohol (*cf., PDR, Micromedex, Nursing Drug Handbook*). This is also true for non-prescription drugs. Elderly who present with hypertension (due to alcohol problems) really do not need any additional medication, but to stop taking alcohol, in order to obtain a normal reading. Depression is the most common accompanying symptom with alcohol problems.[7,12] Metabolism slows down with age causing drugs and alcohol to remain in the body for long periods of time. This slow down increases the risk of drug overdose, alcohol intoxication, and alcohol-drug interaction.

DETECTION (SCREENING) AND DIAGNOSIS OF ALCOHOL USE

Detection of alcohol use in the elderly is not an easy task. The first step toward detecting alcohol use, abuse, and dependence among older patients is to include an alcohol history as a routine part of every history and physical exam. Many patients who are admitted to nursing homes often have alcohol-related symptoms. The nursing home is a place of rehabilitation, and treatment of alcohol problems should be an integral part of rehabilitation. Late-onset alcohol dependence and alcoholism have extremely good recovery potential among the elderly. The symptoms associated with drinking are parallel to those of aging. Some of the physical problems associated with aging may actually be symptoms of an alcohol problem (Table 20-1). Depression, cognitive impairment, malnutrition, frequent falls, incontinence, disruptive behavior, self-neglect, and social withdrawal are all conditions that potentially have their root cause in alcohol. Alcohol use may accelerate the aging process, causing early onset of common conditions associated with aging, such as malnutrition, frequent falls (see Chapter 26), incontinence (see Chapter 14), social withdrawal (see Chapter 27), depression (see Chapter 15), and cognitive impairment (see Chapter 22).[13]

Tools to assess alcohol use are available, though the sensitivity to the elderly has not yet been established. These tools are but one factor in an overall evaluation and assessment of an alcohol problem. Additionally, the tools rely upon the individual's self-report of patterns of drinking that are influenced by guilt, defensiveness, denial, and relative willingness to stop drinking.

The Michigan Alcoholism Screening Test Geriatric Version (MAST-G)[14] is a 24-item questionnaire. The CAGE instrument[15] is a four-question screening tool: Have you ever felt you should **C**ut down on your drinking? Have people **A**nnoyed you by criticizing your drinking? Have you ever felt bad or **G**uilty about your drinking? Have you ever taken a drink first thing in the morning (**E**ye-opener) to steady your nerves or get rid of a hangover?[15]

The MAST-G and the CAGE are both easy to administer, yes-or-no format questionnaires. The CAGE offers the advantage of brevity; the MAST-G provides comprehensive information that is useful for follow-up activities.[16] Both the MAST-G and CAGE are clinically useful assessment tools for geriatric alcohol use. Use of any tool does not guarantee detection of alcohol use, based upon the various relative and influencing factors stated above.

It must be remembered that the alcoholic, especially the elderly, chronic alcoholic, has been using denial, rationalizing, blame, and manipulation to protect his or her drinking pattern. Over the years, the older alcoholic has become a master of using defenses to cover up behaviors that may have led to detection.[17] Alcoholics will do anything to prevent discovery and protect their ability to keep drinking. Individuals with alcohol problems have totally convinced themselves of their right to drink, to use their money anyway they want, and "so what if it kills me" type of mentality. The mind is very clever in its ability to develop good reasons and justifications for maintaining established behavior patterns. The same reasons that people with alcohol problems have been telling themselves for years will be for them the logical explanation as to why it should continue.

TABLE 20-1

Alcohol Abuse Evaluation Protocol

HISTORY

Obtain from family and significant others

Assess for:

- Falls
- Accidents
- Acute onset dementia
- Nutritional deficiencies
- Change in social situation

SCREENING

Alcohol use self-report screening

Depression screening

Nutritional screening

PHYSICAL/LABORATORY PARAMETERS

Complete physical screening

Laboratory evaluation

- SGOT, GGT, CBC (differential), serum albumin, uric acid, HDL, transferrin, ferritin, blood alcohol

Used with permission. Mackel CL, Sheehy CM, Badger TA. The challenge of detection and management of alcohol abuse among elders. *CNS.* 1994;8(3):128-35.

Resistance is to be expected among elderly with alcohol problems. A simple screening test that detects a problem and a health care provider who admonishes the person to stop drinking will do little except provide a new defense strategy for the next encounter. Where there is a difficult patient who apparently is abusing alcohol, a confrontation orchestrated by a professional alcohol counselor may be the only course of action. The professional enlists the aid of family or friends to document occasions of unacceptable behavior. The alcohol abuser, his family or friends, and the counselor have a meeting where the unacceptable behaviors are presented. The alcohol abuser does not respond nor discuss the specific occasions. This is done to break through the denial that exists. Confronted with various and numerous examples of how drinking has interfered with family and social interactions, often for the first time, causes the person to realize the full impact of his or her alcohol problem. Given the difficulty of sorting out geriatric alcohol problems, a comprehensive functional assessment rather than a symptom-oriented one will offer the best means of detection.[18]

TREATMENT

Once the drinking has stopped, withdrawal will be the first consideration. Depending upon the severity of the drinking, medications appropriate to the age and condition of the patient can make this transition to sobriety reasonable for both provider and patient. Delirium tremors accompany heavy abusers, along with delusions, temporary loss of body functions, and other physical manifestations. Shielding the patient from bodily harm is a major priority.

Problems and difficulties precipitating the alcohol problem will now have to be faced. Strong, consistent, supportive family and social support are needed during this transition. For the older alcohol abuser, group therapy may focus more upon age-related losses, depression, boredom, loneliness, negative self-esteem, decreased socialization and rebuilding social support networks, general problem solving, and involvement in community networks.[12] Alcoholics Anonymous is a peer support group offering education, support, and guidance. Local chapters are listed in the phone book. Women for Sobriety addresses women's special needs. Rational Recovery stresses personal responsibility and uses therapy-oriented groups. These are but a few of the established groups offering help.

Educational information is extremely important for family and friends to understand this complex condition. Many groups offer information including the National Council on Alcoholism and Drug Dependence; the National Clearinghouse for Alcohol and Drug Information; and the American Association of Retired Persons (AARP) in Washington, D.C. (Table 20-2).

Follow-up with a patient is a standard nursing routine. We would not hesitate to ask diabetics if they were following their diet and taking their medications. Alcoholism needs to be thought of in the same manner you would think of diabetes, hypertension, or other chronic diseases with a strong lifestyle component. Maintaining a program of sobriety may be easy for those in a controlled situation such as a nursing home or hospital. As with other self-monitored programs, there will periods of poor control or, in the case of alcohol, relapse into destructive behavior patterns. Continued support, renewal of commitment to self-preservation, re-education, and understanding will put the individual back on the recovery program. The natural course of recovery from alcoholism is marked by periods of abstinence that are punctuated by episodes of abuse.[8] A realistic goal of recovery is to shorten the periods of use and lengthen the times of sobriety. Each person is different, and, for some, one relapse will confirm their need for the program, whereas others it may take longer. The longer a person practices the program, the greater chance of remaining sober. It must be noted that alcoholism is a progressive disease. The disease progresses in the sense of decreased tolerance for the drug. If a person stops drinking at age 45 and does not have another drink until age 70, the impact of the last drink will be as if they never stopped. For those with a serious drinking problem or alcoholism, drinking is never an option.

GERONTOLOGICAL NURSING IMPLICATIONS

The long-term consequences of alcohol use indicate a decrease in socialization skills, compromised medical treatment, and overall poor quality of life. In order for nurses to address these issues, a thorough knowledge about the physical, social, mental, and psychological dimensions of alcohol is needed. As our present baby boomers age, we need to be prepared to deal with the impact of recreational drugs more powerful than alcohol. Very soon our need for the long-term consequences of illegal drug use will be the topic of research and chapters in gerontological nursing texts.

TABLE 20-2

Table of Organizations

ORGANIZATION	LOCATION	TELEPHONE
	Resources for Users	
Alcoholics Anonymous (AA)	SASE to PO Box 459 Grand Central Station New York, NY 10163	(check local phone directory for local listings)
Women for Sobriety	SASE to PO Box 618 Quakertown, PA 18951-0618	800-333-1606
Rational Recovery	SASE to PO Box 800 Lotus, CA 96561-0800	916-621-4374 916-621-2667
Secular Organizations for Sobriety (SOS)	SASE to Box 5 Buffalo, NY 14215-0005	716-834-2922
	Support for Family and Friends	
Al-Anon Family Group Headquarters	SASE to PO Box 862 Midtown Station New York, NY 10018-0862	800-356-9996 212-302-7240
National Association for Children of Alcoholics (NACoA)	SASE to 31582 Coast Highway Suite B South Laguna, CA 92677	714-499-3889
Adult Children of Alcoholics (ACA)	SASE to PO Box 3216 Torrance, CA 90510	310-534-1815
National Council on Alcoholism and Drug Dependency, Inc.	12 West 21st Street New York, NY 10010	800-622-2255
National Clearinghouse for Alcohol and Drug Information	PO Box 2345 Rockville, MD 20852	800-729-6686

As nurses, it is important to bear in mind that certain issues impact the older drinker. Grief issues are often present in the older heavy drinker. Loss and grief are part of the universal human experience, and these accumulate with age. Alcohol interrupts the grief process. Heavy use of alcohol may also contribute its own grief to the individual's life. This only compounds the effort required to confront the drinking and the issues that have contributed to its use.[4] Awareness and sensitivity to these factors can open the lines of communication, impact the patient's response to treatment, and restart some important healing processes.

A concept as elusive as alcohol detection in the elderly is the denial that accompanies problem drinking. Denial is insidious and clever in its ability to twist reality, ignore experience, and refuse responsibility. The nurse's ability to instill hope in a patient may assist the patient to overcome elements of denial. Nurses' attitudes such as acceptance, understanding, and promoting mutual trust may promote the denial transcending process.[19] The denial and recovery process are areas for further research and investigation.

When talking with an adult about a possible drinking problem, there are some practices to keep in mind. Treat people as the older adults they are: don't talk down, be direct, and allow them to make their own decisions. Since the goal is to help, don't judge or interrogate the person. Remember grief, guilt, and shame may all be operative. Approach related issues (sleep, personal care, missed appointments) so as not to feed denial or defensiveness. As a self-reporting condition, allow the person to name himself or herself as "alcoholic" or "addict" since we will never thoroughly know the whole life story. Confrontation creates dead ends. The patient's intuition will sense a gentle, caring attitude that offers help and solutions to a problem he or she has been struggling with for years. If the patient is an active drinker, the best time for a reasonable discussion is within a few hours of waking. Remember, it all does not have to be accomplished at one sitting. A little at a time will build the necessary trust and allow you to demonstrate knowledge and skill in dealing with the older alcoholic. Home care nurses should not confiscate alcohol. It can easily be replaced: there may be more hidden, and you make yourself the enemy, rather than a helper. Learn about alcohol. Go to open Alcoholics Anonymous meetings: all are invited. It is the best place to learn the devastating effects of alcohol and how denial can keep people in the disease for years.[20]

Community settings offer the opportunity to develop interagency task forces for establishing community guidelines of care. They also afford practitioners an opportunity to develop educational materials for the practice setting. Established groups like Al-Anon for family and friends provide support and information sharing for those who live, work, or care for people with alcohol problems. Contact with local AA groups may provide support people for the elderly without a family. Along with developing intervention programs for your facility, life-enhancing guidelines and opportunities need to be explored that offer a positive substitution for drinking behaviors. A wide circle of support rooted in compassion, knowledge, sobriety, and experience will draw those with alcohol problems, rather than having to recruit them.[21]

Learning about alcohol and its effects is necessary for professional nursing care. This includes knowing how to negotiate a period when alcohol is eliminated or moderated. Various types of physical, mental, and social assessment tools are available. Some may need only one type, yet the inveterate drinker may need a diverse series. Know how to motivate the patient toward change using internal or external ethics or values. A buddy system approach is used in recovery programs; employ this same tactic for professional guidance, understanding, and support.[19] This is a terrible adventure that is embarked upon, a great period of retroactive development. These survivors have tremendous potential to teach us how to choose well for life. The strength and determination of self-preservation, once tapped, is infectious, life giving, and a profound honor to witness.

REFERENCES

1. Reported epidemic of alcoholism among elderly prompts guidelines. *The Nation's Health.* October 1995:12.
2. Subcommittee on Health and Long-Term Care. *Alcohol abuse and misuse among the elderly.* Publication No.102-852. Washington, D.C.: U.S. Government Printing Office; 1992.
3. A well-kept secret among the elderly: alcoholism. *Tufts University Diet & Nutrition Letter.* December 1993;11(10):1-3.
4. U.S. Department of Health and Human Services. *Health United States 1993.* Hyattsville, MD:May 1994.
5. Willenbring M, Spring WD, Jr. Evaluating alcohol use in elders. *Aging.* Summer 1990;361:22-27.
6. Liberto JG, Oslin DW, Ruskin PE. Alcoholism in older persons: A review of the literature. *Hospital and Community Psychiatry.* October 1992;43(10):975-984.
7. Dufour M, Fuller RK. Alcohol in the elderly. *Annu Rev Med.* 1995;46:123-32.
8. Kettl PA. Detecting problem drinkers in your practice. *Patient Care.* April 1995;29(8):27-34.
9. Welte JW, Mirand AL. Drinking, problem drinking and life stressors in the elderly general population. *J Stud Alcohol.* January 1995; 56(1):67-73.
10. Gomberg ES. Risk factors for drinking over a woman's life span. *Alcohol Health & Research World.* Summer 1994;18(3):220-228.
11. Aging and Alcohol Abuse. *Age Page.* National Institute on Aging. Public Health Service; 1991.
12. Macke CL, Sheehy CM, Badger TA. The challenge of detection and management of alcohol abuse among elders. *Clinical Nurse Specialist.* 1994;8(3):128-35.
13. Thibault JM, Maly RC. Recognition and treatment of substance abuse in the elderly. *Primary Care.* March 1993;20(1):155-165.
14. Blow F. Michigan Alcoholism Screening Test—Geriatric Version (MAST-G). Ann Arbor: University of Michigan Alcohol Research Center; 1991.
15. Mayfield D, McLeod G, Hall P. The CAGE questionnaire: validation of a new alcoholism screening instrument. *Am J Psychiatry.* 1974; 131:1121-1123.
16. Joseph CL, Ganzini L, Atkinson RM. Screening for alcohol use disorders in the nursing home. *JAGS.* 1995;43(4):368-373.
17. Huntington DD. Home care of the elderly alcoholic. *Home Healthcare Nurse.* 1990; 8(5):26-32.
18. Krach P. Discovering the secret, nursing assessment of elderly alcoholics in the home. *J Gerontol. Nurs.* 1990;16(11):32-38.
19. Wing DM. Transcending alcoholic denial. *Image.* 1995; 27(2):121-126.
20. Berkman S. Alcohol abuse among the elderly. *Good Housekeeping.* January 1994;218(1):59-61.
21. Ebersole P, Hess P. *Toward Healthy Aging.* St. Louis:Mosby; 1994.

Chapter 21

Obesity in Older Adults

Henry M. Plawecki, RN, PhD, and Judith A. Plawecki, RN, PhD

OVERVIEW

Many older adults are greatly affected by their cultural heritage, which influences their beliefs about food/diet, health, illness, and traditional healing practices. Many cultures regard being overweight as a sign of health and prosperity, but in the United States, obesity is an increasing national public health problem. Centralized or abdominal obesity is related to the risk of developing health problems such as cardiovascular disease, hypertension, non-insulin dependent diabetes mellitus, osteoarthritis, breast cancer, and gallstones. In order to reduce the rates of obesity in older adults, gerontological nurses must become involved in developing and conducting hospital as well as community-based diet, exercise, and behavior modification programs. The purpose of this chapter is to address those issues that may explain the clinical implications of obesity, review common interventions, and suggest potential strategies that can be used by gerontological nurses to address this ever-expanding health problem.

INTRODUCTION

As a nation, the population of the United States represents a complex multiplicity of interwoven cultures, beliefs, and health practices. Most immigrant groups have brought major portions of their culture to this country. Older adults traditionally have been the caretakers of a group's culture. As a result, cultural preservation is very important to many older adults who were either immigrants themselves or members of the first generation of an American family. Many older adults are greatly affected by their cultural heritage, which continues to influence their beliefs about food/diet, health, illness, and traditional healing practices. In many cases, an older adult's perceptions of being healthy are directly related to culturally accepted beliefs about being overweight/obese. Most cultures of the world regard fatness/obesity as a welcome sign of health and prosperity.[1] In some cultures, the definition of obesity is ultimately linked to cultural perceptions of normalcy, beauty, and health.[1] In contrast to those perceptions, an important precept of American society is individual control and/or the fear of non-control. More specifically, many Americans value self-control and perceive obesity as a visual representation of non-control.[2]

INFLUENCING FACTORS

In order to understand obesity in the older population, one must identify those factors that influence an individual's lifestyle choices. An individual's culture must be recognized as having a significant influence on diet preferences, activity levels, and social expectations. Other societal factors that have influenced the lifestyle patterns of older adults over the past decades have been the mechanization of the workplace, the technical revolution, and the resultant increasing amount of time available for sedentary recreational activities. More specifically, the modernization of society has resulted in lifestyle choices that significantly influenced the increasing rates of obesity among the older adult population. In contrast to many cultural diets that contained an abundance of grains and fruits, the foods ingested by many older adults have become more processed and contain high levels of fat. More specifically, the Westernization of traditional diets involves decreasing the intake of fiber while increasing the intake of fats and sugars.[1] The cumulative consequences of a sedentary lifestyle and the increasing dependence on a high fat diet have contributed to an increasing number of overweight/obese older adults.

Reducing the percentage of overweight/obese adults has been listed as a national health objective in *Healthy People 2000*. Being obese, which is defined as weighing 20% or more than one's ideal weight, may have dramatic health, social, and psychological consequences. As reported in *Healthy People 2000*, approximately 26% of the adult population is overweight.[3] The population's increasing weight problem has occurred in spite of the positive publicity about the increased risk of developing obesity-related illnesses, the availability of reduced-calorie/fat-free foods, and the benefits of exercise/physical fitness activities.

Obesity is non-discriminatory. It affects both genders, as well as all socioeconomic, racial, and ethnic groups.[4] In spite of the increasing prevalence of obesity, the obese continue to experience strong prejudices and have been described as weak-willed, ugly, awkward, self-indulgent, and impulsive.

CLINICAL IMPLICATIONS OF OBESITY

Two methods for the diagnosis of obesity were recommended by the National Institutes of Health Consensus Development.[5,6] These methods included an estimation of relative weight (RW) and the measurement of body mass index (BMI). The BMI is calculated by dividing weight in kilograms by the square of height in meters. A RW that is 20% or more above ideal or desired body weight has been associated with increased health risks, morbidity, and mortality.[6] The BMI is commonly used as a reasonable index of population fatness since it easy to calculate and has been shown to be positively correlated with more direct measures of obesity. It is important to determine an individual's degree of fatness/obesity since many major health problems have been found to be directly correlated with the severity of obesity. In the adult population, overweight is defined as BMI equal to or greater than 27.8 for men and 27.3 for women.[3] Some obesity-related health problems include cardiovascular disease, hypertension, non-insulin dependent diabetes mellitus, osteoarthritis, breast cancer, and gallstones.[7] In addition, the obese older adult has a higher risk for falls as well as decreased longevity.

The degree of obesity and, more specifically, the location of body fat has been identified as an important predictor of health risks. Men and women have general differences in fat distribution. Men are more likely to have a greater proportion of subcutaneous fat at central body sites (eg, chest, back, and abdomen). As men age, their fat stores become more internalized, while the proportion of subcutaneous fat decreases and the amount of fat stored in the abdominal cavity increases.[5] When total body fat increases, there is a tendency for central fat distribution to occur. Central or abdominal fat distribution probably reflects an abnormally large accumulation of intra-abdominal fat, which should be considered an important clinical entity.[7,8] Women have greater proportions of subcutaneous fat at peripheral sites (eg, hips and thighs).[5] Chronic diseases are not closely associated with peripheral body fat.[1] As women get older, especially when post-menopausal, they develop a more centralized type of fat distribution pattern. Women develop more subcutaneous fat and probably more centralized intra-abdominal fat.[5] With increasing age, both sexes acquire an increased ratio of intra-abdominal to subcutaneous fat. A popular measurement of fat distribution is the waist to hip circumference ratio (WHR). Measures of waist and hip circumferences can be used to determine central or abdominal obesity. In order to determine WHR, waist circumference should be measured at the narrowest part as it is viewed from the front. The hip circumference should be measured at the widest portion as it is viewed laterally. A WHR of more than 1.0 in men and more than 0.85 in women is indicative of central or abdominal obesity.[5] A high WHR would indicate a central fat/abdominal distribution. A low WHR would indicate a peripheral distribution of fat in the lower body and extremities. Central or abdominal distribution of fat has been associated with low levels of physical activity, poor physical performance, and decreased lung function. Central fat distribution is a strong predictor for death from all causes in men and, probably, in women.[5] In spite of the belief that smoking increases the basic metabolic rate and produces weight loss, smokers are more likely to develop central fat distribution than non-smokers. In addition, the risk of death for non-smokers was less than that of smokers at all levels of obesity.[5]

Obesity is a multifaceted complex health problem and must be recognized as such by health care professionals. Although the precise physiological mechanism influencing obesity is unknown, several contributing factors have been recognized and include dietary and lifestyle patterns as well as gender and heredity. In the older adult, obesity is associated with decreased activity, which is often due to diminished physical capacities and a progressive decline in caloric requirements for basic metabolic function. The Basal Metabolic Rate (BMR) decreases approximately 2% every 10 years of life while the rate of protein synthesis slowly declines with advancing age.[9]

COMMON INTERVENTIONS FOR OBESITY

Interventions to assist the older adult deal with the problems of obesity must be personalized and directed toward the overall objective of increasing the quality of life and attaining permanent weight control. The efforts should be focused upon reducing health risks while normalizing on an individual basis—one's social, psychological, and functional abilities. The emphasis of any intervention needs to be placed on the qualitative rather than the quantitative changes necessary to improve an individual's health status as well as attain and sustain weight loss.

Personalized intervention strategies must be mutually determined following a comprehensive assessment of the individual's health, physical, dietary, and lifestyle variables. Of particular importance are the determination of the individual's dietary and exercise patterns, social support systems, readiness to take control of lifestyle choices, age of initial onset of obesity, past weight history (ie, previous dieting attempts and episodes of weight cycling), and presenting health risks and medical conditions.[10] Weight management strategies are developed based upon the results of the comprehensive assessment. Programs designed to reduce the degree of obesity generally include interventions in three major areas:

- Diet
- Physical activity/exercise
- Behavior modification/therapy.

Optimal outcomes are achieved when all three areas are implemented into daily long-term lifestyle patterns.

DIET

Many older adults are somewhat knowledgeable about weight loss strategies, such as reducing caloric intake, decreasing fat consumption, and increasing physical activities. However, the strategies for weight reduction/maintenance are poorly understood and rarely integrated into long-term lifestyle patterns. Many people have attempted and succeeded at losing weight by initiating a very low calorie diet. Severely limited caloric intake often produces a rapid initial weight loss, but these diets are difficult to sustain and usually are abandoned in a short period of time. The individual then returns to previous dietary patterns and quickly regains any previous short-term weight loss. To many older adults, the short-term weight loss is perceived as a successful strategy. Unfortunately, the weight that is quickly regained is perceived as a separate event.[2]

Long-term weight reduction programs must be designed to include cultural food preferences, reduction in the caloric intake, decrease in the amount of fat consumed, increase in the amount of dietary fiber, and emphasis on lower calorie food preparation. In addition, diet regimens must meet the recommended daily requirements for protein, vitamins, minerals, and complex carbohydrates. Older adults who initiate weight reduction diets must recognize that long-term weight reduction/maintenance requires a commitment to relearn eating practices. A reasonable long-term diet regimen should include a weight loss objective of about one to two pounds per week.

PHYSICAL ACTIVITY/EXERCISE

Regular physical activity has been commonly accepted as a necessary component of a healthy lifestyle and is directly related to a wide variety of physical and mental health benefits. Exercise is a subset of physical activity that involves the planned, structured, and repetitive bodily movements that are done to improve and/or maintain a component of physical fitness.[11]

It is only recently that the critical role of exercise in weight loss/maintenance programs has been recognized. The relationship of weight loss to exercise is based on the premise that muscles require more energy to function than fat tissue. The planned, structured, and repetitive use of the body's large skeletal muscles burn more calories and promote an overall general feeling of well-being. Regular exercise enhances the body's ability to burn fat rather than carbohydrates, reduces the risk of cardiovascular disease, lowers blood pressure, raises the BMR, and improves psychologic function, ultimately enhancing the individual's self-image and quality of life.[12] Older adults must remember that an exercise program can be as simple as taking a walk.

Many obese older adults generally have developed a sedentary lifestyle and are less physically active than when they were younger. In spite of the fact that they are less active, many older adults have failed to reduce their intake of calories and, consequently, are more likely to gain weight. An individually designed exercise program for an older adult must be based upon his or her readiness to engage in physical activity, abilities/limitations, degree of tolerance, and present health conditions. The mutually agreed upon goals of any exercise program must be to promote feelings of well-being, create positive lifestyle choices, and encourage individuals to continue their participation. Exercise programs must include activities that can be integrated into one's lifestyle, performed regularly, easily tolerated, and enjoyed.

Many older adults recognize the positive relationships between physical activity/exercise, quality of life, and longevity. Consequently, many healthy elderly have attempted to lose weight by increasing their physical activity. Unfortunately, the majority of these individuals fail to recognize that losing weight is a complex long-term process and initiate overly ambitious exercise programs that produce soreness, boredom, or even weight gain. Overly aggressive exercise programs are quickly abandoned, and many discouraged older adults return to a sedentary lifestyle. Low-intensity exercise regimens (ie, aerobic exercises, walking, stretching, and swimming) can be appropriately and successfully added to a weight control program for the older adult. Low-intensity exercises can be tolerated by individuals of all ages, levels of fitness, health status, and athletic inclination. Consequently, low-intensity exercise regimens can be integrated more easily into one's daily activities and produce positive results.

BEHAVIORAL MODIFICATION/THERAPY

Behavior modification, an adjunct therapy, should be in conjunction with the dietary and exercise treatment of the obese adult to improve compliance and long-term results. Keeping records of nutritional/exercise behavior with the use of a diet/activity diary can be very informative for both the older adult and the health care provider. Behavioral changes in diet and/or physical activity will occur more readily when causative factors are self-identified by the older adult. A diet/activity diary should include information about the following: comprehensive list of food and beverage intake, the social/psychological circumstances that stimulated the eating response, an accurate record of all intentional exercise activity, the documentation of successful strategies used to maintain or retain control of the urge to eat, and accurately recording one's weight once each week. In addition, older adults should be encouraged to list any questions that they have about diets, low fat foods, and the labeling of nutritional products.

Within any social context, one must recognize that obesity is an individual's health problem. Social support systems and family members can encourage or assist the individual to modify lifestyle, alter recipes, reduce caloric intake, or increase activity, but, ultimately, each person must accept responsibility for self-control. Reducing one's weight means that the individual must accept the responsibility for following a reduced calorie/fat diet, initiating an increased activity regimen, and making other long-term lifestyle changes. An individual's readiness to take control of and responsibility for lifestyle choices is often preceded by a recognition of the personal, social, or health consequences of maintaining their overweight status. Unfortunately, many weight loss/fitness programs emphasize appearance and have been perceived as unrelated to an individual's health status. Consequently, many older adults perceive dietary/fitness programs as serving only the aesthetic needs of a youth-oriented society.

GERONTOLOGICAL NURSING IMPLICATIONS

Health care personnel, especially gerontological nurses, must recognize the need to evaluate current health/wellness assessment strategies, hospital resources, and the general environmental factors that can be modified to contribute to the well-being of its older, overweight/obese patient population. First of all, the patient assessment process should include an evaluation of the patient's weight/fitness status. Measurement of weight/fitness, such as determining the percent of a person's body fat, can be quickly calculated by using RW, BMI, WHR, or other available electrical, non-invasive devices. These measurements should be added to the standard weight chart to establish baseline data on the patient's degree/level of obesity. Many hospitals routinely conduct estimates of endurance/fitness in their cardiac rehabilitation units. All older obese patients should be referred to those units for a fitness/risk evaluation. Nurses and other health care providers, such as dietitians and physical therapists, could share their expertise about exercise with their colleagues through regularly scheduled staff in-service programs.

The outreach activities of hospitals should include community-based diet/exercise programs for older adults. Non-profit making, but self-financing groups, can be established that are led by dietitians, gerontological nurses, and physical therapists. These health professionals should be able to refer obese individuals to a hospital-based specialist for further investigative advice and/or treatment.[8]

Hospital-based weight loss/fitness programs should be made available to community-dwelling older adults. Programs could be presented during non-peak hours and would produce a needed change in the public's image of a hospital. Low-fat, reduced calorie food should become the standard meal for both hospital patients and staff. Readily accessible convenience foods that are high in fat and calories should only be available through special orders. Community-based educational and exercise programs should be encouraged and tax-supported facilities, such as the public schools, should be made accessible to the older adult population for those purposes. Exercise regimens (ie, walking, swimming), fitness instruction, nutrition classes, and other primary prevention activities could and should be held at public school sites. Obesity must be recognized as a significant community health problem that directly or indirectly affects everyone. Strategies must be developed so that gerontological nurses and other health professionals, as well as all older adults, can benefit from a renewed focus on health promotion activities that reduce the prevalence of obesity.

REFERENCES

1. Brown PJ, Konner M. An anthropological perspective on obesity. *Ann NY Acad Sci.* 1987;499:29-46.
2. Ritenbaugh C. Obesity as a culture-bound syndrome. *Culture, Medicine, and Psychiatry.* 1982;6:347-361.
3. U.S. Dept. of Health and Human Services. *Healthy People 2000: National Health Promotion and Disease Prevention Objectives.* Washington, D.C.: U.S. Dept. of Health and Human Services; 1991.
4. Melkus GD'E. Obesity: assessment and intervention for primary care practice. *Nurse Pract Forum.* 1994;5(1):28-33.
5. National Institutes of Health Consensus Development Conference. Health implications of obesity. *Statement of the 1985 NIH Consensus Conference on Obesity* (Vol 5, No. 9). Bethesda, MD: U.S. Dept. of Health and Human Services.
6. Frankle R. Weight control for the adult and elderly. In: Frankle R, Yang M, eds. *Obesity and Weight Control.* Rockville, MD: Aspen; 1988:361-389.
7. Ashwell M. Obesity in men and women. *Int J Obesity and Related Metabolic Disorders.* 1994;18(Suppl 1):S1-7.
8. Garrow JS. Should obesity be treated? Treatment is necessary. *Br Med J.* 1994;309:654-655.
9. Seim HC, Holtmeier KB. Treatment of obesity in the elderly. *Am Fam Physician.* 1993;47(5):1183-1186.
10. Haus G, Hoerr SL, Mavis B, Robinson J. Key modifiable factors in weight maintenance: fat intake, exercise and weight control. *J Am Diet Assoc.* 1994;94(4):409-413.
11. Pate RR, Pratt M, Blair SN, et al. Physical activity and public health: a recommendation from the Centers for Disease Control and Prevention and the American College of Sports Medicine. *JAMA.* 1995;273(5):402-407.
12. Grubbs L. The critical role of exercise in weight control. *Nurs Pract.* 1993;18(4):20-29.

Chapter 22

Cognitive Impairment and Medication Adherence

Vicki S. Conn, PhD, RN,
Sue G. Taylor, PhD, RN, FAAN, and Rebecca Miller, MS, RN

OVERVIEW

This study examined the relationship between cognitive impairment and medication regimen adherence among non-institutionalized older adults recently discharged from acute care facilities. Cognitive functioning was measured by the Mini-Mental Status Examination; adherence was measured by medication pill counts and verbal self-reports when pill counts were not possible. Twenty percent (*n*=35) of the 178 subjects interviewed were cognitively impaired. Medication regimen adherence was not related to cognitive impairment. Cognitively impaired subjects were more likely than non-impaired subjects to have adult children involved in managing their medications and to have others preparing their medications for administration.

INTRODUCTION AND BACKGROUND

Older adults experience more chronic illnesses and consume more medications than do any other age group. Recent evidence indicates that older adults are consuming increasing numbers of prescribed medications.1 Rates of medication non-adherence, not taking medications as prescribed, among older adults have been estimated at 40% to 75%.2 Medication non-adherence can place older adults at risk for declining health state, increased cost, or avoidable hospital admissions[3-7]; non-adherence has been related to mortality in studies of younger people.8

Older adults may be in danger of non-adherence related to the number of prescription medications they manage, since older adults often must manage multiple medications and there is a inverse relationship between the number of medications consumed and adherence rates.[2,9] Cognitive impairment may also put some older adults at risk for medication non-adherence or mismanagement.[2,10-13] Estimates of the incidence of cognitive impairment in community-residing older adults range from 3% to 20% of the population, depending on the measurement and criteria used to assess cognitive function.[12-15]

Few reported research studies have addressed the relationship between cognitive functioning and medication adherence among older adults. Often cognitively impaired older adults are the very subjects excluded from study. Graveley[16] and Botelho[17] did not find a relationship between cognitive functioning and medication adherence among ambulatory care older adults. Isaac[18] and Palmer[12] found compliance related to selected specific memory functions but not to standard mental status assessment. Methodological limitations prevent drawing conclusions from two other studies because one study used an intervention that would compensate for cognitive impairment[19] and the other study used an inadequate measure of cognitive functioning.[20] Related work found that cognitive functioning was related to knowledge about medications.[21] Studies of cognitive functioning and adherence have not focused on recently hospitalized older adults, despite the possibility that this may be a vulnerable group since they typically have more prescribed medications after discharge than before hospitalization[22] and must cope with the health problem that caused hospitalization.

This study was undertaken to examine the relationship between cognitive impairment and medication regimen adherence among recently hospitalized community-living older adults. It was hypothesized that cognitive impairment would be associated with lower adherence to the prescriptive medication regimen.

METHOD

SUBJECTS

Subjects were 65 years of age or older, were discharged from an acute care hospital to a non-institutional setting, were not having medications prepared by professional health care providers, were on three or more physician-prescribed medications at the time of discharge, and were able to complete an oral interview. The study was approved by the Institutional Review Board for the protection of human subjects. Subjects were identified through discharge records of seven small- and medium-sized private hospitals and two teaching hospitals in two midwestern states. Data were collected 10 to 20 days after hospital discharge.

MEASURES

Cognitive impairment may be defined as decreased capacity to know the world.[23] Cognitive function was measured by the Mini-Mental Status Examination (MMSE) by Folstein.[24] This widely used tool measures orientation, attention, registration, calculation, recall, ability to follow a three-part command, and the use of language. Cognitive impairment is indicated by a score of 23 or below on the MMSE.[25] The MMSE has been used extensively with older adults and has well-documented reliability and validity.[19,25]

Medication adherence is more difficult to measure. Pill counts and self-reports are often suggested by experts.[18,26-28] Both measures of adherence were used in this study. Efforts were made to reduce subject defensiveness prior to the self-report of adherence[29] by saying "People often miss taking some of their medications for a variety of reasons. We are trying to learn more about that experience." Self-report of adherence was calculated based on subjects' responses to the question, "How many pills do you usually miss a week?"

A pill count was conducted for medications prescribed at discharge if the subject had not been on that medication prior to hospitalization. To minimize error, questions were asked about keeping medications in other containers, adding medications to the containers, others consuming medications from the container, and changes in the prescription.

TABLE 22-1

Description of the Subjects*

	COGNITIVELY IMPAIRED			COGNITIVELY INTACT		
Characteristic	**Mean**	**SD**	**Range**	**Mean**	**SD**	**Range**
Age	74.78	6.46	65-101	77.36	8.47	65-97
Chronic illness	2.16	1.07	0-5	2.72	1.21	1-5
Duration of recent hospitalization	8.74	8.92	1-74	12.67	10.85	2-44
Prescribed medications	6.30	2.64	2-14	7.39	3.26	4-16
Adherence scores	.92	.11	.4-1.0	.90	.14	.4-1.0
Mini-Mental Status Exam scores	28.03	1.92	24-30	20.72	20.72	14-23

*N=178.

Subjects were also asked what strategies they used to manage medications and if they received any assistance with medication management. Questions about knowledge of their medications were included. Subjects were asked to describe the cause of missed doses. Demographic data were recorded, including age, gender, chronic illnesses, and living arrangements. The presence of caregivers was not recorded, since it is difficult to classify people as caregivers when subtle types of assistance are provided.

RESULTS

The sample included 85 women (48%) and 93 men (52%). Nine percent (n=17) were black, the remainder were white. Most (n=116, 65%) lived with spouse or other family, 32% (n=56) lived alone, and 3% (n=6) lived with friends, companions, or boarders. The most common chronic conditions reported by the subjects were cardiovascular diseases, joint disorders, and pulmonary diseases. Other sample characteristics are described in Table 22-1.

Self-report of adherence was obtained from all subjects (n=178) for 918 medications. Pill counts were obtained from 114 subjects for 248 medications. Pill counts were used for adherence calculations when available. Self-reports of adherence were used for medications where pill counts were not feasible. Most subject adherence scores (n=114) reflected pill count combined with self-report measurements of adherence. The remainder (n=64, 36%) were based entirely on self-report, 47% of the cognitively impaired subjects' adherence scores were based on self-report only and 34% of the non-impaired subjects' adherence scores were based on self-report only. Since subjects were on varying numbers of medications with different frequencies of administration, a weighted average adherence score was calculated for each subject based on the number of doses to be taken of the specified medication (see Table 22-1).

The relationship between MMSE scores and selected variables are found in Table 22-2. Thirty-five of the 178 subjects (20%) had MMSE scores below 24, indicating cognitive impairment. There was not a significant association between MMSE scores and adherence scores. Since using a correlation may mask important differences between the impaired and unimpaired subjects, further targeted analysis was conducted. When subjects were divided into impaired and non-impaired groups, the adherence scores of the cognitively impaired subjects were not significantly different from the scores of the non-impaired subjects (Wilcoxon Z=-.93, p=.35). There was an inverse relationship between MMSE scores and age, but there was not a significant correlation between age and adherence (r_S=.02, p=.84).

TABLE 22-2

Correlation Between Mini-Mental Status Exam Scores and Selected Variables*

Variable	**CORRELATION WITH MMSE** r_S	p
Adherence	.13	.09
Age	-.29	.008**
Knowing name of medications	.29	.0001**
Knowing purpose of medications	.39	.0001**
Reported "forgetting" doses	.06	.43
Using memory assistive devices	.07	.33
Others assisting with medications	-.35	.0001**
Other preparing medications	-.48	.0001**
Adult child assisting with medications	-.38	.0001**
Spouse assisting with medications	-.03	.70

* *N*=179.
** Significant at the .01 level.

Higher MMSE scores were associated with more knowledge about medications, knowing the name of medications (impaired mean=.73, non-impaired mean=.90), and knowing the purpose of medications (impaired mean=.63, non-impaired mean=.86). Describing the generic or trade name, physical appearance of the medication (such as "the little blue one"), and medication function (such as the "water pill") were accepted as responses correctly naming a medication. Accurately identifying the target organ or body system, naming the function, or describing the diseases, symptoms, side effects of other drugs, or complication of diseases as the intended target of medications were considered as knowing the purpose of medications. Ability to name medications (r_S=.03, p=.70) and identify the medication's purpose (r_S=.05, p=.55) were not related to adherence.

"Forgetting" was the most common reason given for non-adherence (60.2%). Reported forgetting medication doses was associated with lower adherence rates (r_S=-.40, p=.0001). Subjects with lower MMSE scores were no more likely to cite forgetting as the reason they missed medications (see Table 22-2). MMSE scores were not associated with the reported use of memory assistance methods reported by these older adults—timed pill box arrangements, leaving containers in a particular location, taking medications in association with meals or bedtime, using a medication check-off list, writing the number of daily doses on medication container lids, or setting alarm clocks to administer medications. Other much less frequently mentioned reasons for missing medications were that the medication was not perceived as helpful, did not fit in their routine (ie, supposed to take at a time when asleep), and caused side effects.

Subjects with lower MMSE scores were more likely to report others assisting them in medication management (see Table 22-2); only 20% (n=7) of impaired subjects lived alone, compared to 34% (n=49) of the non-impaired subjects. When asked specifically what others did to help with medication management, subjects with lower cognitive scores on the MMSE were more likely to report that others prepared medications for them. Explanations of preparing medications ranged from filling a timed pill box or placing appropriate medication containers by the sink for medications to be taken while the caregiver was away to getting medications out of the containers and handing them to the subject to take at that moment. Those with lower MMSE scores were more likely to have an adult child assisting with medications but there was no relationship between reporting a spouse helping with medications and MMSE scores (see Table 22-2). The percentage of cognitively impaired and non-impaired subjects using memory assistance devices and having assistance with medications are documented in Table 22-3.

TABLE 22-3

Cognitively Impaired and Unimpaired Subjects' Use of Memory Assistive Devices and Assistance from Others with Medications*

	COGNITIVELY IMPAIRED (n=35)		COGNITIVELY INTACT (n=143)	
Variable	%	n	%	n
Medication assistive device	89	32	92	132
Receives help with medications	81	29	41	59
Someone prepares medications for subject	75	27	22	31
Child assists with medications	42	15	5	7
Spouse assists with medications	33	12	28	40

* N=178.

DISCUSSION

Older adults with cognitive impairment are conveniently or systematically excluded from most medication adherence research, perhaps because researchers suspect these subjects cannot give accurate information for research purposes. In this study, older subjects with cognitive impairment (lower MMSE scores) were not more likely to erroneously report adherence scores when pill counts and self-reports of adherence for medications were compared (Wilcoxon $Z=.73$, $p=.46$). One limitation of the study that should be remembered is that these subjects were moderately, not severely, impaired.

The findings of this study are congruent with previous work that found that subjects' knowledge about medication is not necessarily correlated with adherence to medication regimens. This finding does not suggest that patient education about medications is not necessary; adherence to medication regimens is only one aspect of effective self-management of medications. Previous research has demonstrated that knowledge is an essential prerequisite to behavioral change, but is not sufficient to produce the desired change without the corresponding attitude and cue to action.

The measure of cognitive impairment used in this study has been used extensively with older adults in both research and practice settings, including previous studies examining the relationship between cognitive functioning and adherence.[16,17] The MMSE may be more useful as a screening tool for dementia than as a research or clinical tool used to differentiate levels of cognitive ability necessary to manage medications. Management of medically prescribed regimens, such as medications, requires complex cognitive abilities that may not be adequately measured by cognitive impairment screening instruments such as the MMSE. A recent study by Isaac[18] found certain memory aspects related to compliance, but that standard measures of cognitive status among older adults were not closely associated with the type of memory necessary for medication management and compliance. Isaac[18] found visual memory related to medication compliance, which is congruent with clinical experience that many older people learn their medications by shape, size, and color instead of by name.

The association between reported forgetting of medications and adherence is interesting, especially given the lack of relationship found between forgetting and cognitive impairment. Complaints about memory problems are common among older adults but are often exaggerated since memory complaints by older adults do not correlate well with objective measurement on memory tasks.[30,31] These findings are congruent with Isaac's[18] report that memory problems associated with noncompliance were not easily detected on standard mental status tests. The nature and experience of forgetting medications merits further investigation. Asking patients about forgetting medication is easy to do, and many methods of compensating for forgetfulness are available. Recent research indicates that medication administration systems that compensate for forgetfulness are effective in improving medication adherence.[32-35] For example, Murray[33] found a reminder chart significantly increased medication compliance among recently discharged adults.

An important finding of this study is the involvement of caregivers in medication administration among the older adults with decreased cognitive functioning. This finding may provide a potential explanation for other researchers' inability to find a relationship between cognitive functioning and adherence.[16,17] For this study, the presence of caregivers' assistance with medications may mean that the adherence comparison was between cognitively intact older adults and the caregivers of cognitively impaired older adults. It is important to note that the caregiving found in this study was available to cognitively impaired older adults in the period immediately after hospital discharge. This extensive medication assistance may not be available for older adults not recently experiencing hospitalization. The importance of adult children in helping with medications, as compared to spouses, was an unexpected finding.

Compared to some other studies, relatively high rates of adherence were found among this sample. The high rates of adherence may be related to the recent hospitalization of the subjects in this study. When questioning subjects about missing medications, interviewers noted many subjects clarified that they had missed fewer doses *since hospital discharge.* Hospitalization may be a sufficiently salient experience to alter typical patterns of adherence. Patient education about medications may intensify after hospitalization when patients have some new medications, resulting in higher levels of adherence. Since other studies have generally found lower adherence rates among independently living older adults, patient education about medication should probably be at least as intense among those not recently hospitalized. The often held assumption that older adults on the same medication regimen long-term have adequate knowledge about their medications may be a myth.

Discussions of medications among older adults often focus on long-term use of the same medications for chronic conditions. In this sample, 114 of 178 subjects began a new medication after discharge from the hospital. These findings are limited to older adults managing both long-term and newly prescribed medications. Most older adults are not hospitalized in any given year. These subjects' hospitalization experiences and number of chronic illnesses suggest that they were in relatively poor physical health compared to older people in general. The 20% cognitive impairment rate in this sample is not excessive given other estimates of cognitive impairment incidence among older adults and that a sample of recently hospitalized older adults is likely to contain more people at risk for cognitive impairment.

The major findings of the study were that cognitive impairment, as measured by the MMSE, was not associated with adherence and that these cognitively impaired older adults were likely to have caregivers assisting in the administration of their medication in the period immediately after discharge from acute care facilities. These findings suggest nurses cannot assume that standard tests of cognitive functioning will detect older patients who will have difficulty with medications.

GERONTOLOGICAL NURSING IMPLICATIONS

These findings emphasize the need for nursing assessment of the patient's ability to follow the medication regimen and intervention aimed at caregivers of cognitively impaired older adults. This must begin on initial contact. The importance of adult children in helping with medications, as compared to spouses, suggests that nurses should be sure to include adult children in teaching about medications, as well as the older patient and his or her spouse. Nurses should assess family situations of older patients to determine who is providing medication assistance. Phone contact as well as patient education materials for adult children, who may be away from the home when the nurse visits, may be the most convenient way to provide education about medications to caregivers.

Assessment of the instrumental activities of daily living may be a measure to assess for adherence to a medication regimen. If the patient is unable to manage money or prepare a meal, he or she may have difficulty with the administration of medications. Nurses should not rely on simple measures of orientation as indicators that older adults are able to manage medications. Evidence of difficulty with tasks requiring visual memory also should be noted. For example, difficulty identifying seemingly familiar objects, such as car keys compared to house keys, could signal visual difficulties that could hamper medication management. The visual appearance and differentiation of medications is an important component of patient/family education.[18,36]

Patient education should focus on strategies to prevent or compensate for forgetting medications. Nurses should encourage patients and caregivers to use memory aids that not only cue the elder to take the medication, but also provide a way for the older patient to validate that the medication has been consumed. For example, using a timed medication box is probably more effective than placing medication containers in a particular location because the medication containers cannot be easily checked to determine if doses have been administered. Hahn[37] provides an excellent overview of several medication management assistive devices. Another strategy to cue older patients to take medications that has been found to increase compliance is to link medication times with individual daily schedules.[38]

There are few tried and true measures that solve the dilemma of medication adherence among older adults. The challenge that exists is to develop strategies for caregivers when the patient experiences cognitive impairment. Multidimensional interventions, aimed at individuals and families, probably have the highest likelihood of influencing the multifaceted problem of medication non-adherence.

Partial support for this study came from National Institutes of Health Institutional Biomedical Research Support Grant No. RR07053 to the University of Missouri-Columbia.

REFERENCES

1. Stewart R, Moore M, May F, Marks R, Hale W. Changing patterns of therapeutic agents in the elderly. *Age & Aging.* 1991;20:182-188.
2. Salzman C. Medication compliance in the elderly. *J Clin Psychiatry.* 1995;56(Suppl 1):18-22.
3. Col N, Fanale J, Kronholm P. The role of medication noncompliance and adverse drug reactions in hospitalizations of the elderly. *Arch Intern Med.* 1990;150:841-845.
4. Colley C, Lucas L. Polypharmacy: The cure becomes the disease. *J Gen Intern Med.* 1993;8:278-283.
5. Dekker F, Dieleman F, Kaptein A, Mulder J. Compliance with pulmonary medication in general practice. *European Respiratory Journal.* 1993;6:886-890.
6. Hallas J, Harvald B, Gram L, et al. Drug related hospital admissions. *J Intern Med.* 1990;228:83-90.
7. McKenney J, Munroe W, Wright J. Impact of an electronic medication compliance aid on long-term blood pressure control. *J Clin Pharmacol.* 1992;32:277-283.
8. Gallagher E, Viscoli C, Horowitz R. The relationship of treatment adherence to the risk of death after myocardial infarction in women. *JAMA.* 1993;270:742-744.
9. Gilbert A, Luszcz M, Owen N. Medication use and its correlates among the elderly. *Australian J Pub Health.* 1993;17:18-22.
10. Edwards M, Pathy M. Drug counseling in the elderly and predicting compliance. *Practitioner.* 1984;228:291-300.
11. Moore S. Cognitive variants in the elderly: An integral part of medication counseling. *Drug Intelligence and Clin Pharm.* 1983;17:840-843.
12. Palmer H, Dobson K. Self-medication and memory in an elderly Canadian sample. *Gerontologist.* 1994;34:658-664.
13. Stockton P, Jones J. Medication use by the elderly. *Aging.* 1993;5:337-347.
14. Kramer K, German P, Anthony J, Von Korff D, Skinner E. Patterns of mental disorders among the elderly residents of eastern Baltimore. *J Am Geriatr Soc.* 1985;33:236-245.
15. Mortimer J. Epidemiology of dementing illness. In: Mortimer J, ed. *The Epidemiology of Dementia.* New York: Oxford; 1981:2-23.

16. Graveley E, Oseasohn C. Multiple drug regimens: medication compliance among veterans 65 years and older. *Research Nurs & Health.* 1991;14:51-58.
17. Botelho R, Dudrak II R. Home assessment of adherence to long-term medication in the elderly. *Fam Pract.* 1992;35:61-65.
18. Isaac L, Tamblyn R. Compliance and cognitive function: a methodological approach to measuring unintentional errors in medication compliance in the elderly. *Gerontologist.* 1993;33:772-781.
19. Wong B, Norman D. Evaluation of a novel medication aid, the calendar blister-pak and its effect on drug compliance in a geriatric outpatient clinic. *J Am Geriatr Society.* 1987;35:21-26.
20. Wandless I, Mucklow J, Smith A, Prudham D. Compliance with prescribed medicines: A study of elderly patients in the community. *J Royal Coll Gen Pract.* 1979;29:391-396.
21. Mahdy H, Seymour D. How much can elderly patients tell us about their medications. *Postgraduate Med J.* 1990;66:116-121.
22. Gonski P, Stathers G, Freiman J, Smith T. A critical review of admission and discharge medications in an elderly Australian population. *Drugs & Aging.* 1993;3:358-362.
23. Folstein M, Anthony J, Parhad I, Duffy B, Gruenberg E. The meaning of cognitive impairment in the elderly. *J Am Geriatr Society.* 1985;33:228-235.
24. Folstein M, Folstein S, McHugh R. "Mini-mental state": a practical method for grading the cognitive state of patients for the clinicians. *J Psychiat Res.* 1975;12:188-194.
25. Anthony J, LeResche L, Niaz U, Von Korff M, Folstein M. Limits of the "Mini-Mental State" as a screening test for dementia and delirium among hospitalized patients. *Psychological Medicine.* 1982;12:397-408.
26. Craig H. Accuracy of indirect measures of medication compliance in hypertension. *Res Nurs Health.* 1985;8:61-66.
27. Evans L, Spellman M. The problem of non-compliance with drug therapy. *Drugs.* 1983;25:63-76.
28. Westfall U. Methods for assessing compliance. *Topics in Clin Nurs.* 1986;7:23-30.
29. Haynes R, Sackett D, Taylor D. Can simple clinical measurements detect patient non-compliance? *Hypertension.* 1980;2:757-764.
30. Kahn R, Zarit S, Hilbert N, Niederche G. Memory compliant and impairment in the aged. *Arch Gen Psychiat.* 1975;32:1569-1573.
31. Zarit S. *Aging and mental disorders.* New York: Free Press; 1980.
32. Hussey L. Overcoming the clinical barriers of low literacy and medication noncompliance among the elderly. *J Gerontol Nurs.* 1991;17(3):27-29.
33. Murray M, Birt J, Manatunga A, Darnell J. Medication compliance in elderly outpatients using twice-daily dosing and unit-of-use packaging. *Ann Pharmacotherapy.* 1993;27:616-621.
34. Raynor D, Booth T, Blenkinsopp A. Effects of computer generated reminder charts on patients' compliance with drug regimens. *BMJ.* 1993;306:1158-1161.
35. Ware G, Holford N, Davison, J, Harris R. Unit dose calendar packaging and elderly patient compliance. *New Zealand Med J.* 1991;104:495-497.
36. Kelly J. Implementing a patient self-medication program. *Rehabil Nurs.* 1994;19:87-90.
37. Hahn K, Weitor G. Helpful tools for medication screening help prevent dangerous medication errors. *Geriat Nurs.* 1992;13:160-166.
38. Hussey L. Minimizing effects of low literacy on medication knowledge and compliance among the elderly. *Clin Nurs Rese.* 1994;3:132-145.

Chapter 23

Siderails: Rethinking a Standard Practice

Maggie Donius, RN, MN, and Joanne Rader, RN, MN, FAAN

OVERVIEW

Siderails have been in use for many decades. Nurses would never leave a patient's room, particularly an older patient, without first checking to see if the siderails were up. This practice has changed to incorporate needed guidelines on restraint use and patient autonomy. Siderails can be potentially hazardous. This chapter discusses levels of siderail use, provides a decision tree for determining use of siderails and methods to assess the need for siderails.

INTRODUCTION

Using siderails has long been considered standard care for elderly people in health care facilities. However, routine siderail use was based not on demonstrated benefit, but on consensus—the majority "thought" it was a good idea.[1] Rubenstein[1] recommends that a randomized controlled study be conducted to determine whether bedrails constitute protection or a hazard to the average elderly patient. Miles[2] describes situations in which bedrails combined with physical restraints contributed to deaths. In four deaths, people were suspended off the bed and wedged between bedrails. In one case, the body could not be extricated until the bedrail was physically disassembled. The discussion section of this chapter mentions asphyxiation deaths occurring when bedrails fell across the throats of two patients. Corey[3] describes one death attributed to external compression of the left common carotid artery when a patient slipped between the mattress and the siderail of his bed. It is time that siderails receive the attention that other physical restraints have received as being potential hazards rather than universally accepted safety devices. Health care professionals must rethink the use of siderails in light of data implicating siderails as contributing to injury rather than preventing it and the clinical observation that rails often do not prevent falls and increase the distance one falls.

The April 1992, Health Care Financing Administration (HCFA) interpretative guidelines for long-term care facilities identified siderails as a restraint in certain situations; therefore, nursing homes have had to address this issue. Acute care facilities would be wise to rethink siderail use as well. Siderails are not a benign intervention and should not be used without careful consideration. They may have the following negative consequences:

- Increasing the distance one falls from the bed
- Obstructing vision

- Separating the care receiver from the caregiver
- Creating noise
- Causing trauma if the resident's body strikes the siderails or becomes entangled in them
- Pulling on and dislodging tubes during raising and lowering
- Creating the sense of being trapped or jailed
- Imposing bedrest when bedrest may not be desired or desirable.

Questions that should be addressed before implementing siderails include the following:

- Choice: Does the individual want them used?
- What is the intent?
- What is the effect on function?
- Does it prevent or facilitate what the patient wants to do?
- Does the benefit outweigh the burden from the patient's perspective?

For example, a patient may prefer the rail up because he or she feels more secure. It may facilitate turning in bed. A half-rail may be used for support during transfer out of bed. On the other hand siderails can serve as barriers preventing the elderly person from getting where he or she wants to go. Decreased warning time for urination and/or urgency makes it difficult to wait for assistance. Patients may not want to bother staff with something they think they can manage on their own. Bedrest or the immobility that siderails may impose are particularly hazardous to elderly patients. If older people do not use functional or mobility skills, they lose them. Reconditioning takes much longer than deconditioning. Many agree that for each day in bed for a person older than 65, it takes 7 days to recover function. There is little, if any, evidence that bedrest has any therapeutic value, and there is much evidence to the contrary.[4] When a siderail prevents older patients from leaving their beds when they wish, they are more likely to climb over the rails, increasing their risk of injury.

There have been a number of discussions on the issue of autonomy in long-term care.[5,6] The decision about siderails is just one small part of autonomy. Anything providers can do to return control over day-to-day life to the individual will help make the long-term care facility a more desirable place to live. This shifting of control is hard for staff as it flies in the face of the "safety at all costs" and "we know best" mentality that has been pervasive in health care. In light of the new emphasis on autonomy, many common health care practices are being examined. Staff need to be aware of their own comfort level in changing a long-standing practice and facilitating autonomy. Staff may have strong beliefs about the need for siderails to ensure safety; however, this belief is based more on ritual and tradition than on evidence. Currently, when discussing siderail use with a newly admitted person, the staff may not present keeping the rails down as an option, or they may try to influence the choice. Patients who have had siderails in place for a long period of time may be conditioned to believe they "need" them because staff believed they need them. In this situation, patients have the right to continue to use them, even though they may not provide any physical benefit. Ongoing dialogue should occur, providing assessment information to patients or family so that an informed choice can be made and/or a decision changed.

ASSESSING RISK LEVEL

After considering the general issues surrounding siderail use, the individual should be systematically assessed (Table 23-1) and categorized into one of three risk levels. Begin by performing an assessment. Observe the patient getting into and out of bed. If a wheelchair is the person's mode of mobility, observe transfer into and out of the chair, to and from the bed. Document the person's ability or lack of ability. Ask the question, "What may happen if siderails are not used?" If the answer is "probably nothing," the patient is in Level I; if the answer is "a good possibility of something negative," the person is in Level II or III.

TABLE 23-1

Siderail Assessment Documentation Example

- I don't want to wait. Sometimes they don't come when I call, and I don't want to wet the bed.
- Approached bedside in w/c, stood without locking breaks, got into bed supporting self on bedside stand. Got to supine without difficulty, unable to come from supine to sitting. Raising the siderail on the wall side for support facilitated this position change. Was unable to retrieve the w/c, which rolled out of reach during transfer to bed. When asked about the brakes, patient was unaware.
- Staff report w/c brakes have been explained multiple times but not remembered by patient.
- Safety of independent transfer is questionable related to not locking brakes of w/c, but patient may be able to use a stationary commode next to bed. Wall siderail facilitates supine to sitting position change.
- Assess patient's ability to safely use commode if left at bedside and discuss with patient, family, and staff.

Level I—Low Risk: Siderails Serve No Purpose

Patients in Level I include those who are able to get into and out of bed safely without assistance and those who do not move without staff assistance (eg, someone in a persistent vegetative state whose position is changed by staff on a schedule and is found in the same position upon staff's return). Patients who do not move can be positioned on their sides in the center of the bed rather than at the edge of the bed and the rails left down. A facility has reported that positioning was done better and more carefully when siderails were not used (M. Hughes, personal communication, 1993).[7] Documenting the observation that the patient is able to get into and out of bed safely or is unable to move provides evidence that siderails serve no purpose.

Level II—Moderate Risk: Patients Cannot Get In or Out of Bed Safely

This group has some perceived safety risk and therefore needs a safety plan. Siderails may or may not be part of that plan. Patients in Level II may exhibit behaviors that appear to put them at risk for negative consequences (eg, wandering into rooms of others uninvited, falling, etc.). These patients may need their whereabouts monitored or need assistance during transfer

(Figure 23-1). A conference including patients and/or family may be needed to discuss risks and develop a safety plan other than siderails or to decide that siderails are needed.

Level III—High Risk: For This Group, Siderails Are Used to Restrict Movement

Patients fall into this group because there are no alternatives, alternatives have failed, or the benefit of using siderails outweighs their burden. Some patients with delirium (acute confusional state) may benefit from short-term siderail use. For example, a patient who has an IV and tries to leave for the bathroom without the IV pole may benefit from a siderail as a reminder to call for help, unless he or she is likely to try to crawl over it, in which case it becomes a hazard.

FORMULATING A SAFETY PLAN

Check your assessment of risk level with the perceptions of others, including staff on other shifts. Discuss the assessment and staff consensus with the patient. Include the family if the patient is unable to participate and seek their input. Remember a patient's rights override the family's desires. If all agree that the rails can be left down, this should be noted on the plan of care and the plan carried out. Because siderail use has been an accepted yet unexamined standard of practice, it may be necessary to note on the plan of care that siderails will not be used. Documentation of the assessment process used and factors in decision-making should be described clearly. When the standard of practice has changed, it should not be necessary to document when rails are not used, only when they are. After the decision to keep siderails down has been agreed upon, a gradual process can be instituted if indicated. The siderail can be lowered on a schedule tailored to the patient, or the rails can be put down for a short time initially and the periods gradually lengthened.

If the patient or family disagrees with the staff's assessment, a conference can be helpful to sort out the issues and develop a plan that is agreeable to all parties. This often can be done by phone. It is important to include significant others in the decision, especially when standard practice is being changed.

Facilities with policies requiring siderail use should revise them before instituting this change to prevent legal difficulties resulting from acting in conflict with their own policy. Fear of litigation often encourages staff to be overly restrictive, but as Greenlaw[8] points out the importance of freedom of movement requires that each patient be evaluated so the least restrictive means of ensuring safety will be employed.

INTERVENTIONS

There are a variety of alternatives that can be implemented when siderails are not wanted or desired and a safety plan is needed. Alternative interventions can be environmental, physiological, and psychosocial. Interventions should be evaluated considering the benefit as well as the burden the intervention may impose from the patient's point of view. Interventions should be implemented only when the benefit outweighs the burden.

ENVIRONMENTAL INTERVENTIONS

When a patient is suffering from a dementing illness, behavior often cannot be controlled or changed. The environment should therefore be modified whenever possible to accommodate the behavior. A low bed without rails is an environmental intervention that can enhance patients' safety. Low beds can facilitate getting into and out of the bed independently or with increased safety because the patient's feet will touch the floor when he or she is sitting on the bedside. This provides a firm base of support to come to standing or to pivot for a transfer. For other patients, a low bed will put them so close to the ground that they are unable to stand. Depending on the patient, being "stuck" on the bed may cause them to call for help and/or decrease the risk of injury should they fall because the distance of the fall will be decreased. Pads can be placed on the floor to cushion a potential fall. A periodic cleaning plan is needed if this intervention is used. Placing the mattress on the floor may be the safest option for some. Currently, fire regulations may prohibit this in some states, but if a satisfactory individualized evacuation plan is developed, regulators can be consulted for an exception.

A siderail on one side of the bed can facilitate a position change, which makes transfers into and out of bed safer for some patients. One half-rail may provide the support needed to stand and/or to get into a chair. A transfer pole placed in a strategic location may serve the same purpose.

A pillow or rolled blanket under the mattress edge that creates a lip may provide a less confining "bumper" to prevent the patient from accidentally rolling out of bed if this is likely to occur. This intervention is less likely to cause accidental skin trauma than a siderail.

A number of alerting devices are available that can be helpful in certain situations. These devices alert staff to a position change in progress by setting off an auditory alarm, or some can be set up to turn on the call light. Some devices are worn around the thigh; others go on the bed, detecting a position or the weight/pressure change of the patient when he or she leaves the bed. Another device allows the caregiver to clip a cord to the patient's clothing; when the patient goes beyond the length of the cord, the alerting unit sounds. A listening device, such as a nursery monitor, can alert staff that a patient is stirring. Some call light systems, when disconnected from the wall, will sound/light. The call light can be pinned or fastened to the patient's clothing; if he or she goes beyond the reach of the call cord, it will be pulled out of its socket and sound. These signals alert staff to check on the person immediately.

Non-skid rubber-backed rugs at the bedside can prevent slips if urine loss on standing is a problem. These rugs can be treated with the appropriate cleaning chemicals when necessary and hosed off. A rug at the bedside can also provide firm footing or traction for those who attempt to leave the bed in bare feet or slippers without traction. For those who find themselves inadvertently on the floor at bedside, a rug prevents them from being on the cold floor until they are assisted. These interventions are only a few ways in which the environment can be modified to enhance safety and eliminate siderails when they are not wanted or pose a hazard to patients.

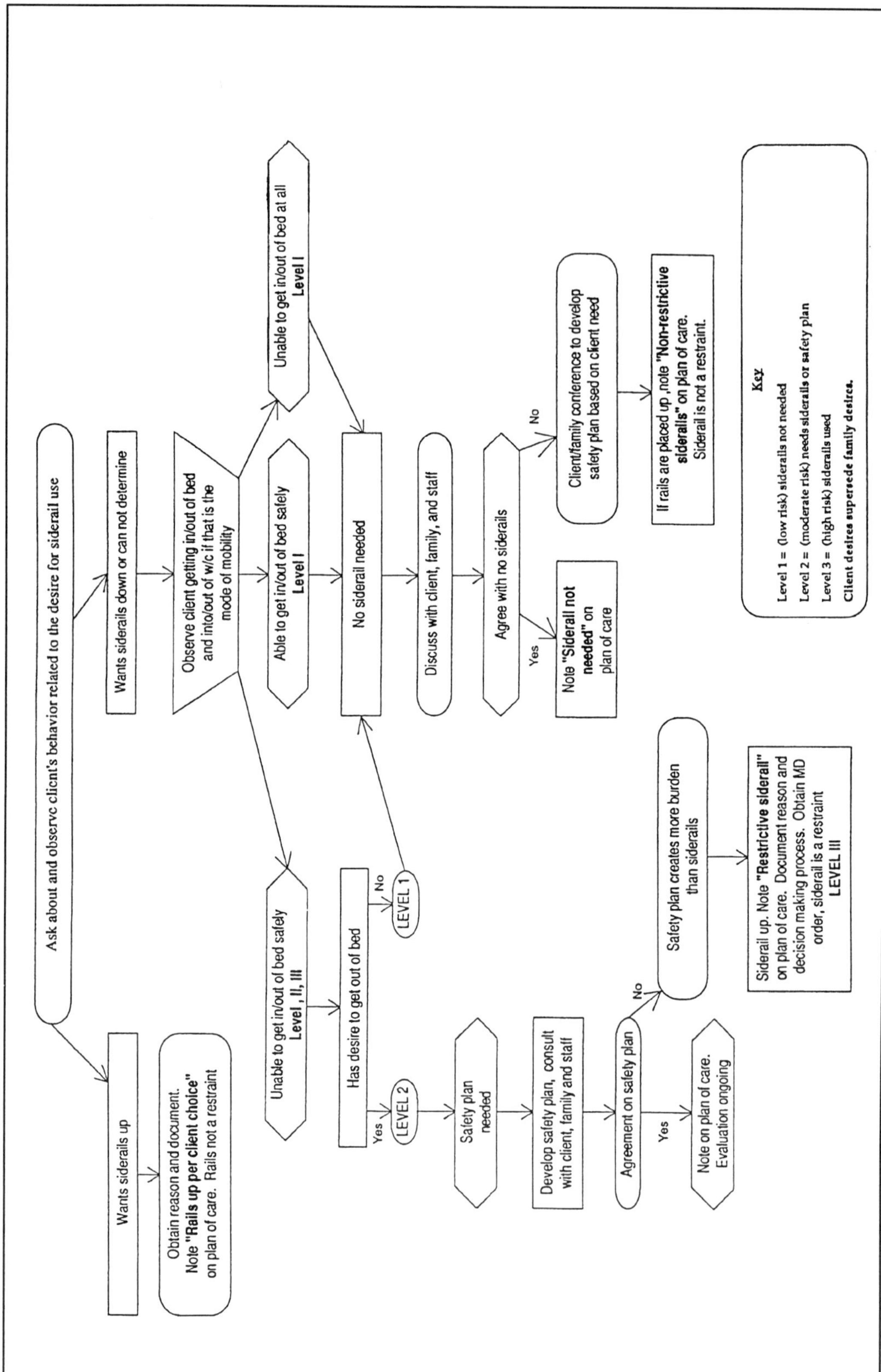

Figure 23-1. Flow chart to determine siderail use. Copyright © 1995 Maggie Donius, RN, MN.

Physiological Interventions

Physiological interventions include those that address health and comfort needs. The patient may be suffering from an acute illness (ie, urinary tract infection) or flare up of a chronic illness (ie, congestive heart failure) that could be causing him or her to leave the bed. Treating or managing these illnesses may eliminate or decrease this behavior. Family members or sitters may be willing to stay with patients suffering from delirium to provide reassurance and safety monitoring. The person could be too warm or cold, hungry, thirsty, or in pain and be unable to communicate these needs. Meeting these needs may decrease or stop unassisted transfers. The patient may have been in bed too long. Getting a person up when he or she is not sleepy and want to leave the bed will prevent unassisted exit. Expecting patients to stay in bed, day or night, when they are "slept out" is an unrealistic expectation. A toileting schedule may be helpful in preventing unassisted exiting. A bedside commode, urinal, or female urinal may facilitate independent elimination, which is safer when a patient will not or cannot wait for help. Most people will attempt toileting without assistance rather than be incontinent.

Psychosocial Interventions

A person may attempt to leave the bed because he or she is fearful. Placing the person in a lighted area, staying with the person, or putting him or her with others (at the nurses' station) so he or she is not alone may alleviate fear and the behavior. It is wise to discuss these fears with the patient, as they may require a simple remedy.

When Is a Siderail a Restraint?

According to the April 1992 HCFA interpretive guidelines for long-term care facilities, siderails are restraints if they restrict freedom of movement by preventing a resident from getting into or out of bed voluntarily. Whether or not patients are able to do so safely does not alter the fact that it is a restraint. A physician's order is necessary when siderails restrict freedom of movement.

Siderails are not restraints when patients choose to use them. A restless sleeper might need siderails to prevent him or her from falling out of bed; however, since the patient does not intend to get out of bed, the siderails are not restraints. In such cases, a physician's order is not required. If patients cannot make their preferences known, the family should be consulted and assessment information used to determine whether or not to use siderails. The reason for siderail use should be recorded on the plan of care (ie, "rails up—lots of involuntary movement during sleep"). Documentation should indicate that use is based on the patient's preference or consultation with the family.

GERONTOLOGICAL NURSING IMPLICATIONS

Nurses caring for frail older people in all health care settings need to rethink siderail use. Siderails should be considered an optional intervention that could help or hurt rather than a routine dictated by facility policy or tradition. Gerontological nurses, advocating for the patient, must first ask him or her about siderail preference. A siderail assessment needs to be performed, and the outcome discussed with those involved. This assessment is important for the patient's health as siderails have the potential to help or hinder. Consideration must be given to whether siderails provide the least restrictive environment possible, maximize the older person's ability, and promote quality of life from the patient's point of view.

The goal is not to eliminate all siderails. The goal is to maximize autonomy and individualize siderail use—to use them only when they truly increase the safety, security, and mobility of patients in our care. If a patient is going to climb over the rails, the siderail will increase, not decrease, the risk. In such cases, siderail use cannot be justified in any setting.

REFERENCES

1. Rubenstein HS, Miller FH, Postel S, Evans HB. Standards of medical care based on consensus rather than evidence: the case of routine bedrail use for the elderly. *Law, Med and Healthcare.* 1983;11(6):271-276.
2. Miles S, Irvin P. Deaths caused by physical restraints. *Gerontologist.* 1992;32(6):762-766.
3. Corey TS, Weakley-Jones B, Nichols GR, Theuer HH. Unnatural deaths in nursing home patients. *J Forensic Sci.* 1992;37(1):222-227.
4. Creditor MC. Hazards of hospitalization of the elderly. *Ann Intern Med.* 1993;118(3):219-223.
5. Gamroth LM, Semradek JK, Tornquist EM. *Enhancing Autonomy in Long-term Care.* New York, NY: Springer; 1995.
6. Kane RA, Caplan AL. *Everyday Ethics Resolving Dilemmas in Nursing Home Life.* New York, NY: Springer; 1990.
7. Hughes M. personal communication; 1993.
8. Greenlaw J. Failure to use siderails: when is it negligence? *Law, Med and Health Care.* 1982;125-128.

Chapter 24

Documentation of Adult Vulnerability, Abuse, and Neglect

Marlene Frost, PhD, RN, and Karen Willette, MS, RN

OVERVIEW

The factors that contribute to abusive or neglectful situations have been examined in the past, but no studies have explored the documentation of adult vulnerability to abuse/neglect. The researchers reviewed the documentation of 60 home health charts to identify the following:

- What is currently documented
- The influence of increased awareness of the need for documentation
- The influence of an in-service on subsequent documentation.

Results included increased documentation as nurses were provided more information. Charted data focused on the physical and cognitive realms with little psychosocial documentation. There was minimal documentation on support systems or caregiver capabilities. Implications for clinical practice are discussed.

DOCUMENTATION OF ADULT VULNERABILITY, ABUSE, AND NEGLECT

Elder abuse/neglect is an increasing problem in our society. Estimates are that 500,000 to 1.5 million individuals are victims of elder abuse or mistreatment every year[1-5] with only one in every five cases being reported.[6] This is of great concern due to our aging population, the chronicity that accompanies aging, and the decreasing length of hospital stays by which individuals are returning to the community more vulnerable than ever before.[7,8]

Despite the increased concern for elder abuse/neglect, documented research on this topic is lacking. The purposes of this study are:

- To explore what is currently documented in a home care agency regarding adult vulnerability, risk, and abuse/neglect
- To examine the influence of increased awareness (ie, discussion groups, audits, charting changes) of the need to document adult vulnerability on subsequent documentation.

Identification and assessment of suspected abuse can be difficult, underscoring the importance of nurses' understanding of the complexities.[9,10] A sense of hopelessness, helplessness, or powerlessness is noted in dealing with elderly abuse/neglect because of the complexity of the situation, the strong emotions it elicits, and societal norms for privacy.[11,12] Defensive avoidance was often used by providers because of potential negative consequences for the patient.[12] Obstacles to intervention include lack of evidence, lack of cooperation by patient and family, lack of governmental response or resources, unclear reporting requirements and fear of involvement were noted as reasons for not reporting elder abuse, and lack of training for assessing elder neglect.[13,14]

Accurate diagnosis is hindered by the reality that much abuse/neglect occurs in the home of an individual where few health professionals have access.[15] The elderly's fear of reprisal or being placed in a health care facility, as well as the caregiver's reluctance to share, are concerns because of public opinion and legal prosecution.[16] Furthermore, cultural values and beliefs influence the definition of abuse/neglect.

Adult vulnerability is closely related to that of elder abuse/neglect. Defining vulnerability, the Minnesota state statute[19] identified the vulnerable adult as anyone 18 years or older who is a resident or inpatient of a facility licensed to serve adults, who receives home care services, or who regardless of residence or type of service is unable or unlikely to report abuse or neglect. This definition varies by state. Generally, vulnerable adults are presented as at risk for physical, mental, or emotional impairment. Rose[20] cautions that risk and vulnerability are at times used interchangeably; however, risk refers to hazards or stressors in the environment, vulnerability to characteristics of the individual. Highly vulnerable people can be of concern in a low-risk environment; individuals who have low vulnerability often function well under poor conditions. Times of biological, social, and psychological transitions make individuals more vulnerable.[21] Variations in definitions and the ambiguity of what comprises vulnerability and abuse/neglect is an impediment to a clear depiction and understanding of this problem.[5,10,14,22]

A variety of factors are identified as contributing to adult vulnerability or risk for abuse/neglect including being older than 65,[23,24] being a white woman,[7] and having significant physical, psychological, or mental impairments that create increasing dependence for meeting daily needs.[3,5,7,18,25]

Contributing caregiver factors include alcoholism; chronic medical problems; financial concerns;[18] lack of support systems or social isolation;[10] excessive stress; sudden, unwanted, or unexpected dependency;[10,17,26,27] demands exceeding abilities;[3,18,22,26] and a lack of knowledge concerning elders' needs.[26]

Client and caregiver interpersonal risk factors include[18] lack of role delineation,[28,29] generational role conflicts,[17,28] competition for authority,[29] family norm of violence,[10,18,22,26] not understanding aging and its associated losses,[17,28-30] and ignoring the aged's social needs.[28]

Indicators of abuse/neglect include unexplained, poor skin integrity, contractures, decubiti, dehydration, impaction, poor nutrition, over- or undermedication,[14,31] bruises, fractures, burns, fear, unusual listlessness or withdrawal, violation of rights,[26,31] inappropriate clothing, failure of response to obvious disease, surveillance failure,[14] poor hygiene,[14,31] sexually transmitted diseases, extreme mood changes, and depression.[26]

Mandatory reporting laws and Medicare regulations for suspected elder abuse, neglect, or mistreatment mandate documentation including the assessment of adult vulnerability.[32] Few research studies indicate a thorough documentation of elder abuse. Phillips[15] had 34 public health nurses assign 74 elders into an abuse/neglect relationship therapy group or a positive relationship group. Nurses agreed on group assignments of all but 12 subjects. In another study by Phillips,[12] the researchers concluded that health care providers assessed the quality of the caregiving situation while overlooking the quality of the client-caregiver relationship. A vacillation cycle was apparent in which the care provider would try to make a decision while making verbal justifications for not being able to decide. The decision maker would often stall at this stage, not proceeding to an actual diagnosis. A third study, Phillips[15] reported the lack of established procedures for dealing with or following up reported mistreatment cases. If the caregiver was perceived as doing the best he or she can, being charming, appearing overworked, or socially prominent, then the situation was often not identified as abusive.[15] These studies need to be replicated to validate additional data. In the agency from which data were collected, risk factors for abuse/neglect were included under the definition of adult vulnerability. Thus, the use of the term adult vulnerability in the remainder of this chapter will refer to both vulnerable characteristics of the individual and risk factors outside the individual.

METHODOLOGY

Data were gathered retrospectively from 60 home health agency charts from a moderate sized non-teaching hospital in the Midwest. The 60 charts were reviewed during three different time periods, which corresponded to increased information that the nursing staff received on adult vulnerability. Charting procedures also changed during the three different data collection times as a means to increase documentation awareness. Twenty charts were reviewed prior to a visit by Medicare for accreditation purposes (data collection period one). Nurses were aware of the need to chart on vulnerability at this time but had not been given information on vulnerability assessment. During this time, the only charting procedure was to place an asterisk by areas on a general assessment tool that indicated vulnerability. The term vulnerability was not included on the tool.

The second data collection period followed the Medicare accreditation visit. At this time, informal information was introduced through staff discussions about adult vulnerability. Two additional changes were added to the previous charting practice of placing the asterisk by areas increasing the risk of adult vulnerability and potential vulnerability.

Data collection period three began after in-service education on the vulnerability of older adults, highlighting the characteristics of the abused and abuser, state reporting laws, and charting procedures. The 2-hour class was led by a master's prepared home care nurse manager (see Table 24-1 for the class outline). Twenty charts were reviewed during this period.

Current documentation on adult vulnerability was explored by randomly selecting 20 charts of clients older than 21 from each of the three data collection periods. Charts were examined for the following:

- Nursing diagnoses identified as areas that would increase individuals' vulnerability or risk for abuse/neglect
- Assessment data documenting factors putting individuals and caregivers at risk for abusive or neglectful situations

- Assessment of various support systems.

The data were then classified according to these three areas. Documentation in each of the data collection periods was analyzed with respect to the influence of awareness of the need for documentation as well as the educational intervention.

FINDINGS

Patients ranged in age from 55 to 94 years with a mean of 75 years of age. Fifty individuals were receiving Medicare; 10 were not. Thirty-two participants were men; 28 were women. The majority of the primary diagnoses (*n*=50) represented chronic conditions; the remaining diagnoses (*n*=10) represented acute conditions. The aforementioned data were comparable across data collection times.

TABLE 24-1

Vulnerable Adult Inservice Content

- Definitions and descriptions of vulnerable adult, abuse, neglect, and family caregiver.
- Definitions of types of abuse and neglect: physical, psychosocial, sexual, and financial.
- Home care employee responsibilities related to the vulnerable adult: (1) knowledge of agency policies, (2) what to assess, (3) agency documentation forms and procedures, (4) development and evaluation of abuse prevention plan, and (5) abuse and neglect reporting procedures— internal reporting, external reporting (state requirements).
- Case studies of the vulnerable adult, abuse, and neglect.

Charting on the 60 clients was completed by 12 registered nurses. Charting was completed by six nurses during the initial data collection period, seven nurses during the second data collection period, and eight during the third data collection period.

NURSING PROBLEMS

Nursing diagnoses were reviewed for factors that would increase adult vulnerability as well as for data on actual abuse or neglect. Fewer nursing diagnoses suggesting possible vulnerability of a client were noted during data collection period one (*n*=7 on six charts) than during the following two data collection periods (*n*=29 on 18 charts, *n*=44 on 19 charts, respectively). As time progressed and the nurses were increasingly exposed to the notion of adult vulnerability, the number of nursing diagnoses on charts and the variety of diagnoses expanded. There seemed to be increased understanding of what adult vulnerability means, with decreased designation of medical diagnoses as areas increasing vulnerability (*n*=3, *n*=3, *n*=0 during data collection periods one, two, and three, respectively).

Comparing the focus of the nursing diagnoses across data collection periods, the majority of nursing diagnoses were physiologically based. It wasn't until data collection periods two and three that psychosocial diagnoses were identified. Diagnoses related to caregivers' needs appeared first in data collection period three (Table 24-2).

TABLE 24-2

Areas Identified from Documented Nursing Diagnosis as Increasing Client Vulnerability

PROBLEM IDENTIFIED BY NURSING DIAGNOSIS	TIME PERIOD 1*	TIME PERIOD 2*	TIME PERIOD 3*
Physiological			
Decreased Endurance/Weakness	1	1	3
Immobility/Limited Range of Motion			2
Potential for Falls/Injury/Unstable Ambulation		4	9
Decreased Cardiac Output and Ineffective Airway	1		
Shortness of Breath with Minimal Exertion			2
Unstable Blood Glucose			1
Inability to Speak		1	
Limited Vision		1	
Poor Nutritional or Fluid Intake		2	5
Incontinence			1
Break or Potential Break in Skin Integrity			3
Potential Infection			1
Numbness			1
Dizziness			1
Cognitive			
Knowledge Deficit	2	7	3
Signs of Brain Dysfunction/Poor Memory/ Confusion		2	2
Psychosocial			
Lacks Confidence in Self-Care Abilities		2	
Loneliness		1	
Overwhelmed by Treatment			1
Depression			3
Anxiety about Caregiver's Health		1	
Caregiver			
Dependence on Caregiver with Limited Physical Abilities		1	
Dependence on Caregiver with Limited Mental Abilities	1		
Need for Caregiver Respite			2
Unacceptance of Caregiver			1
Miscellaneous			
Noncompliance with Medical Regimen	1		
Self-Care Deficit	1	6	4

* Areas noted as increasing client vulnerability were reported on 6 of the 20 charts during time period 1, 18 of the 20 charts during time period 2, and 18 of the 20 charts during time period 3. More than one area may have been recorded on a chart.

ASSESSMENT DATA

Assessment data were reviewed for factors that would increase adult vulnerability as well as for data on actual abuse/neglect. There was an increased number of charts with assessment data related to actual or potential vulnerability after the first data collection period (*n*=12, *n*=20, *n*=18 charts data collection periods one, two, and three, respectively). During data collection period one, there were two types of actual abuse or neglect documented for five different clients. These included medication neglect and physical abuse or neglect. Although documented as assessment data, there was not an accompanying diagnosis of abuse, neglect, or increased vulnerability. Additionally, four charts contained assessment of bruises and abrasions, with one chart noting an individual who had several bones broken in the past few years. Although the causes could be related to aging or illnesses, they could also be related to abuse or neglect. Assessment documentation was lacking for a woman who had a diagnosis of osteoporosis and had a husband who was belligerent and agitated at times. This individual had documented petechiae, a fractured shoulder 3 years before, a back injury from a fall 2 years before, and a hip injury from a fall just 2 months before the current need for home care for an infected leg ulcer. There was no documentation of assessment data regarding the cause of these falls or to any questioning of family members concerning abusive behaviors.

Assessment data regarding cases of abuse or neglect charted during data collection period two was missing; there were two documented cases of actual neglect during data collection period three. There was no corresponding nursing diagnoses; however, referrals and interventions were instituted.

The assessment data related to vulnerability during data collection period one reflected environmental, physical, and cognitive factors. During data collection periods two and three, sparse psychosocial assessment documentation was evident. Assessment data related to anxiety and lack of support were noted during data collection period two; depression data during collection period three (Table 24-3).

There was a significant increase in the number of charts that contained vulnerability assessment data from collection period one to period two; there was a slight decrease from data collection period two to period three. There was an increase in the number of diagnoses indicative of increased vulnerability during data collection period three. This may be reflective of a change in charting on the assessment form. The vulnerability area was removed from the assessment form, but was added as the initial diagnosis to the care plan.

There was documentation of the assessment of support systems on 16 of the 20 charts reviewed during the first data collection period, 19 of the 20 charts during the second data collection period, and 17 of the 20 charts during the third data collection period (Table 24-4).

Although there was an increase in the documentation of assessment data of support systems during data collection period two, the most frequently assessed area of support remained physical assistance with care. There was an increase in the amount of documentation of informational support, social support, and economic support during data collection period two.

During data collection period three, physical assistance with care was noted less frequently than during the previous data collection times. Other areas of support were comparable to chart review during data collection period two (see Table 24-4). Across the data collection periods, there were several charts (*n*=4, *n*=5, *n*=7 data collection periods one, two, and three, respectively) in which there was documentation of with whom the individual lives while not noting the individual's ability to assist with care.

TABLE 24-3

Most Frequently Documented Assessment Data* Noted as Increasing Client Vulnerability

ASSESSMENT DATA	TIME PERIOD 1**	TIME PERIOD 2**	TIME PERIOD 3**
Physiological			
Mobility	√	√	√
Shortness of Breath Interfering with Self-Care	√	√	√
Ecchymosis	√		
Poor Nutrition		√	
Decreased Endurance/Weakness		√	√
Break in Skin Integrity		√	√
Poor Vision		√	
Inability to Visualize Wound		√	
Environmental			
Environmental Factors Creating Safety Concerns	√	√	√
Cognitive			
Knowledge Deficit	√	√	√
Signs of Brain Dysfunction/Poor Memory/Confusion	√	√	√
Psychosocial			
Anxiety		√	
Lack of Social Support		√	
Depression			√
Miscellaneous			
Noncompliance with Medications			√
Self-Care Deficits	√		√
Need for Physical Assistance	√	√	√

* Only categories of assessment data noted on four or more charts are reported here.

** Assessment data noted as increasing client vulnerability were reported on 12 of the 20 charts during time period 1, 20 of the 20 charts during time period 2, and 18 of the 20 charts during time period 3. More than one assessment category may have been recorded on a chart.

CONCLUSIONS

The documentation for potential vulnerability did not give a holistic picture of the level of patients' vulnerability. Providing a specific area on the assessment form often elicited one or several factors that may increase a patient's vulnerability. Resources and abilities of the individual to deal with these problem areas were frequently not noted. All individuals are potentially vulnerable to a certain degree when there is a care need. Nurses need to make decisions about the extent of an individual's risk based on vulnerability, risks in the environment, and available resources.

The identification of environmental hazards in this study as increasing vulnerability or risk for abuse/neglect may, at times, be inappropriate. Although some environmental hazards, such as scatter rugs and cluttered rooms, may increase the risk for injury, they don't necessarily increase the risk for abuse/neglect. Other environmental hazards, such as loose railings needed to access bathroom facilities, may result in not being able to adequately care for hygiene needs, leading to an assessment of neglect.

TABLE 24-4

Support System Assessment

TYPE OF SUPPORT	TIME PERIOD 1	TIME PERIOD 2	TIME PERIOD 3
Physical Assistance	15*	19*	15*
Informational Support	8	12	12
Social Support	5	9	8
Economic Support	2	2	2

* Charting on four charts from time period 1, five charts from time period 2, and seven charts from time period 3 noted who was available for physical assistance without providing information regarding the abilities of the caregiver to provide the care needed.

There is a need to clearly delineate factors that increase vulnerability and risk as compared to factors that may indicate actual neglect or abuse. For instance, ecchymosis was identified as a factor increasing adult vulnerability or risk. However, ecchymosis could be a sign of actual abuse, not a factor that increased adult vulnerability or risk. Further refinement of the definition of vulnerability will aid this delineation as well as assist in the development of assessment tools.

LIMITATIONS

This study was based on the review of a limited number of charts from one institution. A significant limitation with chart review is that data may have been gathered but not charted. It was not possible to analyze the differences in charting based on educational preparation due to the limited number of nurses' charts reviewed.

Definitions of vulnerability, abuse, and neglect vary considerably, resulting in possible variations in categorization of data by other researchers. Cultural background may influence the decision-making process as to factors that indicate abuse/neglect. The covert nature of the dynamics between the vulnerable adult and potential abuser can result in cases of abuse/neglect not being reported. *There is likelihood for an underestimation of the number of cases of abuse/neglect.*

GERONTOLOGICAL NURSING IMPLICATIONS

The findings of this study point to the need to educate nurses about the identification, evaluation, and documentation of vulnerability and actual or potential abuse/neglect. An educational program should include a comprehensive orientation on the policies of the agency and the laws of the state; definitions of vulnerability, abuse, and neglect; and risk factors, as well as assessment and documentation requirements. Case studies are useful in stimulating discussion and clarification of vulnerability, abuse, and neglect issues. Nonjudgmental discussions of ambiguous situations should be encouraged during routinely scheduled conferences. A multidisciplinary team approach allows for varied perspectives. A second opinion is desirable and can be accomplished by having another team member observe the questionable situation. Discussions should focus on weighing the factors creating vulnerability, individuals' environmental risk factors, caregiver and client needs, and supportive resources. Interviews should be conducted individually with the client and the caregiver to allow freedom to discuss issues.

Psychosocial factors such as interpersonal relationships and emotional states need to be emphasized in addition to the physical and cognitive factors. Findings about nurses' decision-making processes should be reviewed to increase awareness of biases and to stimulate discussion. All[25] suggests assessment of the level of dependency on the caregiver, a mental status examination, and direct questions about abuse. The caregiver's perceived level of burden and stress, as well as types of support, should be assessed.

Charting procedures and forms should be organized into a concise, easily understood format. Chart audits at regular intervals may reveal weaknesses in the process and could be a helpful tool for providing learning experiences and in planning future in-service programs. Active involvement of staff nurses in reviewing and improving documentation may stimulate a feeling of responsibility and provide a greater understanding of nurse involvement.

There is a need for the development of assessment tools that give a holistic perspective on individuals' level of vulnerability. An area on the assessment form that asks the nurse to address physiological, mental, psychological, caregiver, interpersonal, as well as other environmental factors that may contribute to the increased risk is a helpful tool for documentation. This followed by the resources (physical, informational, social, and economic) available as well as an evaluation of the resources' ability to assist the patient and caregiver is needed. This provides information on whether the level of risk warrants a nursing diagnosis and where intervention is essential. Assessment tools found in the literature[2,3,32] provide a beginning foundation for clinical practice.

Jewell[33] notes that patients may leave hospitals without the support services they need, placing them and their families who are caring for them in a vulnerable position. The decreased lengths of stay in hospitals demand that discharge planning begins with admission so that vulnerability will be minimized. Coordinating care between patients, families, and community health providers facilitates the anticipation and prevention of potential problems.

REFERENCES

1. Fulmer TT. Mistreatment of elders: Assessment, diagnosis, and intervention. *Nurs Clin North Am.* 1989;24(3):707-716.
2. Fulmer TT. Elder mistreatment assessment as a part of everyday practice. *J Gerontol Nurs.* 1992;18(3):42-45.
3. Hamilton GP. Using a family systems approach: Prevent elder abuse. *J Gerontol Nurs.* 1989;15(3):21-26.
4. Ozmar B. Encountering victims of interpersonal violence: implications for critical care nursing. *Crit Care Nurs Clin North Am.* 1994;6(3):515-523.
5. Weiler K. Elders vulnerable to telemarketing fraud and abuse. *J Gerontol Nurs.* 1995;21(2):11,43.
6. Ashley J, Fulmer TT. No simple way to determine elder abuse. *Geriatr Nurs.* 1988;9(5):286-288.
7. Delunas LR. Prevention of elder abuse: Betty Newman health care systems approach. *Clin Nurse Spec.* 1990;4(1):54-58.
8. Magilvy JK, Congdon JG, Martinez R. Circles of care: home care and community support for rural older adults. *Adv Nurs Sci.* 1994;16(3):22-33.
9. Criner JA. The nurse's role in preventing abuse of elderly patients. *Rehab Nurs.* 1994;19(5):277-280.
10. Kingston P, Penhale B. A major problem needing recognition: assessment and management of elder abuse and neglect. *Professional Nurse.* 1994;9(5):343-347.
11. Holland LR, Kasraian KR, Leonardelli CA. Elder abuse: an analysis of the current problem and potential role of the rehabilitation professional. *Physical and Occupational Therapy in Geriatrics.* 1987;5(3):41-50.
12. Phillips LR, Rempusheski VF. A decision-making model for diagnosing and intervening in elder abuse and neglect. *Nurs Res.* 1985;34(3):134-139.
13. Clark-Daniels C, Daniels RS, Baumhover LA. The dilemma of elder abuse. *Home Healthcare Nurse.* 1990; 8(6):7-12.
14. Fulmer T, Ashley J. Clinical indicators of elder neglect. *Appl Nurs Res.* 1989;2(4):161-167.
15. Phillips LR. Elder abuse—what is it? Who says so? *Geriat Nurs.* 1983;4(3):167-170.
16. Fagg J. Detection of abuse. *Nurs Times.* 1994;90(37):66-68.
17. Hudson MF, Johnson TF. Elder neglect and abuse: a review of the literature. *Ann Rev Gerontology and Geriat.* 1986;6:81-134.
18. O'Malley TA, Everitt DE, O'Malley HC, Campion EW. Identifying and preventing family-mediated abuse and neglect of elderly persons. *Ann Intern Med.* 1983;98:998-1005.
19. *Minnesota State Statute.* 1989: Statute no. 626.557.
20. Rose MH, Killien M. Risk and vulnerability: a case for differentiation. *Adv Nurs Sci.* 1983; 5(3):60-73.
21. Wolf RS. Elder abuse: Scope, characteristics, and treatment. *Nurse Practitioner Forum.* 1990;1(2):102-108.
22. Galbraith MW, Zdorkowski RT. Teaching the investigation of elder abuse. *J Gerontol Nurs.* 1984;10(12):21-25.
23. Midenberger C, Wessman HC. Abuse and neglect of elderly persons by family members: a special communication. *Physical Therapy.* 1986;66(4):537-539.
24. Baillie V, Norbeck JS, Barnes LE. Stress, social support, and psychological distress of family caregivers of the elderly. *Nurs Res.* 1988;37(4):217-222.
25. All A. A literature review: assessment and intervention in elder abuse. *J Gerontol Nurs.* 1994;20(7):25-32.
26. Hickey T, Douglass RL. Mistreatment of the elderly in the domestic setting: an exploratory study. *Am J Public Health.* 1981;71(5):500-507.
27. Beck CM, Ferguson D. Aged abuse. *J Gerontol Nurs.* 1981;7(6):333-336.
28. Sayles-Cross S. Profile of familial elder abuse: a selected review of the literature. *J Comm Health Nurs.* 1988;5(4):209-219.
29. Podnieks E. The victimization of older person. *Can J Psychiatric Nurs.* 1987;28(1):6-11.
30. Spence DM. The elder assessment team: protecting elders from abuse and neglect. *Nurs Admin Quarterly.* 1990;14(2):24-28.
31. Fulmer TT, Cahill R. Assessing elder abuse: a study. *J Gerontol Nurs.* 1984;10(12):16-20.
32. Phillips LR, Morrison EF, Chae YM. The QUALCARE Scale: developing an instrument to measure quality of home care. *International J Nurs Stud.* 1990;27(1):61-75.
33. Jewell SE. Discovery of the discharge process: a study of patient discharge from a care unit for elderly people. *J Adv Nurs.* 1993;18(8):1288-1296.

Chapter 25

Nursing Process: Teaching Elderly Patients

Cheryl Dellasega, GNP, PhD, Darlene Clark, RN, MS, Amy Helmuth, RN, MS, Delores McCreary, RN, MS, and Patricia Schan, RN, MS

OVERVIEW

Patient education is one of the many recognized roles of the gerontological nurse. Teaching elderly adults in any health care setting requires special approaches to accommodate the many age-related changes that influence the ability to learn and retain new information. Although specific content will vary, use of the nursing process can assist gerontological nurses with planning, implementing, and evaluating effective teaching programs for their elderly patients in both institutional and community settings. The stages of the nursing process are outlined as they specifically address the development of a patient education program.

INTRODUCTION

Older people are primary consumers of care. Nurses in any health care setting are in frequent interaction with elderly patients who need patient education related to various aspects of their health care regimen. Nurses, having expertise in gerontological health issues, are in an ideal position to teach elders and their families how to adopt behaviors that lead to optimal health. A survey of nurse administrators confirmed that "development of patient education programs specific to the needs of the elderly patient" is seen as a key nursing role in both acute and long-term care facilities.[1] Furthermore, education is a key intervention in preventing adverse drug reactions in older adults.[2]

Education of older patients requires the same principles; however, incorporating the knowledge of gerontology is imperative. In the present age of cost cutting and discharging patients early from acute care settings, education is not necessarily considered a priority. It is not uncommon for this to take place the day of discharge or at the elevator when the patient is leaving. Nurses, as well as other members of the team, are frustrated by this. Developing a teaching plan on admission can eliminate a last-minute approach.

Patient education is always individualized, and applying guidelines about specific needs of older individuals can provide the basis for an effective teaching plan. Awareness of common physical and psychosocial changes occurring during the later years, as well as incorporating the nursing process, can equip the gerontological nurse with the necessary skills to educate elderly patients on a variety of topics.[3]

Many age-related changes have the potential to affect an older person's ability to learn new material. Modification of traditional teaching approaches to address special needs of older patients will enhance the effectiveness of the teaching plan. For example, alterations in short-term memory may make it difficult for an older person to learn and retain new information unless educational strategies are structured accordingly.

Sensory impairments, specifically decreased vision and hearing, may alter an elderly patient's ability to learn and retain new information. Musculoskeletal limitations may affect the ability to carry out skills, as can a generalized slowing of nerve conduction, which delays reaction time.

Motivation is key to any patient education program developed for older people. It is important before beginning any program to ascertain from patients if they desire to improve[4] (see Chapter 21, *Obesity in Older Adults*). Creating an environment of trust as well as a desire to improve in the face of major chronicity is a difficult challenge that must be undertaken. Sociocultural factors, such as loss of support systems and financial difficulties, also can affect the ability of older people to learn new behaviors.

Since teaching is more than the mere giving of information, it requires a well-developed program for each individual patient. The steps of the nursing process—assessment, nursing diagnosis and goal setting, planning, intervention, and evaluation—provide nurses with the natural progression to develop an individualized patient education program.[5]

THE NURSING PROCESS

ASSESSMENT

Assessment of the older person's learning needs and motivation to change behavior should be carried out by the gerontological nurse. It is important to list any age-related changes that may influence the patient's ability to learn and act upon new information. Include both physiological and psychological. Screen for changes in sensory function, as well as cognitive status. Physical limitations, such as arthritis or impaired mobility, that might prevent the patient from achieving treatment outcomes should also be noted. A general evaluation of overall health can enable the gerontological nurse to recognize other conditions that might impair learning.

Other information about the older individual that can provide valuable insight for the nurse/teacher includes educational level and the patient's ability to read. Asking about prior experience in reference to learning style and what has proven effective will provide the basis for the teaching plan and eventual intervention strategies. For example, does the person learn best by doing, seeing, or reading? It also is important to ascertain the patient's baseline knowledge about the topic that is being developed. Older people have many personal experiences with the health care system and have developed misconceptions about particular medications or illnesses from their peers.

Available support systems should be included in the initial pre-teaching assessment. Family members are often in the position of providing partial or complete care for an aged individual. Attitudes toward older family members are also important and offer insight on whether the family will encourage individuals to care for themselves or foster dependency. Sociocultural values that are meaningful to both the patient and family, such as religious beliefs, food choices, and ceremonies celebrated, should be identified; these factors greatly influence both the synthesis and eventual success of any teaching plan.

Assessing for financial resources is important prior to developing a teaching plan; there may be monetary constraints that require that the nurse identify for the patient creative alternatives to costly methods of care. The living situation and attendant resources—both in the home and community—need to be described in order to develop realistic goals.

Finally, as previously stated, patient motivation and interest in learning are of paramount importance. Situational factors, such as the learning environment along with personal instincts and developed skills, contribute to motivation and should also be assessed.[4] If the patient shows signs of being uninterested or unreceptive to teaching efforts, even the best attempts at education are destined for failure. Identification of possible barriers to learning, such as pain, discomfort, denial, or fear, may provide a logical first step for nursing intervention prior to implementing the plan.[5,6]

Diagnosis/Goals

The information derived from the assessment now serves as the blueprint for building a teaching plan. Using nursing diagnoses to structure the plan enables the nurse to establish individualized goals that are both measurable and achievable. Careful consideration of what is realistic for older people should be considered, as traditional outcomes may not always be the most appropriate. For example, an older person with many chronic illnesses may not be able to regain lost function; however, he or she may be able to preserve current function and ability. A guiding principle for the gerontological nurse is to support behaviors that maximize the individual's capacity for self-care. This approach not only encourages independence and autonomy in the elderly who desire it, but also promotes a sense of self-esteem.[7]

Plan/Intervention

Several factors related to the actual teaching plan must be taken into consideration before actual implementation occurs. These include the learning environment, subject matter and presentation, attributes of the teacher, and strategies that can enhance compliance.

A comfortable, familiar environment is a vital first step in enhancing the older person's educational experience. If possible, teaching in the patient's own home can provide such a setting.[8] A discharge education program is needed to provide continuity. Home care nurses will reinforce the teaching plan developed.

Physical needs should be provided for by making sure that the patient is not in pain and can comfortably sit and move as desired during the session. Adequate lighting will facilitate communication for those who may be visually or hearing impaired; small intense lights that avoid glare are preferable.[9,10] Temperature and noise levels should be adjusted to desirable levels and privacy ensured. Avoiding interruptions and distractions can further enhance the patient's ability to focus on the nurse/teacher. Modification of the environment to provide comfort and compensate for age-related changes not only facilitates learning, but demonstrates the gerontological nurse's concern for and interest in the patient.

The content of the teaching plan will be shaped not only by the assessment but also by resources that are available to the patient. Incorporating tangible and intangible resources is important. Having a significant other and any needed prompts (audiovisuals, etc.) are equally important.

For an older person, new material is best processed if it is presented in small increments at frequent but manageable intervals.[11] Continual assessment of the patient's energy level is an important consideration; often, the time of day can influence learning ability. Pacing the presentation should allow for both questions and mutual feedback between the teacher and learner to guarantee effective communication. In this way, continuous evaluation of the patient's understanding is apparent.[12] Content selected for inclusion in the teaching plan should initially focus on priorities and have some flexibility to allow for a degree of behavior change. Actively involving the patient in the teaching process can be accomplished by having the patient recite necessary information and demonstrate techniques taught.

Wording and terminology should be carefully chosen; often, medical jargon and slang are potential sources of confusion and misunderstanding. Preview any audiovisual material for readability and comprehension level. Many older people are given preprinted materials that are illegible or unintelligible to them.[13,14] Nurses act as interpreters for the patient. They will need time to process the information and often have questions at a later time. Providing a phone number is helpful in the event, post-discharge, the patient has a question about altering a technique or time for treatment. Providing for questions and concerns to be addressed is very important.

Nurses need to be aware that their attitudes about older people can enhance or inhibit the effectiveness of the teaching plan.[15] From the moment of first contact with a patient, the nurse's credibility can influence subsequent interactions.[9,14] Nurses, often younger than the elderly patients they must teach, are challenged to develop a spirit of motivation and caring about the future health of their patients. Nurses teaching older people must be aware of their own age-related attitudes. Stereotyping or infantilizing an older patient will be counterproductive. Instead, nurses need to be interested in working with the elderly and believe older adults can learn new behaviors and have the ability to care for themselves. One example of an ageist belief system is the assumption that patients who are going from an acute care or community setting to a long-term care facility do not require any type of health education.

A professional appearance can enhance the nurse's credibility. Older people may have difficulty identifying with colored dress, sneakers, and jewelry that is often an acceptable dress code in some facilities. If possible, the same person should follow through on all aspects of the teaching process in order to foster a therapeutic relationship and promote a consistent approach. In addition to considering external attributes, several other internal characteristics of the nurse are important to consider. The ability to be flexible when teaching is important; the most thoroughly prepared efforts may not proceed according to plan. Unanticipated needs, time constraints, lack of interest on the part of the learner, or other unforeseen crises are all possibilities. By constantly assessing the learner's receptiveness and progress, the nurse can modify teaching strategies appropriately.

Knowledge of age-related changes can help the gerontological nurse to use special teaching skills during the actual presentation. Speaking in a lower tone of voice and at a slower pace; being visible; making sure the patient has needed prostheses, such as glasses and/or hearing aids; and allowing increased time for responses are all measures that can offset circumstances that detract from the individual's ability to learn using traditional methods. Appropriate use of touch can also be a helpful reinforcer and means of communication.

Experience of the nurse is another variable that must be considered when implementing the teaching plan. Education of the elderly, who are likely to have complex health care needs, requires special skill and preparation; therefore, a nurse with advanced preparation, such as a gerontological nurse clinician, is the most qualified person to carry out this process. If a gerontological nurse clinician is not available to provide the direct teaching, the nurse developing the plan should have it appraised by a supervisor prior to its implementation.

EVALUATION

Any teaching plan should be thoroughly evaluated at its conclusion in order to determine whether the learner has understood and retained desired material. Clues about the effectiveness of learning can be obtained immediately from the types of questions the patient asks, as well as statements and/or comments made. In addition to subjective feedback, nurses can ask the patient to demonstrate new skills, which provides an observable behavior indicative of learning. These same observations can and should be made of family members and significant others who are involved in the teaching process and who will assist with care in the home setting.

The initial goals that were established early in the teaching plan can provide a measurable standard for teaching effectiveness. If the goal was not reached, the home care nurse may have the responsibility of setting more realistic goals. Ongoing evaluation of the patient's health status by nurses in varied settings offers clues about the effectiveness of initial teaching efforts and provides for continued identification of learning needs.

The effectiveness of a teaching plan is reflected in the physical and psychological well-being of the patient. Nonadherence is a signal to the nurse that an intentional or unintentional breakdown has occurred in communication between the professional and patient. For older individuals, unintentional nonadherence is more often the case and often results from physical barriers (eg, being unable to open pill bottles or read labels) or social factors (eg, having financial limitations or living alone).[16]

If the patient is returning to a community setting, feedback from the local pharmacist can offer valuable insight into the patient's ability to adhere to a medication schedule. Another helpful resource is the primary care provider, who may be receiving telephone calls or visits from the patient, which indicate that the patient did not fully understand the needed self-care behaviors related to the treatment plan.

The older person who is being discharged from an acute care facility also needs to be closely evaluated and frequently reassessed during the initial discharge period, because hospital-induced delirium may persist into the post-discharge period.[17] Delirium, a temporary alteration in cognition that is likely to affect elderly patients in the hospital setting, interferes with the ability to learn new information.[18] Often a return to a familiar environment can bring about a dramatic improvement in mental status.

The evaluation component is very important to begin re-assessment for better health and prevention of exacerbation and possible recidivism. Monitoring and reassessment after discharge from the acute care setting can be accomplished with a daily telephone call to the patient as a means for evaluating cognitive status. An instrument developed[19] makes assessment of mental status by telephone feasible. Home visits by the nurse will provide first-hand evaluation of how the patient is readjusting and coping post-discharge. Referrals to home health agencies are another important resource for older patients who require follow-up care and continued teaching once they leave the institutional setting.

GERONTOLOGICAL NURSING IMPLICATIONS

Patient education, often an afterthought in the patient treatment plan, is the key to opening a door to promotion of health and the further prevention of disease. That door must be opened for older patients. Nurses caring for older people have a responsibility to initially set the stage for the patient to view what is on the other side of the door. It could be walking, painlessness, restoration of ability once thought lost, or just a feeling of well being.

Promoting adherence to a patient education/health care regimen is the ultimate goal to be achieved. The older patient must see value in the plan, which is the incentive to achieve health. Gerontological nurses must present a realistic picture for their older patients and identify desired behaviors needed to achieve the goal.

Support systems to reinforce continued use of the behavior also should be employed. Involve peers who have had similar experiences or significant others directly involved in care.[20] Both the individual and significant others need to know the value of continued positive reinforcement.[21,22] If significant others value continued independence in the older loved one, then the patient will also value the dependence to be achieved. For example, use of a pre-discharge medication schedule can enhance independence in patients post-discharge.[23] If an organized system for use in the post-discharge setting can be developed, adaptations that may need to be made in the home environment can be carried out. Patients should describe possible barriers they might anticipate that would affect their performance with the prescribed regimen. The gerontological nurse can then develop alternative strategies.

Communicating with members of the health care team is necessary to enhance effectiveness of the plan as well as obtain needed feedback. Referrals to appropriate others should be made to provide continued follow-up and reassessment. Referrals are made to home care agencies by the case manager/discharge planner. Follow-up is important as the patient and family must not feel abandoned in their "new beginning" toward health.

Preparing the patient to deal with possible setbacks once he or she is more independent can prevent frustration and promote adherence. Although the goal is for patients to be able to care for themselves to their utmost ability, the nurse should stress that ongoing assistance from health care professionals is always available.

Health teaching is an ongoing process, requiring application of all aspects of the nursing process. A recognized expert in gerontological nursing is the most appropriate person to assume responsibility for education of the elderly patient. The role of the nurse as teacher is a role that can enable older patients not only to participate as fully as possible in their care, but also to experience a quality life in their later years.

REFERENCES

1. Heine C. The gerontological nurse specialist: Examination of the role. *CNS.* 1988;2(1):6-11.
2. Stewart T, Cooper J. Polypharmacy in the aged: practical solutions. *Drugs and Aging.* 1994;4(6):449-461.
3. Mackay L. The nurse's role in giving nutritional advice. *Professional Nurse.* 1995;10(7):427-428.
4. Ford D. *Humans as Self-Constructing Living Systems: A Developmental Perspective on Behavior and Personality.* State College: Ideals, Inc.; 1994.
5. Simmons J, Nelson E, Roberts E, Salisbury L, Kane-Williams E, Benson L. A health promotion program: staying healthy after fifty. *Health Ed Quarterly.* 1989;16(4):461-472.
6. Welch-McCafferty D. To teach or not to teach? Overcoming barriers to patient education in geriatric oncology. *Oncology News Forum.* 1986;13:25-31.
7. Burnside I. *Nursing and the Aged: A Self-Care Approach.* (3rd ed.). New York: McGraw-Hill; 1988.
8. Dellasega C. Self-care for the elderly diabetic. *J Gerontol Nurs.* 1990;16(1):16-20.
9. Collette C. Assessing the patient education needs of the elderly. *Medical Times.* 1988;116:95-99.
10. Stanton M. Teaching patients: some basic lessons for nurse educators. *Nursing Management.* 1985;16:59-62.
11. Gress L, Bahr R. *The Aging Person: A Holistic Perspective.* St. Louis: Mosby; 1984.
12. Knowles M. *The Modern Practice of Adult Education.* Chicago: Follet; 1980.
13. Streiff D. Can clients understand our instructions? *Image.* 1986;18:48-52.
14. Potter P, Perry A. *Fundamentals of Nursing: Concepts, Process, and Practice.* (2nd ed.). St. Louis: Mosby; 1989.
15. Demuth J. Patient teaching in the ambulatory setting. *Nurs Clin N Amer.* 1989;24(3):645-654.
16. Richardson J. Perspectives on compliance with drug regimens among the elderly. *J Compliance Health Care.* 1986;1(1):33-45.
17. Lipowski Z. Delirium (acute confusional states). *JAMA.* 1987;258:1789-1792.
18. Pousada L, Leipzig R. Rapid bedside assessment of perioperative confusion in older patients. *Geriatrics.* 1990;45,59-64.
19. Brandt J, Spencer M, Folstein M. The telephone interview for cognitive status. *Neuropsychiatry, Neuropsychology, and Behavioral Neurology.* 1988;1,111-117.
20. Allen J. New lives for old: lifestyle change incentives among adult adults. *Health Values.* 1986;10:8-18.
21. Hassey L, Gilliand K. Compliance, low literacy, and locus of control. *Nurs Clin N Amer.* 1989;24(3):605-615.
22. King K. Selected behavioral strategies for the health educator. *Health Ed.* 1982;13:35-37.
23. Esposito L. The effects of medication education on adherence to medication regimens in an elderly population. *J Adv Nurs.* 1993;21(5):335-343.

Chapter 26

Geriatric Falls: Prevention Strategies for the Staff

Rebecca Brady, BSN, RNC, CNA, Francis R. Chester, MPA, RN, CPQA, Linda L. Pierce, MSN, RNC, CRRN, Judith P. Salter, MSN, RN, CRRN, Sharon Schreck, RN, and Rosanne Radziewicz, MSN, RN, CS

OVERVIEW

It is estimated that by the year 2030, 21.2% of the population in the United States will be 65 years or older.[1,2] Aging, and many of the disorders common in late life, can increase the risk for falling. Falls among the elderly are the second leading cause of accidental death.[3] Another complication of falls is a significant incidence of "fear of falling," which results in a negative effect on self-confidence, self-efficacy, and independence.[4]

Hospitalized patients account for up to 90% of all reported falls that occur.[5] Furthermore, the risk for falling is noted to be significantly greater in the hospitalized elderly than in other hospitalized age groups.[6] Annually, about 50% of institutionalized elderly patients will fall. Many of these patients will fall several times. Repeat falls in institutions are a serious problem.[7] This hazard provides a significant risk for nurses, health care personnel, and institutions caring for the geriatric population. Inpatient falls, besides having a negative effect on the people caring for these patients, are also costly to all parties involved.

This chapter will describe quality improvement efforts to decrease the incidence of geriatric falls. These efforts were developed following research at the MetroHealth Center for Rehabilitation in Cleveland. Presented is the protocol for the program and a staff inservice program designed to heighten awareness of falls.

INTRODUCTION

There is an abundance of literature regarding patient falls. Most studies focus on risk factors and populations that have a higher incidence of falls. Consistently reported intrinsic variables that increase risk for falls include a history of previous falls, increased age, and gait problems.[8,9]

One-fourth to one-half of hospitalized patients who fall have experienced a previous fall, either prior to or during their admissions.[10-12] A number of authors have noted that the risk of falls increases as a person ages.[11] Johnson[10] states that multiple falls and injuries are more prevalent among the elderly older than 75. A significant relationship between gait problems and falls has been established.[13] Other personal characteristics that have been found to increase the risk for falls are agitation, confusion, impaired mental status, impaired gait and balance, sensory impairment, urinary and bladder dysfunction, and medical diagnostic categories, including cancer and cardiovascular, neurologic, and cerebrovascular diseases. Polypharmacy, substance abuse, certain drug classifications, and psychosocial issues also contribute to increasing the risk for falls.[7,12,14-17]

Falls in the population aged 60 to 75 years can be attributed to the interaction between age-related changes and environmental factors. Falls in this age group are largely attributed to slipping and tripping. In contrast, adults older than 75 years fall due to a combination of disease and medical-related factors.[7] The literature cites extrinsic characteristics that place patients at risk for falls. Environmental factors such as unstable furniture, elevated bed positions, smooth floors, poorly soled or unsafe footwear, and dim lighting in rooms and hallways are identified as contributors to patient falls.[18]

In general, studies of time-related factors reveal few significant relationships between falls and time of day, or day of week, month, or season.[19] When falls do occur, it is often during the first week of hospitalization and again after the third week.[11] Despite the multiple risk factors identified for falls in the elderly, no high-risk profiles have been developed with adequate sensitivity and specificity to be useful as a predictive tool.[18]

METHODS

Elderly patients admitted to MetroHealth Medical Center for Rehabilitation exhibited many of the characteristics associated with falls. Statistics showed an increased rate of geriatric falls. In addition to claims for injuries related to falls, there were additional expenses incurred from increased lengths of stay, diagnostic/treatment procedures, and emotional suffering of both the patients and the nursing staff.

Retrospective Chart Review

A baseline regarding patient falls was established by a retrospective chart review (*n*=71 cases) conducted in a quality improvement effort on a 28-bed geriatric rehabilitation unit. Falls were examined during a 10-month period. A fall was defined as an uncontrolled and undirected occurrence in which the patient comes to rest on the floor.[17]

The greatest incidence of falling occurred during the first (23%) and the fifth (26%) weeks of hospitalization. The highest percentage of falls occurred during the day shift, with 6% at 8 a.m. and 15% occurring between 2 p.m. and 3 p.m. Eight percent of evening shift falls happened at 10 p.m. During the night shift, 8% of the falls occurred between 5 a.m. and 6 a.m. The remaining percentage of falls revealed no specific trend.

Falls most frequently occur in the patients' rooms or bathrooms when they are on their own. Analysis of the 71 total number of falls reveals a group of 36 patients. The largest percentage of fallers from this group were in the 70 to 79 age range; men were predominant. The largest percentage of women were also in this age group. The activity that patients were trying to accomplish at the time of the fall included attempting to get into the bathroom, leaning forward in their chairs, and transferring in and out of bed.

Quality Improvement Activity

A review of the retrospective chart audit results revealed that patients whose needs are anticipated and met fall less. The results showed that the need to toilet, seek rest, or obtain nutrition and hydration were activities prevalent at peak fall times or at the time of an actual patient fall. A quality improvement monitor was designed to provide proactive nursing interventions to reduce potential falls during four peak fall times based upon patient care needs identified in the audit.

The four peak fall times were chosen to implement the nursing interventions. Thirty minutes before these times, a nursing staff member asked each patient on the unit if there was a need for toileting, assistance in and out of bed or wheelchair, or fluids/nourishment. The nursing staff intervened to meet identified needs and reinforced calling for assistance for future needs. Examples of questions and interventions were included on the data collection form to ensure conformity of approach to each patient (Figure 26-1).

Twenty-five patients were included in this quality improvement monitor, which was conducted over a 2-week period. Staff compliance with the interventions during this same time was 86%. The outcome criterion, to decrease patient falls without injury by 50% for a 2-week period, was met. A comparison between falls occurring during the monitor period and the same time frame for the years 1989 and 1990 showed an 80% and 88% decrease in falls, respectively. The success in reducing the number of falls through proactive nursing interventions supported the belief that patients whose needs are anticipated and met fall less.

Fall prevention was clearly the focus of this program, rather than an identification of characteristics or risk factors associated with falls. The falls prevention program is clearly an outgrowth from previous literature and the need to improve the life of older people at risk for falling. Development of the MetroHealth Falls Prevention Program incorporated these practice measures in conjunction with identified risk factors.

THE FALLS PREVENTION PROGRAM

A nursing task force was convened to address patient falls at the Medical Center. Membership consisted of staff nurses, unit managers, and clinical nurse specialists from rehabilitation and acute geriatric units, as well as representatives from education and quality assurance. The Falls Task Force agreed that the approach to decrease patient falls would be simply to focus on nursing interventions and reduce risk factors for falls within a nurse implementation model. Every attempt was made to work within the present staff workforce. The task force worked on two nursing units and produced the Falls Prevention Protocol.

Protocol

The Falls Prevention Protocol was developed to outline the nursing responsibilities and management for a patient at risk for falls (Figure 26-2). Protocols were classified as dependent, independent, or interdependent.[20] Results from a quality improvement falls study historically find that staff nurse actions include all independent functions and orders. This Falls Prevention Protocol is classified as independent, to reflect autonomous nursing actions and functions that require only a nursing order to implement.

Quality Assurance Data Collection Form
Standard: Potential for injury
Nursing Diagnosis (Indicator): Sensory/Motor/Cognitive deficits
Outcome Criteria:
Decrease patient falls without injury by 50% for a 2-week period.
Nursing will document evidence of proactive interventions to reduce potential falls during peak activity times.
Process Criteria:
Note: If patient transfers to another unit, please discontinue this form and place in an envelope.
Ask need for and/or assist with toileting
Offer fluids and/or nourishments
Ask need for and/or assist with transferring patient in/out of bed or wheelchair
Reinforce verbally to call for assistance
Indicate any fall(s)
Indicate if restraints of any type are being used
Process Criteria Format (example of Questions and Interventions to Follow):
Toileting Needs "Do you need to go to the bathroom?" Offer appropriate means—bedpan, urinal, bedside commode, or assist to bathroom. Remind patient with Foley catheter, "Mrs. S, remember you have the catheter to drain your urine. It will go into this bag." Offer to show bag and/or tubing.
Fluids and/or Nourishment Needs "Would you like anything to drink?" Try to keep water pitcher full and offer snacks, if appropriate. For patients with fluid restriction: "Mrs. S, you are on a fluid restriction, but I will bring you a drink of water or juice at 1 P.M."
Patient in Need of Assistance When leaving room, always ask if there is anything else that you can get for them or that they need. Remind them to call the nurse and that you will help them. For ambulating patient (ad lib): "Please call if you need anything and I or another nurse will assist you if you do not feel well." For patient on bed rest: "Please do not try to get out of bed without assistance due to (possible weakness, dizziness, equipment, etc.) Please call and I or another nurse will assist you so you do not hurt yourself." Ensure that the following duties are carried out: call light, bedside stand, over-the-bed table, and other necessary items are within easy reach; side rails are up; and lights are on or off, as appropriate.

Figure 26-1. Form for quality assurance data collection.

Assessment, intervention, reportable conditions, patient/significant other instruction, and documentation were the areas addressed in the nursing intervention section of the protocol. According to the protocol, the nurse is responsible for assessing the cognitive, sensory, and mobility status of patients on each shift. The criteria for degree of risk for falls are based on a level system focusing on these assessment areas. Level 1 patients would demonstrate no deficits, while Level 2 patients would demonstrate a deficit in one or more areas.

The intervention section focuses on strategies the nurse would implement for each patient level. The interventions content in Level 1 include basic nursing interventions, such as placing the call bell within the patient's reach and lowering the bed. Examples of Level 2 interventions include addressing the potential for injury through the standard nursing care plan (Potential for Injury) or through another related nursing care plan, reinforcing patient calls for assistance, and offering assistance for toileting.

Additionally, Level 2 interventions to alert the staff were developed by the Falls Task Force and had not previously been used at MetroHealth Medical Center. Included in these interventions are placement of a yellow wrist band on the patient and posting of yellow signs that indicate implementation of the falls program above the bed and outside the patient's room. Note that Level 2 patient interventions incorporate all Level 1 patient interventions.

Reportable conditions include any patient fall or change in cognitive, sensory, or mobility conditions. Instruction to the patient and/or significant other is an orientation and reinforcement of the falls program. To help accomplish this task, a simple, easy-to-read handout was developed that explains the program and contains guidelines for preventing falls. In the documentation section, the nurse is directed to document assessments in the medical record and/or applicable flow sheets. Initiation or the discontinuation of Level 2 interventions is based on ongoing patient assessment.

AWARENESS CAMPAIGN

Although the literature strongly supports increased nursing awareness to reduce patient falls, few articles suggest involvement of other professional and nonprofessional staff members.[14,15,17,21] The Task Force agreed that, to be successful, the program must include the support and assistance of all individuals who have contact with a patient during hospitalization.

Two types of education programs were designed: one for nursing staff members and one for other professional and nonprofessional staff members. The nursing staff education component consisted of orientation to and implementation of the protocol. The non-nursing staff was introduced to the Falls Prevention Program by focusing on what must be done to assist patients at risk for falls. Notifying the area staff when a patient, identified at risk for falls, is brought to or returned to the area is an example of such assistance.

The awareness campaign was designed to heighten consciousness of the staff, regardless of the type of patient contact. Included was a week-long falls prevention poster presentation given at key times in the employee cafeteria. A one-page brochure describing the Falls Prevention Program was distributed to employees at this time.

Falls Prevention Protocol

Initiated	Discontinued
Date: Time: RN:	Date: Time: RN:

Purpose: To outline nursing responsibilities and management for a patient at risk for falling.

Level: Independent (requires nursing order only).

Supportive Date: A fall is defined as an uncontrolled and undirected occurrence in which the patient comes to rest on the floor. All patients are at risk for falls by virtue of hospitalization and treatment. Two levels for falls are identified. As the levels progress, the potential for falls becomes greater.

NURSING INTERVENTIONS

Assessment

1. Perform admission assessment and every 8 hours in the following areas: cognitive, sensory and mobility
2. Assess degree of risk for falling according to the following criteria:
   - Level 1 patients: Demonstrate no cognitive, sensory, and mobility deficits.
   - Level 2 patients: Demonstrate a deficit in one or more areas: cognitive, sensory or mobility (ie, untreated visual impairment, impaired judgment, unsteady gait, disorientation); and/or a previous history of falls.

Intervention

3. If patient is assessed as Level 1:
   Ensure the call bell is in reach
   Lower the bed
   Lock the wheels of beds and wheelchairs, as appropriate
4. If patient is assessed as Level 2:
   Address potential for injury through standard care plan or other related nursing care plans
   Alert all care givers and staff of the patient's potential for falling by:
      Replacing patient's identification band with yellow ident-a-band
      Placing yellow signs indicating implementation of the falls program over the patient's bed and outside the patient's room
      Assess cognitive, sensory and mobility deficits every shift
   Every 4 hours as necessary:
      a) Implement Level 1 interventions
      b) Ensure the side rails are up
      c) Reinforce calling for assistance
      d) Offer assistance for toileting
      e) Offer fluids and nutrition
      f) offer transfer assistance

Reportable conditions

5. Any patient falls
6. Any significant changes in cognitive, sensory, or mobility conditions

Patient/significant other instruction

7. Orient to and reinforce falls program

Documentation

8. Record initiation of falls prevention protocol on progress note in the medical record
9. Record changes in assessment findings in the medical record
10. Initiate or discontinue the intervention levels based on ongoing patient assessment

Figure 26-2. Falls Prevention Protocol. Adapted from Dallaire LB. Reducing patient falls. *Nursing 89*. 1989;19(5):78-79; and Hendrich AL. An effective unit-based fall prevention program. *Journal of Nursing Quality Assurance*. 1988;3(1):28-36.

GERONTOLOGICAL NURSING IMPLICATIONS

Implications for the practice of gerontological nursing include minimizing unsafe patient activity to provide a conducive environment that is less restraining. Autonomy and self-esteem are supported if the geriatric patient, already dealing with multiple losses, is spared the additional loss of freedom. The nurse can maintain a sense of control over patient safety without the ethical and legal concerns of restraining.

While only 5% to 6% of falls result in serious injuries, there exists the added consequences of embarrassment; a loss of confidence (fallaphobia); restricted activity; a sense of fragility and vulnerability; and depression that nursing interventions must attempt to prevent.[7] The age-old belief that the elderly fall as an inevitable result of aging must be challenged by gerontological nurses. Educating geriatric patients and their families to the reality that falls can be minimized, if not prevented, is an important part of teaching.[2,7] Resources, such as the call light and the phone, which permit access to assistance and support, can provide a psychological safety net and alleviate the need for unsafe activity on the part of patients. Simple trust-building behaviors on the part of the nurse, such as returning to the patient at a promised time, letting the patient know preventing injury is a goal, can also enhance the patient's sense of safety and limit unsafe behaviors in the unfamiliar clinical setting.[22]

Planned interventions throughout the shift have implications for time management. Allowing for nursing interventions at prearranged times alleviates responding to multiple patient calls for assistance in the midst of other work activities or the more time-consuming response to a fall.

Any measures to reduce falls directly impacts health care expenditures, which decrease the burden to society and the health care system. Nurses must take the lead in assessment for falls risk and intervention for the prevention of falls for the geriatric patient. Development and implementation of falls prevention programs are crucial in decreasing health care costs. This responsibility for education and prevention extends not only to patients and families, but also to all health care providers. In this time of rapid change, improving quality of services to geriatric patients could easily be lost in the pressures for reorganization, budget cuts, and managed care. Using an assessment method that is grounded in the perceptions of the staff delivering services within an organization and implementing a team approach to solve the problems of geriatric patients can prove to be worthwhile not only from the patients' point of view, but also from the organization's point of view.

Implications for further nursing research into falls are multiple. Clinical decision-making variables that impact on nursing behaviors associated with preventing patient falls need further investigation. Nurses must develop the ability to combine their observations/assessments with clinical knowledge in a way that fosters anticipatory and proactive nursing interventions, which prevent falls in the geriatric inpatient population.[22] Exploring systems that focus on nursing interventions in populations susceptible to falls, in combination with the identified risks of fallers, may be the key to further eradication of preventable falls. It is imperative that health care organizations formulate actions to improve the quality of services and continue to implement new and innovative programs, especially in times of overwhelming change and chaos.[23]

REFERENCES

1. Liptzin B. The geriatric patient and general hospital psychiatry. *Gen Hosp Psychiatry.* 1987;9:198-202.
2. Miller CA. *Nursing Care of Older Adults: Theory and Practice.* Glenview, IL: Scott, Foresman/Little, Brown Higher Education; 1990.
3. National Safety Council. *Accident Facts.* Chicago: NSC; 1987:9-11.
4. Tinetti M, Powell L. Fear of falling and low self-efficacy: a cause of dependence in elderly person. *Journal of Gerontology.* 1993; 48:(Special Issue)35-38.
5. Raz T, Baretich M. Factors affecting the incidence of patient falls in hospitals. *Med Care.* 1987;25(3):185-195.
6. Rhymes J, Jaeger R. Falls: Prevention and management in the institutional setting. *Clin Geriatr Med.* 1988;4(3):613-622.
7. Miller JM. Falling and the Elderly. In: Stanley M, Beare P, eds. *Gerontological Nursing.* Philadelphia: F.A. Davis Co.; 1993:281-296.
8. Gross YT, Shimamato Y, Rose CL, Frank B. Why do they fall? Monitoring risk factors in nursing homes. *J Gerontol Nurs.* 1990; 16(6):20-25.
9. Maciorowski L, Munro B, Dietrick-Gallagher M, et al. A review of the patient fall literature. *J Nurs Quality Assurance.* 1988;3(1):18-27.
10. Johnson E. Accidental falls among geriatric patients: can more be prevented? *J Natl Med Assoc.* 1986;77:633-639.
11. Tack K, Ulrich B, Kehr C. Patient falls: profile for prevention. *J Neurosci Nurs.* 1987;19(2):83-89.
12. Miller C. Mobility and Safety. *Nursing Care of Older Adults: Theory and Practice.* Philadelphia: J.B. Lippincott Co.; 1995.
13. Tinetti M, Williams T, Mayewski R. Fall risk index for elderly patients based on number of chronic disabilities. *Am J Med.* 1987; 80:429-434.
14. Grant J, Hamilton S. Falls in a rehabilitation center: a retrospective and comparative analysis. *Rehabilitation Nursing.* 1987;12:74-76.
15. Hill B, Johnson R, Garrett B. Reducing the incidence of falls in high risk patients. *JONA.* 1988;18(7/8):24-28.
16. Lamb K, Miller J, Hernandez M. Falls in the elderly: causes and prevention. *Orthopaedic Nurs.* 1987;6(2):45-49.
17. Mion L, Gregor S, Buettner M, et al. Falls in the rehabilitation setting: incidence and characteristics. *Rehabilitation Nurs.* 1989;14:17-21.
18. Whedon MB, Shedd P. Prediction and prevention of patient falls. *Image.* 1989;21(2):108-114.
19. DeVincenzo D, Watkins S. Accidental falls in a rehabilitation setting. *Rehabilitation Nursing.* 1987;12:248-252.
20. Smith-Marker C. *Setting Standards for Professional Nursing: The Marker Model.* St. Louis: C.V. Mosby; 1988.
21. Hendrich A. An effective unit-based fall prevention plan. *J Nurs Quality Assurance.* 1988;3(1):28-36.
22. Turkoski B, Schreck S, Salter J, Radziewicz R, Pierce LL, Guhde J, Brady R. Clinical nursing judgment related to reducing the incidence of in-patient falls among the elderly. *Unpublished research.* 1994.
23. Rantz M, Davis ND, Tapp RA. Assessing elderly acute care services: improving quality amid chaos. *J Nurs Care Quality.* 1995;9(3):1-9.

Chapter 27

Providing Social Support for Disabled Long-Term Care Residents: Choice and Unit-Based Activities

Winifred WindRiver, RN, MSN

OVERVIEW

Social isolation, and the loneliness that usually results, seldom appear on a list of health problems requiring nursing diagnosis. Yet they flourish in every long-term care institution and may result in physical deterioration, mental illness, and even death.[1-3] Gerontological nurses in long-term care must make it a high priority to detect and assess social isolation and undertake a plan of systematic intervention drawn from the growing body of research about the human necessity for social support (see Chapter 6, *Gerontology, Spirituality, and Nursing*). In the words of St. Francis of Assisi, "Where there is despair, let me sow hope; where there is darkness, let me sow light; where there is sadness, let me sow joy."

INTRODUCTION

Those who require institutionalization are usually surrounded by people with whom they feel little commonality. *Social loneliness* results from the lack of a group with which to affiliate and identify as an accepted member. This can cause feelings of boredom, aimlessness, and marginality that may lead to an anxious, compulsive search for activities or groups. *Emotional loneliness* results from the lack of a close, intimate attachment to one other person, such as a spouse or confidant. Choice, mutuality, reciprocity, trust, and delight develop cumulatively as intimacy between them matures. Separation from this person increases the likelihood that depression may accompany such challenging events as institutionalization and declining health, as well as separation through death.[4] Isolation from family (emotional) and friends (social), these two ways of being "lonely in a crowd," may exist separately or together, and can result in shame, self-doubt, withdrawal, and even rage.[1,5,6]

Interventions that provide adequate social support are essential for any person's health and longevity, especially the lonely. Norbeck describes social support as "a network of communication and mutual obligation."[3] This includes emotional intimacy, one-way or mutual assistance, an exchange of information, and companionship.[7] Powers found that an

TABLE 27-1

Patient Assessment of Social Support

EVALUATE THE ABILITY TO SOCIALIZE

Consult the medical record, direct patient assessment:

- Mental functioning
- Communication skills
- Vision
- Mobility
- Independence

Preference for isolation or discomfort with social integrations:

- Less able to socialize
- Attentive family
- Values self-reliance

EVALUATE EXISTING SUPPORT*: CONSULT THE RESIDENT, SIGNIFICANT OTHERS, THE MEDICAL RECORD, AND DIRECT OBSERVATION

Quality of support (resident's view):

- Negative/Positive
- Emotional support
- Information
- Gifts, material exchanges
- Assistance
- Who gives, who receives
- Length of the relationship
- Subjective meaning of the relationship

Quantity of support:

- Intensity of interactions
- Frequency of contact

Social network type:

- Institution-centered
- Small cluster
- Kin-centered
- Balanced

EVALUATE THE NEED FOR ADDITIONAL SUPPORT

Look for the warning signs:

- Recent loss
- Failed social initiative
- Aggression, interpersonal problems
- Poor self-image, depression
- Confusion, difficulty making decisions
- Feeling confined or deserted
- Suicide thoughts or attempts

Ask patient his or her preference:

- Group activities
- One close friend
- Solitary activity

* Sources outside the institution include friends, relatives, neighbors, church members, and formal and informal group associations. Sources inside include friends, roommates, interdisciplinary staff members, and mealtime companions.

adequate network of support enhances self-esteem and provides assistance in coping with stress.[8]

ASSESSMENT AND PLANNING

For each resident who exhibits symptoms of social isolation, the gerontological nurse must assess 1) the existence and availability of social support, 2) the need and desire for particular patterns of supportive relationships, and 3) the ability to establish and maintain social contacts (Table 27-1). Information about social support that is available can be obtained from the resident, the family, medical records, the Activities Director, and the Social Worker. The nurse will have ultimate responsibility to identify problems of social isolation and develop a plan of care.

EXISTING SUPPORT

The resident is the best person to appraise the quality of support a particular relationship provides. Both the positive and negative aspects of relationships must be evaluated. It is important to identify the entire network of existing relationships both outside and within the institution. Previous studies suggest that the longer a person resides in a long-term care facility, the fewer visits and the fewer visitors they receive from outside the facility.[9] "The issue for nursing practice is how to accurately monitor the fluctuations in levels and types of support available and accessible to clients over time."[8]

The type of social networks residents have chosen is determined by the extent and nature of all of their interactions. Samples of various networks follow, with none of them being an exclusive behavior pattern. For example, residents with institution-centered networks have a few friends with whom they make connections infrequently, and they value being self-reliant; residents with small-cluster networks form a small, rather exclusive group of friends with whom they spend a great deal of time and who spend time with each other. Residents with family-centered networks prefer to engage emotionally and spend social time with their own relatives. Residents with balanced networks have large numbers of people with whom they interact in a variety of ways, including family, outside friends, staff, and other residents.[10,11]

Institutionalized individuals exhibit different social needs and preferences; these differences are particularly pronounced for elders who have spent more years developing distinctive characteristics. A few people who previously lacked adequate mothering may have developed strong defenses against social contacts to avoid the pain of expected rejection.[6] Self-reliant residents may prefer only low-intensity friendships. Residents with family-centered networks often prefer not to develop significant relationships with people within their institution nor to participate in its structured activities.[11] However, when self-reliant residents or those preferring family-centered networks lose their associations with significant others, or when physical health deteriorates, they may eventually turn to staff to fill some of their increased needs for dependency and social support. Until clear signs of wanting institutional relationships are revealed, it may not be useful to intervene.[10] Long-standing interpersonal relationships enhance well-being more profoundly than new friendships, especially for elders.[3,11] It is important to determine whether a lonely resident is feeling a need for more companionship with a peer or with staff, and whether a one-to-one relationship or a close-knit group of friends is preferred. Residents who desire and seek close relationships, but fail in their effort, face an even greater risk for depression and loneliness.[12]

Social isolation is such a painful experience that a resident may not verbalize it directly. This diagnosis should be considered if a resident exhibits the following:

- Aggression or other interpersonal problems
- Poor self-image or signs of powerlessness
- Confusing the past with the present
- Difficulty setting goals and making decisions
- Complaints about feeling confined or deserted
- Suicidal thoughts or actions.[1,2,5]

The assessment must evaluate the duration and intensity of support required (Table 27-2). A new resident with a good self-image and strong social skills may need only short-term intervention; others will require it continuously. The nursing care plan should indicate whether minimal intervention will suffice or if a higher level of intervention intensity is required, as may be needed following a loss, relocation, or during acute illness.[3]

Few friendships develop in the structured, sterile environment of most long-term care institutions for a variety of reasons. Throughout life, people carefully choose a small percentage of human acquaintances as friends. When a person is disabled and institutionalized, only the few people in their immediate environment are accessible; probably few of them will share interests, experiences, and needs. Pre-institutional friendships usually include an exchange of resources, material aid, skills, money, and gifts. Institutionalized people have little access to such resources; what they can access may not be valued by the residents and staff they encounter.[11]

Patients entering an institution have suffered multiple losses over time, including losses in health, competence, love, independence, freedom, and choice. Elders, knowing they and their institutionalized companions are at high risk for illness, death, and additional loss, have a significantly reduced motivation for forming meaningful relationships. The disorientation and stress that frequently accompany initial adjustment to institutional life further reduces the energy needed for developing new friendships.[7,11] In addition, institutional structures provide few opportunities for exercising personal choice (see Chapter 4, *Nursing Home Quality Perceptions*). There is a risk of a downward spiral after entering an institution. Loss of control can lead to social isolation, and the resulting loneliness can result in cognitive impairment and further deterioration of an already fragile condition.[7]

The resident's social abilities may be adversely affected by reductions in mental functioning, communication ability and skill, vision, mobility, and by his or her increased needs for personal assistance. Such deficits will be discovered through careful observation and are amenable to compensatory interventions. A sociable resident with mental deficiencies will need arranged contacts with someone who can appreciate these limitations, or who has a similar level of intellectual functioning. When the ability to speak has been damaged, a speech therapist can provide devices, techniques, and alternative methods of communication. People with visual handicaps need tactile activities and assistance from a better-sighted person; having a friend provide this assistance could provide a bonding experience. Assistive listening devices for the hearing-impaired might significantly enhance their relationships[13] (see Chapter 16, *Cerumen Impaction and Hearing Impairment Among Nursing Home Residents: Nursing Implications*). Residents unable to move themselves require transportation assistance from staff, relatives, or other residents. However, psychosocial deficits such as discomfort interacting with people or attending structured activities, inherent to the residents' personality, are not easily compensated.[6]

TABLE 27-2

Duration and Intensity of Social Support Required for Institutionalized Elders

DURATION OF SUPPORT REQUIRED	INTENSITY OF SUPPORT REQUIRED		
	Low	**Medium**	**High**
Short-term			Support needed for acute stressors or illnesses
Intermediate		Support needed for managing life changes and transitions and for facilitating rehabilitation for major illnesses or surgery	
Long-term or continuous	Support needed for day-to-day living for individual well-being and performance in the major social roles	Support need to cope with chronic stressors or illnesses	

Adv Nurs Sci. 1981;3(4):50. Copyright © 1981 Aspen Publishers, Inc.

FACILITY-BASED ACTIVITIES

When residents first enter a long-term care institution, they should be assisted to comprehend its unique and complex social environment. They should be guided to remember ways they have coped with difficult adjustments in the past so they can draw on already-developed strengths.[11] Unlicensed Assistive Personnel (UAP) provide much of the direct patient care and are an excellent resource for generating valuable intervention ideas. Team and staff meetings should be held regularly to evaluate each patient's adjustment. Consensus among staff is important since each and every personality interacts differently depending upon the circumstances, the topic, and the people involved.

CHOICE

Everyone needs to have a sense of choice and control. Consumer responsibility is one of the principals of *Nursing's Agenda for Health Care Reform.* It emphasizes the importance of making decisions that can ultimately affect the quality of one's life.[14] For residents in a nursing home, this is very important. Residents' functional decline, coupled with rigid structures resulting from the institution's need for economy, severely limits the choices available to long-term care residents.[7] A recognized intervention for loneliness is to provide opportunities and assistance in making choices, setting goals, and making decisions that enhance self-esteem.[1] Research has shown that treasured activities for long-term care residents include such things as doing chores for themselves, keeping in touch with interesting ideas, deciding how they will use their time, helping others and being companionable, and contacting and visiting their families and friends. However, the resident may feel incapable of achieving these valued goals in an institution and may not try. Staff should be encouraged to learn more about the residents' desires for life in an institutional setting. State laws and insurance policies offer some restrictions about what residents can and cannot do. Emphasis should be placed upon what they can do, if they choose. Residents should be given verbal, auditory, and visual exposure to ideas they want to know more about. Assistance in making social contacts, by introductions, reminders about activities, and made to feel part of a group are common social graces. Providing such resources constitutes a departure from currently accepted dependence-oriented care. It requires a dramatic shift in agency guidelines and management strategies, and major deliberately planned institutional change, which will lead to improved morale among the residents.[7]

Structured activities programs, organized at the institutional level, have benefited highly functional residents, encouraging initiative and greater participation. However, disabled residents are likely to be overwhelmed by these same activities.[15] They may rarely be taken off their unit, but transported only as far as their own lounge or dining room where there is severely limited opportunity for interesting activity. The constant television viewing, in such areas, discourages eye, hand, and brain activity and severely impedes social interactions. Most institutionalized people have few resources of their own to occupy their time, to share with friends, or to contribute in response to the needs of others. It is the rare institution that provides such resources on the units where the most disabled residents spend their days. A nursing diagnosis of diversional activity deficit is appropriate for such residents. Since boredom, loneliness, and lack of choice could be considered "epidemic" in institutions, it is reasonable to experiment with interventions that might reduce these factors.

UNIT-BASED ACTIVITIES

A block of time each day should be designated for staff to assist impaired residents to engage in social or solitary activities of their own choosing. People who are severely disabled will participate more readily in events that involve smaller numbers of people, and where familiar staff take some initiative and establish greater rapport with each of them.[15] Scheduling times when residents can have fun together might have a positive effect.[16]

Grouping social interactions among residents, according to preference, can be accomplished through proper assessment. Some residents will prefer intimate one-on-one companionship, some will enjoy a small consistent group of people, and others who are self-reliant or focused on their families may prefer solitary activities.[11] Thorough introductions are essential for new residents and may require several repetitions for the cognitively impaired. Seating two residents by themselves in a small room will enhance their relationship more than if they are seated together in a highly populated lounge. They are more likely to interact when they have privacy, choices, and a sense of control over their environment.[15] Offering them preferred refreshments may provide a greater feeling of their pre-institutional social experiences.

Happily engaged people appear more attractive, feel better about themselves, and are more successful in making friends. Opportunities to make and do things for others contribute to happiness.[8] Productive involvement seems to be infectious; active residents stimulate activity in others.[15] Each unit should be equipped by the Activities Director with games; materials for art, crafts, construction, cooking, and sewing projects; videos; large-print books; magazines; and mellow musical instruments, as well as assistive listening devices. Walls could be decorated with residents' art work. Groups of residents could listen to music of their choice, and sing along or join the production by playing percussion instruments. Reminiscence groups, for sharing life experiences, might promote social connections. Such an environment would provide more enjoyable choices, enrich solitude, and enhance relationships with other residents, staff, and visitors.

GERONTOLOGICAL NURSING IMPLICATIONS

Gerontological nurses are in a unique position to assess for social isolation of residents and develop a therapeutic plan that includes unit-based as well as individual resident-chosen activities. Nurses must initiate the structural and personnel changes necessary to support such innovations and be challenged to meet the needs of the residents who are disabled. The interventions must be outcome oriented and researched in order to maximize the effectiveness of the intervention initiated.

Of the four foundational elements of nursing theory and practice, person, environment, health/illness, and nursing intervention, environment has been least studied and theoretically developed. Research in the area of social support in long-term care is needed. Public attention has been drawn to the deep inadequacies in the quality of the institutional environment. Studies that test specific nursing interventions for a diagnosis of loneliness are exceedingly rare, yet essential for improving the quality of life for the many people in our society requiring long-term care.

Developing a positive attitude toward the work place and the people can be infectious. The long-term care setting provides a unique opportunity for this infectious care, which is often referred to as holistic care. The body/mind connection is just as strong in the elderly as in anyone else. Keeping the mind active, providing a supportive caring environment for each other will supplement all the therapies and medications, and may also eliminate the need for some prescriptions. Choosing to be alone is one thing, but being lonely is rarely a positive experience. A kind word, an encouraging touch, a thoughtful introduction all contribute to decreasing loneliness and isolation and an increase in community and wholeness.

REFERENCES

1. Copel LC. Loneliness: a conceptual model. *J Psychosoc Nurs.* 1988;16(1):14-19.
2. Brant BA. The suicidal patient in long-term care institutions. *J Gerontol Nurs.* 1990;16(2):15-18.
3. Norbeck JS. Social support: a model for clinical research and application. *ANS.* 1981;3(4):43-49.
4. Russell D, Cutrona C, Rose J, Yurko K. Social and emotional loneliness: an examination of Weiss's typology of loneliness. *J Pers Soc Psychol.* 1984;46(6):1313-1317.
5. Meddaugh DJ. Before aggression erupts. *Geriatr Nurs.* May/June 1991;12(3):114-116.
6. Welt SR. The developmental roots of loneliness. *Arch Psychiatr Nurs.* 1987;1(1):25-32.
7. Bowsher JE. A theoretical model of independence for nursing home elders. *Scholarly Inquiry for Nursing Practice.* 1994;8(2):207-224.
8. Powers BA. Social networks, social support, and elderly institutionalized people. *ANS.* 1988;10(2):40-58.
9. Greene VL, Monahan OJ. The impact of visitation on patients' well-being in nursing homes. *Gerontologist.* 1982;22:418-423.
10. Powers BA. The roles staff play in the social networks of elderly institutionalized people. *Soc Sci Med.* 1992;34(12):1335-1343.
11. Powers BA. The meaning of nursing home friendships. *Adv Nurs Sci.* 1991;14(2):42-58.
12. Murphy E. Social origins of depression in old age. *Br J Psychiatry.* 1982;141:135-142.
13. Thibodeau L. Facilitating communication in nursing homes through the use of assistive listening devices. *Nursing Homes.* October 1989;38:25-28.
14. American Nurses Association. *Nursing's Agenda for Health Care Reform.* Washington, D.C.: American Nurses Publishing; 1993.
15. Lemke S, Moos RD. Personal and environmental determinants of activity involvement among elder residents of congregate facilities. *J Gerontol.* 1989;44(4):S139-S148.
16. Golander H. Chronically ill, old, and institutionalized: being a nursing home resident. *Fam Community Health.* 1995;17(4):63-79.

Chapter 28

Predicting Discharge Planning Needs

Ann Blaylock, RN, CS, MNSc, and Carolyn L. Cason, RN, PhD

OVERVIEW

The Blaylock Risk Assessment Screen (BRASS), developed as part of a discharge planning program to meet the needs of hospitalized older adults, identifies those patients who most benefit from aggressive discharge planning. It can be used with ease by advanced practice nurses and staff nurses. It has proven effective in referrals to other departments as well as coordinating the future care of the patient. This tool has demonstrated reduced admission rates, decreased lengths of stay, and improved quality of care. Continued research will be needed to promote the reliability of this tool.

INTRODUCTION

As early as 1885, Sir Thomas Loch recognized the need for discharge planning and its pivotal role in continuity of care when he said, "There is a need for someone at the hospital to direct the patient, to represent the patient and his interests ... someone instructed as to all existing means of preventing and treating illness. He should help to make those who can become self-reliant or obtain help for those who need it or else the medical care may fail of its good purpose."[1] Today, the standards of the Joint Commission on Accreditation of Health Care Organizations (JCAHO), the regulations of the Health Care Financing Administration (HCFA), and the legislative mandates of the Omnibus Budget Reconciliation Act of 1986 speak to its importance.[2-4]

Growing concern about spiraling health care costs has prompted the development of managed care systems, which emphasize efficient resource use. Institutions must have efficient discharge planning systems in order to acquire a health maintenance organization (HMO) or a preferred provider organization (PPO) and other types of managed care contracts. To be competitive within a market where Medicare is the largest single payer for health care, the discharge planning program must be especially responsive to the needs of people 65 years of age and older.

Older adults make up 31% of hospital admissions and account for 42% of patient care days.[5] The literature suggests that older adults are at higher risk than other adults for increased lengths of stay.[6-10] Comprehensive discharge planning programs, including early identification of those at risk, can alter these statistics.[8,11-16]

Screening inventories to identify those patients at risk have been available for many years.[10,17-19] Most consist of a list of criteria, which, if met, flag patients who need social service assessment. These criteria include the patient's age, residence, lives alone, hospital admissions, and degree of disability. If the patient meets one or more of these criteria, the social worker or nurse case manager begins planning for discharge. Tools, such as the Continence, Ambulatory, Age, Social Background and Thought Process (CAAST)[20] and the Katz Index of Independence in Activities of Daily Living,[21] assess functional abilities and predict the discharge planning needs of the elderly. In addition, the Long Term Care Information System includes an initial assessment that translates the patient's discharge needs into services available to meet those needs.[22] Unfortunately, these tools are not specific to the needs of the elderly, are not comprehensive enough, and are not practical for nurses to use at the bedside. The Blaylock Risk Assessment Screen (BRASS) was developed to address these deficiencies.

The BRASS was developed as part of a discharge planning system with special concerns for older adults. The literature associated with their needs served as the primary basis for identification and selection of content for the tool. The review of the literature resulted in identifying seven factors: age,[14,23,24] functional status,[6,7,14,25-27] cognition,[14,26] social support,[14,28] living situation,[29] number of previous admissions/ER visits,[6-9] and number of medical problems.[6,9] Behavior patterns, mobility, sensory deficits, and number of medications were added because of their relevance to the elderly.[7]

THE BLAYLOCK RISK ASSESSMENT SCREEN

The BRASS, administered as part of the admission assessment, identifies patients at risk for prolonged hospital stay and in need of discharge planning resources. The tool assesses 10 characteristics of the patient (Table 28-1). To use the tool, the clinician circles the assessment options that best match the patient. For functional status and behavior pattern, the clinician circles each option that matches the patient. For the other characteristics, the clinician circles a single option. Each option has a numerical value that represents the degree to which the characteristic indicates the need for discharge planning. Total scores, computed by summing across all characteristics, range from 0 to 40. Low scores (less than 10) suggest that the patient has few needs for discharge planning or resources and indicates a low BRASS Risk Index Score (RIS). A moderate RIS (10 to 19) suggests that the patient has more extensive problems and requires extensive discharge planning resources probably without institutionalization. A high RIS (greater than 19) suggests that the patient has extensive problems and requires extensive discharge planning resources, including probable institutionalization or rehabilitation.

VALIDITY AND RELIABILITY

To evaluate the adequacy of the BRASS in identifying those patients who needed discharge planning resources, data were collected on 206 patients (ages 16 to 85) admitted or transferred to a 23-bed general medical nursing care unit in a 400-bed tertiary care teaching hospital. Within 48 hours of the patient's arrival on the unit, a staff nurse completed the BRASS and computed the RIS.

BRASS total scores ranged from 0 to 28 and correlated significantly with age (r=.40) and length of hospital stay (r=.35). Patients with low RISs had an average age of 48 (SD=16) with an average hospital stay of 8 days. Those with moderate RISs had an average age of 58 (SD=14) with an average hospital stay of 14 days. Those with high RISs had an average of 69 years (SD=11) with an average hospital stay of 19 days.

Using length of stay as the criterion variable and all other variables as predictors, regression analysis yielded five statistically significant predictors: meal preparation and medication administration (options of functional status), confusion and appropriateness of behavior (associated with behavior pattern), and the body system affected by the illness. These five variables accounted for 30% of the variability in the BRASS scores.

Independent ratings by 14 staff nurses and one control nurse were completed on 49 patients. The BRASS scores obtained by the staff nurses correlated well (r=.84) with those obtained by the control nurse. Consistency among raters was also significant (intraclass correlation coefficient of .87).

DISCUSSION

These results suggest that the BRASS can identify patients needing discharge planning as well as the appropriate resources. With only brief instruction, staff nurses were able to administer the tool with ease and completed a patient assessment within 3 to 5 minutes.

Previous studies have not identified dependence in meal preparation or medication administration, especially important variables to be considered when assessing for discharge planning needs. However, studies have associated functional decline in activities of daily living and physical ability with higher incidences of nursing home admission and increased lengths of stay.[14,25,26] Both meal preparation and self-medication administration are considered instrumental activities of daily living. The results of this study suggest that meal preparation and self-medication administration play a more important role than previously thought and should be included in the assessment for discharge planning.

Findings also indicate that 26% of the patients returned to the hospital within 2 months of discharge. Although others report equivalent rates,[30] the rate indicated a need for examining patient outcomes following hospitalization. By visiting patients who had moderate RISs on admission within 72 hours of discharge, we were able to evaluate the discharge plan in action and determine the patient's preparation for home care.[31] The most frequent care problems encountered were in the area of medication management.

CONCLUSIONS

The BRASS tool meets all of the criteria identified as important for inclusion in an effective discharge planning tool.[19] It is short, simple, and guides staff in early planning for referral. Additionally, it identifies those patients who need discharge planning resources and thus permits more economical use of scarce or limited resources. The data it provides permit nurses to improve the care outcomes for the patient while in the hospital and in the patient's transition to home care.

Its implementation as part of an admission assessment meets JCAHO's requirement for a mechanism to identify those at risk for and in need of discharge planning resources. Given the nature of the items, its results can provide useful information to the hospital health care team as well as planners and providers of post-hospital care. Early initiation of discharge planning for hospitalized patients, if coordinated, can result in desired cost savings outcomes and possible shortened hospital lengths of stay.

The usefulness of BRASS data in managed care environments requires further research. Investigation and evaluation of risk will identify the effects of early assessment for home care and track readmission rates. Nurses in managed care community settings have a challenge to develop research studies that will protect the quality of care given older people. Patients at moderate to high risk in this study indicate that appropriate use of the BRASS yields quality patient care with cost-efficient use of health care resources.

GERONTOLOGICAL NURSING IMPLICATIONS

The simplicity and ease of administering the BRASS make it an ideal assessment tool for use by both nurses in advanced practice and staff nurses. For the advanced practice nurses, it targets patient care needs and facilitates prioritization of care resources. For staff nurses, it quickly identifies those needing referral to other specialty services.

As a medical record form, the BRASS meets the JCAHO criteria for initiating discharge planning on admission and helps in care planning for patients while hospitalized. For example, knowing that the patient has difficulty with meal preparation and self-medication early in the hospitalization permits the nurse to identify ways to meet the patient's needs more effectively following hospitalization. Since medication administration is a common problem in home care, early preparation/instruction is important. When the patient arrives home, it may be necessary to evaluate and revise the original teaching plan. Such nursing actions help decrease readmissions associated with medication mismanagement and improve the quality of home care (see Chapter 19, *Screening for Polypharmacy in a Nursing Home Care Unit*).

The BRASS provides important baseline data that facilitate care planning and management. For example, assessment of the patient's cognition shortly after admission permits nurses to observe the effects of hospitalization on the patient. Nurses can easily identify changes in cognition during the hospital stay, explore contributing factors, and develop appropriate interventions and referrals.

The BRASS also may reveal other needs of the patient. For example, nurses in this study caring for a 70-year-old man admitted for an abdominal aortic aneurysm repair discovered that he served as the primary caregiver for his wife who had Alzheimer's disease. The nurses made a referral to social services, which found a caregiver for his wife. This action alleviated this man's emotional distress about care for his wife while he was hospitalized and facilitated a timely discharge.

TABLE 28-1

Blaylock Discharge Planning Risk Assessment Screen

Admission Date: Transfer to Floor Date:

CIRCLE ALL THAT APPLY AND TOTAL
REFER TO RATING SCALE FOR RISK FACTOR INDEX AND INSTRUCTIONS*

Age:
0 = 55 or younger
1 = 56-64 years
2 = 65-79 years
3 = 80+ years

Living Situation/Social Support:
0 = Lives with spouse only
1 = Lives with family
2 = Lives alone with family support
3 = Lives alone with friends support
4 = Lives alone—no support
5 = Nursing home/Residential Care

Functional Status:
0 = ADL&IADL Independent
Dependent In:
1 = Eating/Feeding
1 = Bathing/Grooming
1 = Toileting
1 = Transferring
1 = Incontinent of bowel function
1 = Incontinent of bladder function
1 = Meal preparation
1 = Responsible for own medication admin.
1 = Handling own finances
1 = Grocery shopping
1 = Transportation

Cognition:
0 = Oriented
1 = Disoriented—some spheres some time
2 = Disoriented—some spheres all time
3 = Disoriented—all spheres some time
4 = Disoriented—all spheres all time
5 = Comatose
Spheres (Person, place, time, self)

Behavior Pattern:
0 = Appropriate
1 = Wandering
1 = Agitation
1 = Confusion
1 = Other

Mobility:
0 = Ambulatory
1 = Ambulatory with mechanical assistance
2 = Ambulatory with human assistance
3 = Non-ambulatory

Sensory Deficits:
0 = None
1 = Visual deficits or hearing
2 = Visual and hearing deficits

Number of Previous Admission/ER Visits:
0 = None in the past 3 months
1 = 1 in the past 3 months
2 = 2 in the past 3 months
3 = More than 2 in the past 3 months

Number of Active Medical Problems:
0 = 3 medical problems
1 = 3-5 medical problems
2 = More than 5 medical problems

Number of Drugs:
0 = Less than 3 drugs
1 = 3 to 5 drugs
2 = More than 5 drugs

Total Score:

*Risk Factor Index
Score of 10: At risk for home care resources
Score of 11 to 19: At risk for extended discharge planning
Score of more than 20: At risk for placement other than home

If patient's score is 10 or greater, refer Patient to Discharge Planning Coordinator/Discharge Planning Team

Nurse Signature:

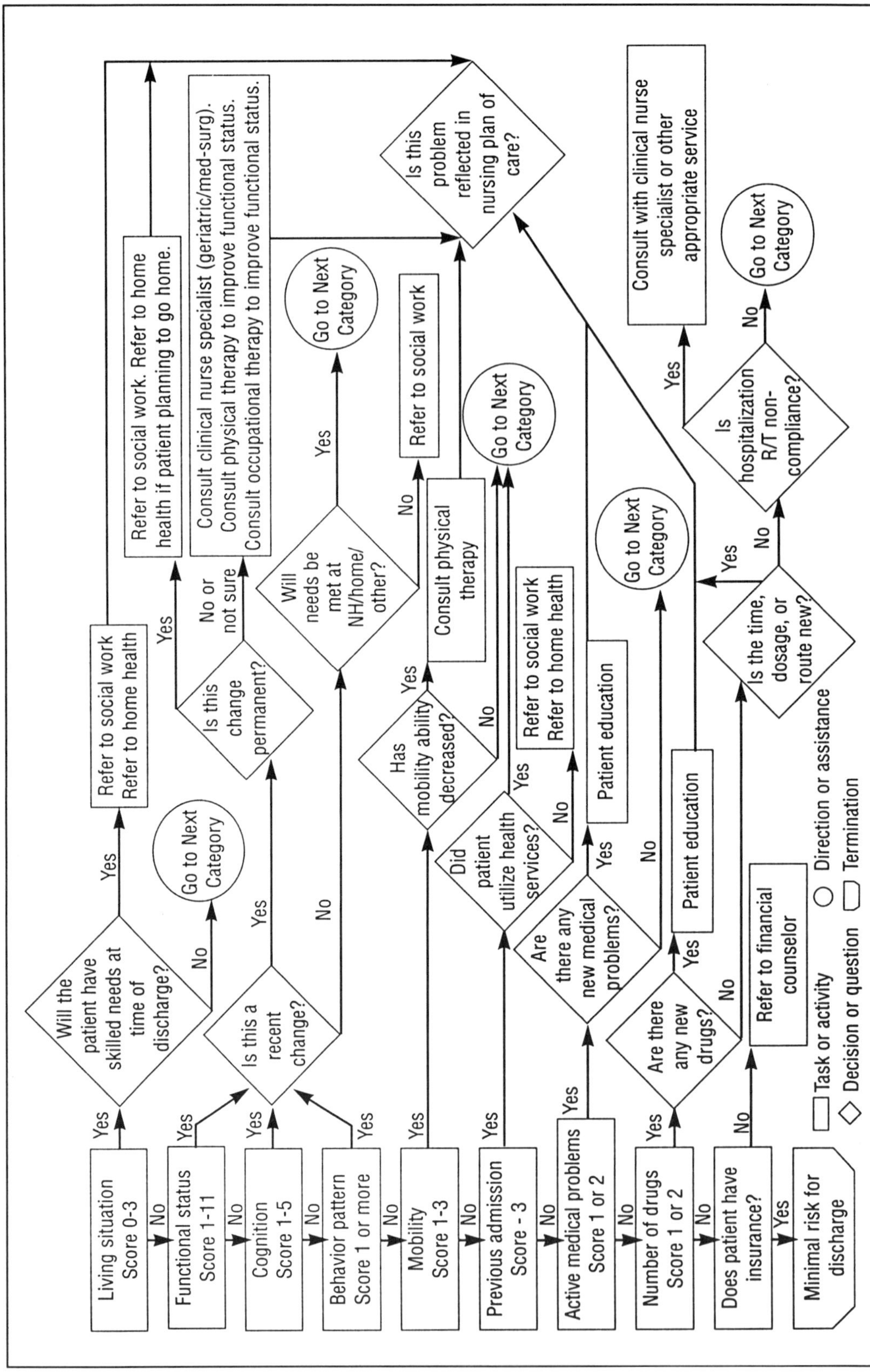

Figure 28-1. Use Decision Tree in conjunction with Blaylock Risk Assessment Screen.

Although intended for use by nurses, others can administer the BRASS. Social workers can use it for disposition planning. For example, changes in ability to perform activities of daily living independently following admission serve as indicators for extended or skilled care planning and alert the social worker to begin plans for placement. Physical therapists can effectively use the scores associated with activities of daily living in setting the patient's rehabilitation goals.

A decision tree assists in the organization of data. Appropriate interventions in the plan of care can be easily decided upon and evaluated (Figure 28-1).

In managed care environments, BRASS data can be used in clinical pathway development. The RIS or changes in individual variables can serve as indicators for referral. For example, a patient who loses the ability to independently perform activities of daily living because of physical needs may need referral to rehabilitation services. When used in this way, the path should indicate the schedule for re-administering the BRASS.

The BRASS tool used in concert with the decision tree enhances the bedside nurse's ability to effect quality care. As hospitals and other in-patient care settings revise care delivery systems to become more patient focused and cost-efficient, nurses at the bedside will provide an invaluable service in planning post hospital care.

REFERENCES

1. Sharmansky S, Boase J, Horn B. Discharge planning: yesterday, today, and tomorrow. *Home Health Care Nurse.* 1984;2(3):14-18.
2. *Accreditation manual for hospitals.* Chicago: Joint Commission on Accreditation of Health Care Organizations; 1984.
3. Birmingham J. Quality discharge planning requires timely documentation of all phases. *HPR.* 1987; Spring:3-5.
4. *Omnibus Budget Reconciliation Act.* Washington, D.C.: U.S. Government Printing Office; 1986.
5. Fowles DG. *A profile of older Americans.* Washington, D.C.: Program Resources Department of the American Association of Retired Persons and Administration on Aging, U.S. Department of Health and Human Services; 1988.
6. Anderson GF, Steinberg EP. Hospital readmissions in the Medicare population. *N Engl J Med.* 1984 ;311:1349-1353.
7. Andrews K. Relevancy of readmissions of elderly patients discharged from a geriatric unit. *J Am Geriatr Soc.* 1986;34:5-11.
8. Cable EP, Mayers SP. Discharge planning effect on length of hospital stay. *Arch Phys Med Rehabil.* 1983;64:57-60.
9. Goodling J, Jette A. Hospital readmissions among the elderly. *J Am Geriatr Soc.* 1985;33:595-601.
10. Inue TS, Stevenson KM, Plorde D, Murphy I. Identifying hospital patients who need early discharge planning for special dispositions: a comparison of alternative techniques. *Med Care.* 1981;19:922-929.
11. Lamont CT, Sampson S, Matthieas R, Kane R. The outcome of hospitalization for acute illness in the elderly. *J Am Geriatr Soc.* 1983;3:-282-288.
12. Kennedy L, Neidlinger S, Scroggins K. Effective comprehensive discharge planning for hospitalized elderly. *Gerontologist.* 1987;27:577-580.
13. Naylor MD. Comprehensive discharge planning for hospitalized elderly: a pilot study. *Nurs Res.* 1990;39:156-161.
14. Wachtel TJ, Fulton JP, Goldfarb J. Early prediction of discharge disposition after hospitalization. *Gerontologist.* 1987,27.98-103.
15. Evans RL, Hendricks RD. Evaluating hospital discharge planning: a randomized clinical trial. *Med Care.* 1993;31:358-370.
16. Lockery SA, Dunkle RE, Kart CS, Coulton CJ. Factors contributing to the early rehospitalization of elderly people. *Health & Social Work.* 1993;19(3):182-191.
17. Cunningham LS. Early assessment for discharge planning: adopting a high-risk screening program. *QRB.* 1984;10:561-565.
18. Kitto J, Dale B. Designing a brief discharge planning screen. *Nurs Management.* 1985;16(9):28-30.
19. Rasmusen L, Buckwalter KC. Discharge planning tools: development implementation and evaluation. In: McClelland E, Kelly K, Buckwalter KC, eds. *Continuity of Care: Advancing the Concept of Discharge Planning.* Orlando: Grune & Stratton, 1985:93-103.
20. Glass RI, Weiner MS. Seeking a social disposition for the medical patient: CAAST, a simple objective clinical index. *Med Care.* 1976;14:637-641.
21. Katz S, Downs TD, Cash HR, Grotz RC. Progress in development of the index of ADL. *Gerontologist.* 1970;10:20-30.
22. Falcone AR. Using the long-term care information system for effective community care. *Home Health Care Services Q.* 1981;2:83-97.
23. Blake R. What disables the American elderly. *Generations.* 1984;8(4):14-17.
24. Floyd J, Buckle J. Nursing care of the elderly. *J Gerontol Nurs.* 1987;13(2):20-15.
25. Waters KR. Discharge planning: an exploratory study of the process of discharge planning on geriatric wards. *J Adv Nurs.* 1987;12:7-83.
26. Narain R, Rubenstein LZ, Wieland D, et al. Predictors of immediate and 6-month outcomes in hospitalized elderly patients: the importance of functional status. *J Am Geriatr Soc.* 1988;3-6:775-783.
27. Holloway CM, Pokorny ME. Early hospital discharge and independence: what happens to the elderly? *Geriatric Nurs.* 1994;15(1):24-27.
28. Davis C, Moore D. *Interdisciplinary discharge planning in the elderly.* Little Rock, AR: University of Arkansas for Medical Sciences; 1987.
29. Roy AW, Folman SJ, Ford AD. *The elderly and risk factors for institutionalization: evidence from the Cleveland GAO study.* Cleveland, OH: Case Western Reserve University;1989.

30. Wennberg JE, Freeman JL, Shelton RM, Bubola TA. Hospital use and mortality among Medicare beneficiaries in Boston and New Haven. *N Engl J Med.* 1989;321:1168-1173.
31. Rhoads C, Dean J, Cason C, Blaylock A. Comprehensive discharge planning: a hospital-home healthcare partnership. *Home Healthcare Nurse.* 1992;10(6):13-18.

Chapter 29

Health Risk Behaviors Of Older Adults

Johannah Topps Uriri, MNSc, RNP, CS,
and Rozanne Winger, PhD, RNP, C

OVERVIEW

Approximately 80% of older adults suffer from at least one chronic illness, and by the year 2000, an estimated 50% of health care expenditures in the United States will be devoted to their health care. Health promotion and illness prevention programs are important for addressing lifestyle behaviors that can contribute to illness. Usually these programs target younger adults and emphasize preventing disabilities or chronic diseases later in life. Data indicate that chronic disease morbidity and mortality in the older adult population could be reduced through prevention, including lifestyle behavioral changes. Consequently, the chronically ill older adult who maintains good health habits will have a more highly functional and enjoyable life. This chapter will detail the results of a research study that sought to identify risk behaviors of older people using the Health Risk Appraisal (HRA). Gerontological nursing implications resulting from this study are discussed.

INTRODUCTION

Health promotion and disease prevention for older adults is imperative. By the year 2000, the term older adult will take on new dimensions as the population older than 85 doubles in number. Their needs for wellness and "good health" pose major implications for service delivery systems as well as for providers. Presently, health care services funded by Medicare typically focus on treatment, cure, or both, instead of illness prevention. This focus is compounded by providers being disease oriented. With the escalation of health care costs, the focus has now shifted toward health promotion and illness prevention for older adults. This shift has produced programs that include education about healthy living and methods to change health behaviors specifically for older adult participants. These programs reflect the goals of *Healthy People 2000* objectives for older adults to promote healthy lifestyles and the quality of one's older years.[1-6]

Reports of the effectiveness of health promotion programs for older adults show a variety of results. Not all reports are based on empirical data, and those that are frequently do not use standard instrumentation to measure results. The desired outcome of health promotion and illness prevention activities was to assist the older adults in sustaining or increasing functions deemed necessary for them to live independently and optimally in the community.

LITERATURE REVIEW

Health Risk Appraisal (HRA) uses an individual's self-reported health behaviors, age, sex, certain physiological measures, and health risk history to estimate a person's risk of dying within a given period of time. Estimates are based on the Framingham and other epidemiological studies. Several different types of HRA exist. Robbins and Hall, in 1960, developed one of the first HRAs entitled the "Health Hazard Appraisal" as part of the emerging emphasis on prevention in medical practice.[7] They advocated using the health hazard appraisal to help practitioners focus on disease prevention as well as cure.

In the 1970s, the HRA became popular with private industry and business, where employees completed HRAs receiving feedback regarding their major health risks. Corporations frequently offered exercise or fitness programs in conjunction with the HRA programs. Employers liked the HRA because they inferred that it stimulated employees to engage in healthier behaviors that could decrease absenteeism and save the company money. Some programs have demonstrated cost savings in the company's health care plan for employees.[8,9]

In the 1980s, several senior citizen programs designed health promotion activities specifically for older adults. Dychtwald compiled reports of these programs in *Wellness and Health Promotion for the Elderly*.[10] Most of these programs focused on group sessions of exercise, nutrition information, smoking cessation, and some aspect of mental health, often stress reduction. Evaluation of the programs seldom involved a pre-participation measure of the participant's health behaviors making an evaluation of changes to healthier behaviors difficult to accomplish.

Few researchers have reported studies that focused on health risk behaviors along with health promotion and education interventions. Bamberg found statistically significant improvement in the health behaviors of 55 subjects ages 21 to 68 years.[11] After a 13-month period, subjects scored lower on saturated fat in their diets and blood cholesterol levels. They scored higher on exercise, seat belt use, and colorectal examinations. The authors concluded that the HRA provided instructions and stimulus for people to incorporate positive health behaviors, thereby reducing their risk for disease and illness. A variety of methods for stimulating older adults to modify or change their lifestyles to reduce risky behaviors have been used. In all attempts, education appears to be the force motivating seniors to change behavior. The comment, "I've done it this way for 73 years, and I haven't suffered any ill effects yet," is very real among many older adults. Showing the older participant some concrete evidence of his or her risk for suffering "ill effects" has been thought to be helpful. To that end, the health risk appraisal has shown some success. Ellis analyzed data from 247 HRAs completed by adult volunteers. Respondents were grouped by age as younger than 60 and age 60 and older.[12] Older respondents judged the HRA as significantly more helpful than did younger respondents and were significantly more likely to change their health behaviors in response to the information learned from completing the HRA. Other investigators found similar results or indicated that the addition of counseling improved the success of changing participants' health behaviors.[8,13-15]

Measuring outcomes poses a challenge, particularly quantifying outcomes to reduce morbidity and mortality. The interest of these researchers was in outcomes that are somewhat more immediately identifiable; that is, the behavioral steps along the pathway to reducing morbidity and mortality. In a Health Care Financing Administration (HCFA) project (n=1800), the San Diego Medicare Preventive Health Project, the HRA was used on selected modifiable risk behaviors. Researchers found that preventive services were well-received by participants.

METHODOLOGY

In this quasi experimental study, the investigators monitored the health behaviors of subjects who attended a community-based clinic for 1 year. Clinic patients completed the HRA as part of their initial clinic assessment (baseline). Patients who volunteered to participate in the study completed the HRA again at 6 months post-baseline (Test I) and 12 months post-baseline (Test II). The investigators compared the data obtained from baseline with the responses obtained during Test I and Test II. The Human Research Advisory Committee approved the study, and the investigators assured all patients that their willingness or unwillingness to participate in the study would in no way affect their care at the clinic.

Of the 68 subjects, there were 55 women and 13 men, 46 blacks and 22 whites. Most subjects were black women. Subjects' ages ranged from 65 to 98 years. Most subjects were between the ages of 74 and 85 years (41%), with a mean age of 79 years.

INSTRUMENT

The investigators used the Healthier People Health Risk Appraisal developed by the Centers for Disease Control in Atlanta. This HRA identifies risky health behaviors and provides suggestions for correcting those behaviors and incorporating healthy behaviors into one's lifestyle. Healthier People, a 45-item, self-administered questionnaire, consists of open-ended and multiple-choice questions, along with physiologic measurements such as blood pressure, weight, height, and cholesterol level.

Foxman found that the Healthier People HRA could accurately identify risky health behaviors in younger adults.[16] An assessment of the reliability of the HRA found that only the category related to physical activity fell below the desired .80 correlation (.65).[17] Test-retest reliability (4-week interval) with a sample of 51 older adults ages 65 to 91 years indicated that older adults responded to the instrument consistently on repeat testing (r=.87).[18] Others have established initial validity of the Healthier People HRA for coronary heart disease and heart attack risk.[19]

Healthier People identifies controllable factors that can contribute to the development of chronic illness and provides information that will encourage the respondent to work on changeable lifestyle habits. Some Healthier People items ask for health history information to calculate the subject's overall risk level. The investigators excluded these items from the data analysis. They analyzed data only from items that measured health behaviors the subjects could feasibly change. Those items were rectal/prostate examination, last mammogram, self-breast exam, professional breast exam, high fiber diet, dietary fat, exercise, seat belt use, and perceived physical health.

PROCEDURE

All subjects were enrolled in the North Little Rock Community Seniors Health Services (NLRCSHS) project. Health care services included health maintenance, promotion, education, and prevention using a multidisciplinary team managed care model.[20] Upon enrolling in the project, patients completed the HRA as part of their initial assessment to assist in identifying lifestyle and health behaviors. Along with health history and other examination data, the team used the computerized HRA results to design individualized care plans for patients. In addition to the individualized health maintenance/promotion interventions, the team offered a health promotion program with a different topic and activity each month. The team encouraged patients to participate in these programs along with their individual activities.

Six months after completing the initial HRA (baseline), those patients who volunteered for this study completed the HRA again (Test I). Twelve months after baseline, subjects again completed the HRA (Test II). For both Tests I and II, the investigators contacted the subjects by phone and made appointments to visit them at home to complete the HRA. The questionnaire took 30 to 45 minutes to complete depending on the amount of assistance needed. Poor eyesight or reading skills accounted for most of the assistance required. During the visit, the investigator measured the subject's weight and blood pressure. Previous studies have concluded that measuring the values rather than relying on self-reports increased reliability of these physical indicators.[17] After the home interview, the investigators reviewed the subject's medical record to verify the accuracy of demographic data.

ANALYSIS

The investigators used the paired *t* test to compare subjects' HRA responses on the nine selected health behaviors at baseline with responses at Test I and Test II. Results showed no significant changes from baseline to Test I on any of the nine health behaviors. However, analyses revealed statistically significant changes (p=.0001) in six of the nine health behaviors from baseline to Test II, indicating positive changes in health behaviors of the subjects.

The one item to which only men responded asked about the length of time since they had last had a rectal or prostate exam. At baseline, 25% of the men reported never having had a prostate exam. At Test II, that percentage decreased to 16% (p=.0001), with more of the men reporting having had a prostate exam less than a year ago.

Only women responded to two items. One asked about their use of mammograms. Results revealed that the percentage of women who had never had a mammogram decreased from 53% at baseline to 31% at Test II (p=.0001). On the other item, women were asked about the frequency of breast examinations. Monthly self-breast exams increased 5% from baseline to Test II (p=.0001), and the percentage of women reporting "rarely or never" performing self-breast exam decreased by 9% over the same time period (Figure 29-1). The percentage of female subjects reporting breast exams by a professional within the year increased from 32% at baseline to 48% at Test I and remained the same at Test II (p=.0001) (Figure 29-2).

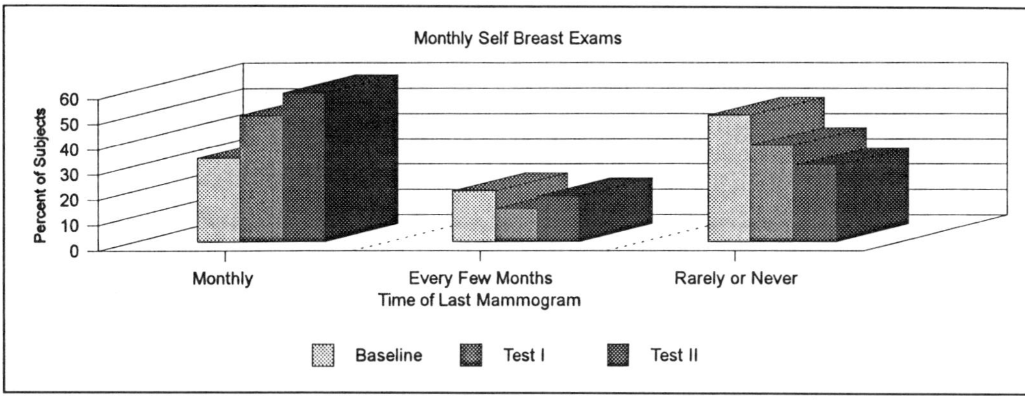

Figure 29-1. Percentage of monthly self-breast examinations performed.

When asked about daily consumption of some food high in fiber, most subjects reported already eating foods high in fiber (90%) at baseline. Nevertheless, this behavior increased to 97% at Test II (p=.18) (Figure 29-3). The frequency of eating foods high in fat decreased from 83% at baseline to 70% at Test II. The percentage of subjects eating a diet low in fat stood at nearly 30% at Test II (p=.04) (Figure 29-4).

In an average week, the number of times subjects reported engaging in 20 minutes of nonstop physical exercise "at least three times" increased from 38% at baseline to 69% at Test I, but decreased to 58% at Test II. The lower frequency of engaging in physical exercise "1-2 times a week" increased from 20% at baseline to 25% at Test II (p=.002) (Figure 29-5). The subjects who reported fastening their seat belts 100% of the time increased from 38% at baseline to 70% at Test II (p=.0001) (Figure 29-6).

Subjects rated their own physical health as excellent, good, fair, or poor in response to the question, "Considering your age, how would you describe your overall physical health?" The percentage of subjects responding "good" increased from 42% at baseline to 47% at Test II (p=.0001) (Figure 29-7).

HEALTH RISK APPRAISAL AND BLACK AMERICANS

The United States is experiencing an increasing racial and ethnic diversity. To influence lifestyle and behavior, health care providers must consider the diverse values, attitudes, culture, and life circumstances of patients when implementing health promotion and disease prevention programs. The four major groups of minorities are non-whites: Asian/Pacific Islanders, blacks, Hispanics, and Native Americans. Currently, blacks are the largest minority group, yet Asian/Pacific Islanders are the fastest growing population in the United States.[21,22]

The growth of the minority population of older adults is rapidly increasing, and it is predicted that non-whites will out-number whites in America. Studies reveal that blacks overall have the highest mortality rate of the four minority groups. Also, black older adults' health status is markedly worse than white older adults, experiencing a greater increase of chronic illnesses. A prevention of major risk factors prevalent in blacks can be achieved by a change in health behaviors and practices. Therefore, health promotion programs offer immense potential for preventing or lessening the severity of chronic illness in minorities[22] (Table 29-1). Further compounding the problem of chronicity nationally, health care providers often render substandard health care services to black older adults. For example, providing less patient education, data collection, diagnostic test, therapeutic interventions, and monitoring especially when acutely ill.[22-25]

TABLE 29-1

Higher Risk for Minorities

If you are Hispanic American, you are at higher risk for:	**If you are black, you are at higher risk for:**
• High blood pressure • Diabetes	• Heart disease • Stroke • High blood pressure • Diabetes • Cancer • Cirrhosis of the liver
If you are an American Indian or Alaskan native, you are at risk for:	**If you are a Pacific/Asian American, you are at higher risk for:**
• Heart disease • Malignant neoplasm • Diabetes • Accidents • Chronic liver disease • Cirrhosis • Pneumonia/influenza	• Heart disease • High blood pressure • Diabetes • Cancer

Adapted from American Association of Retired Persons. *Perspectives in Health Promotion and Aging.*

A large number of blacks participated in the study necessitating a secondary analysis of the data to look specifically at the health behaviors of minority participants. A comparison was made of the health behavior changes of black older adults to white older adults. The outcomes showed some differences that may be useful to others planning programs, especially for black elders.

Health behaviors of older blacks show similar characteristics. The difference in the literature seems to be that health behaviors of older blacks have been studied as single factors, rather than as groups of health promotion/prevention behaviors. For example, Haber's health promotion program targeted high blood pressure in a group of low-income older blacks.[26]

Surage focused on pap testing and mammography behaviors in Mexican-American and black women.[27]

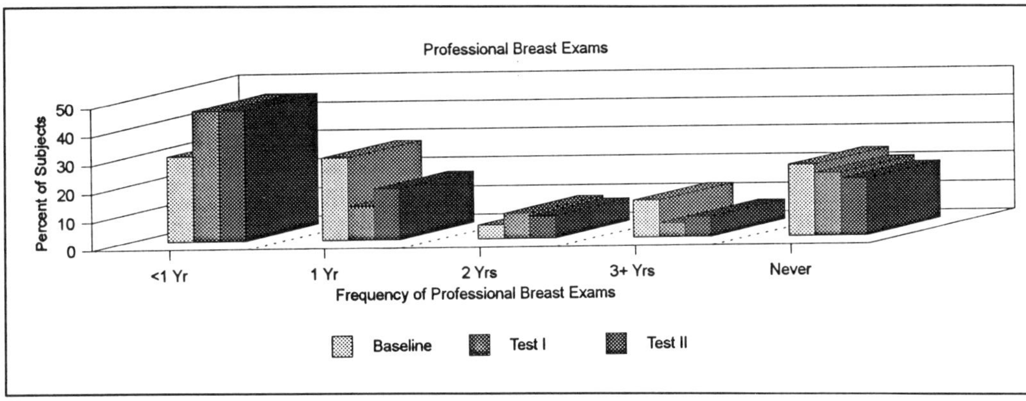

Figure 29-2. Percentage of professional breast examinations performed.

RESULTS

A paired *t* test was used to compare subjects' HRA responses on the nine selected health behaviors at baseline with responses at Test I and Test II. No significant changes occurred during the period from baseline to Test I on any of the nine health behaviors. However, analyses revealed statistically significant changes in six of the nine health behaviors from baseline to Test II, indicating positive changes in health behaviors of the subjects. A closer look revealed that most of the changes had occurred for the black subjects. Indeed, seat-belt use was the only statistically significant health behavior change in the white subjects. Results from black and white subjects were then analyzed separately to identify health behavior changes specific to the elder blacks.

In obtaining annual mammograms, the percent of blacks reporting this health behavior increased from 28% at baseline to 43% at Test II (p=.003). More white women initially reported having annual mammograms; however, their increase from baseline to Test II was from 34% to 41%, and not statistically significant. In this study, the number of women obtaining mammograms did increase during the 12-month interval, with the greater increase seen among the black women.

At baseline, 30% of black women reported doing self-breast exam. That number increased to 57% by Test II. For white women, 41% reported this health behavior at baseline, and that increased to 50% by Test II (p=.001). Thus, the older black women changed their practice of this health behavior to a greater extent than did the white women.

Having had a breast exam done by a health care professional within the past year was reported by 28% of the black women at baseline. Twelve months later, at Test II, 48% of black subjects reported having had a professional breast exam done in the past year. For white subjects, the percentage reporting a professional breast exam did not increase from baseline to Test II, but rather remained the same at 65%.

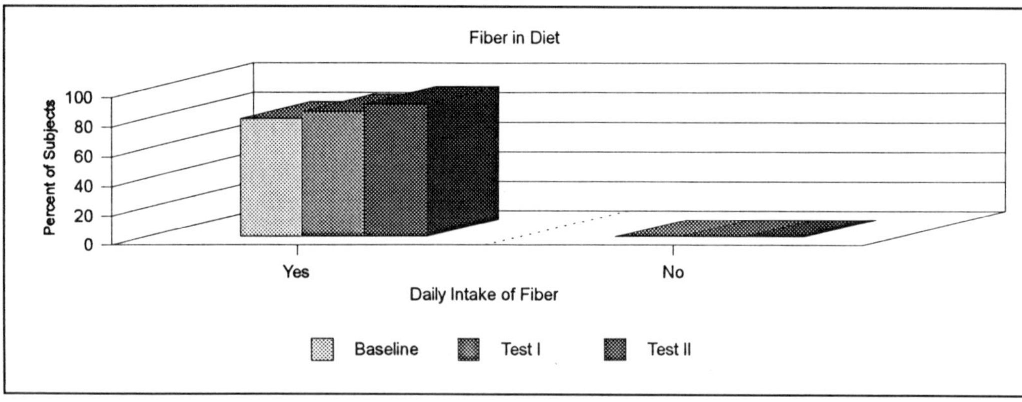

Figure 29-3. Percentage of subjects' daily intake of fiber.

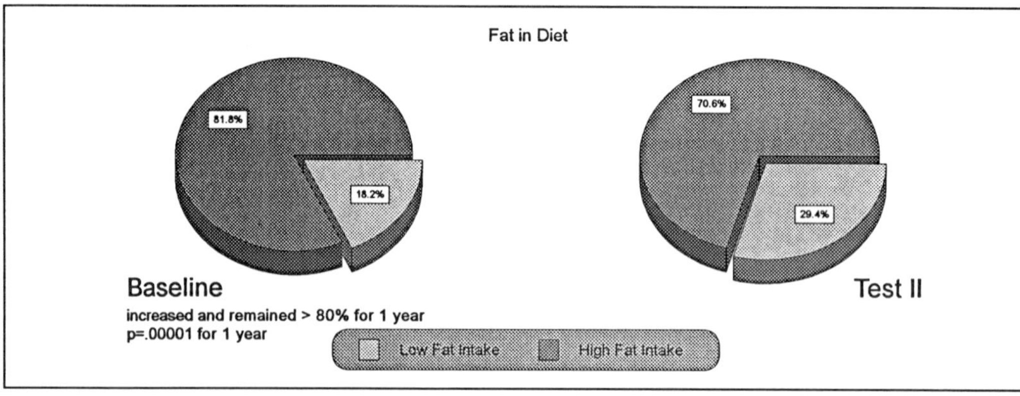

Figure 29-4. Percentage of fat in diet.

Eating foods high in fiber at least daily was reported by most subjects. At baseline, 89% of black subjects and 95% of white subjects so reported. The percent of black subjects increased to 96% by Test II (p=.05) while the percent of white subjects eating high fiber foods daily did not change from the 95% at baseline.

When asked about eating foods low in fat, 61% of blacks responded positively to this item at baseline, with an increase to 80% at Test II (p=.01). The percentage of white subjects reporting a diet low in fat was high at baseline, 91%, and remained at that level at Test II.

In an average week, the number of times subjects reported engaging in physical exercise "at least three times" increased from 30% at baseline to 52% at Test II for blacks (p=.0l) and from 50% to 64% for white subjects (p=.12).

The percent of subjects who reported using seat belts 100% of the time was 38% at baseline and increased to 70% at Test II (p=.0001). Although there was an increase in this health behavior, we regard the significance of this change with suspicion. In the 12-month time interval between testing periods, the Arkansas state legislature passed a mandatory seat belt law. Again, the new law may have influenced how black subjects responded to this item.

Subjects were asked to rate their overall physical health as excellent, good, fair, or poor. The majority of subjects rated their health as good or fair. Black subjects increased their choice of this rating from 41% at baseline to 50% at Test II (p=.18). The percentage of white subjects reporting their health as "good' remained at 47% at both testing periods.

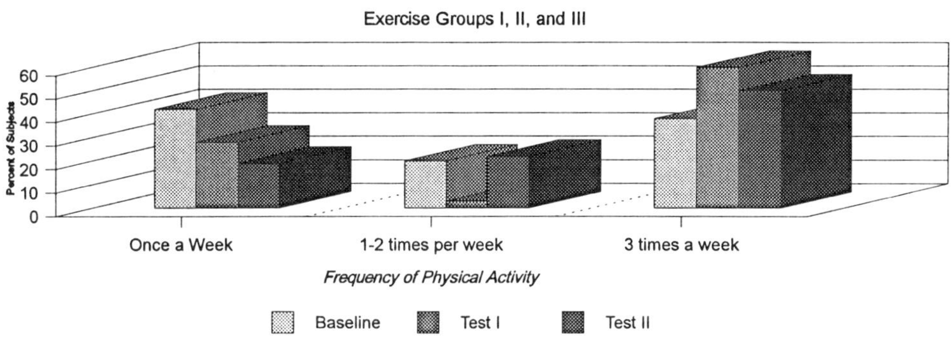

Figure 29-5. Graph showing subjects' frequency of physical activity.

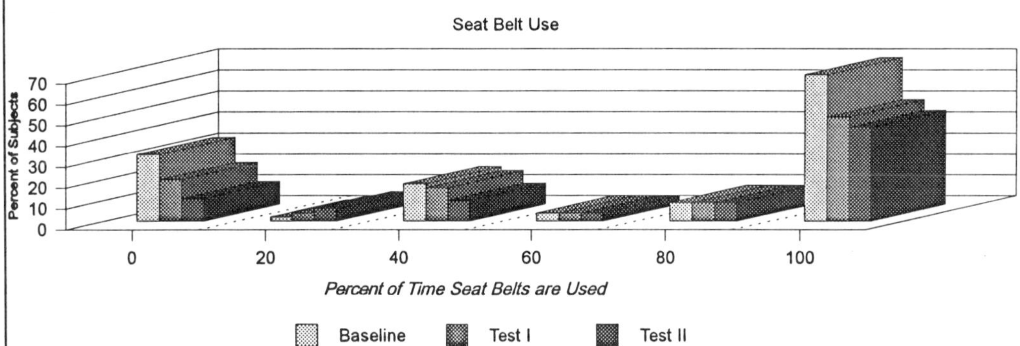

Figure 29-6. Percentage of frequency of seat belt use.

Our findings of few changes at the 6-month interval, Test I, followed by significant changes at the 12-month interval, Test II, indicate that our older participants required time to modify their health behaviors. This may be a demonstration that, as researchers, sometimes we are too eager to see the results of our efforts, the outcomes of our projects, and begin measurements prematurely. Yet, we know that older learners require more time to assimilate information.

Based on this study, the HRA appears to be useful not only for assessing older patients' health risks, but also for measuring changes in their health behaviors. Healthier People was easy to administer and highly comprehensible by the subjects. Comments made during data collection indicated that subjects were familiar with behaviors we asked them to focus on and that they thoughtfully considered their responses to each HRA item.

We cannot say to what extent using the HRA motivated our subjects to change their health behaviors. It is likely, however, that it did increase the subjects' awareness of what their health behaviors were and, to some extent, of when those behaviors were risky to their health. This awareness, combined with the combination of health promotion/education interventions used, worked together to move the participants toward changing their health behaviors.

DISCUSSION

The results of this project demonstrate some very positive indications that older adults can and will modify their health behaviors, given active health promotion, education, and illness prevention interventions. In this project, all of those modalities were used. Patients had individualized care plans that were implemented by a multidisciplinary team using a managed care model of service delivery. No standard time frame for clinic visits was followed; rather, each patient was seen as indicated by his or her needs. Individualized health education was planned and implemented by the team member or members who were the most appropriate, based on the type of education needed. The health promotion programs were considered an integral part of a patient's care plan, and attendance was highly encouraged by the providers. Some topics undoubtedly were not highly pertinent to every patient, and not all patients participated in all health promotion activities. Nevertheless, positive changes in health behaviors were demonstrated.

Comparing the health behaviors of older adults with baseline measurements at two testing times—6 months and 12 months—researchers saw the greatest changes occurring over the time span of 12 months. This suggests that older adults will change lifestyle behaviors, but will make the changes slowly. It would appear that the HRA increased the subjects' awareness of what their health behaviors were and, to some extent, when those behaviors were risky to their health.

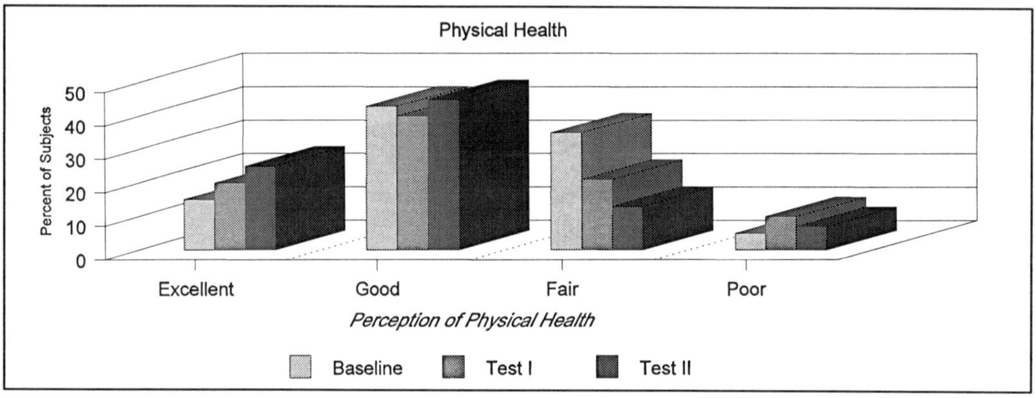

Figure 29-7. Perception of physical health.

This study indicates that women are more likely to perform self-breast examinations instead of obtaining examinations from medical professionals. According to Kane, women themselves detect 80% to 90% of primary breast cancers, and self-breast examination has been promoted as an inexpensive way to detect cancer.[28] In this study, the number of women obtaining mammograms increased over time.

A legal factor may have artificially influenced the finding that seat belt use increased dramatically to 70% usage. Subjects completed the last questionnaire after the Arkansas Legislature passed a mandatory seat-belt-use law. Another factor related to this finding is that the senior citizen buses, which many of the subjects rode regularly, do not have seat belts available for use.

Exercise in these older adults increased after participation in the project. Often the subjects exercised by walking in groups. This health behavior may keep older adults out of the hospital, decrease the length of a hospital stay, or both.[29] Further, physical activity is related to reduced incidence of various chronic diseases and conditions striking the older population.[5]

Almost half of the subjects reported that their health was good, but this may involve the use of coping mechanisms. According to Kane, older adults generally report their health as "good," although they have more chronic conditions and impairments than younger adults.[30] This disparity highlights older adults' use of coping mechanisms thus adapting to problems by ignoring or denying them.

Although the number of subjects was small and did not represent all older adults, the findings are consistent with other studies that used the HRA on younger adults.[11,12]

Cultural Implications

The high percentage of white subjects responding to positive health behavior items at baseline suggests that the white subjects may already have had more information about what constitutes a healthy lifestyle than did black elders. That finding also suggests that a need exists to develop directed efforts to help older blacks learn about promoting and maintaining their health. It is likely that cultural differences may affect an older person's acquisition of health information and healthy lifestyle behaviors. Thus, to be effective, gerontological nurses must identify and use culturally oriented methods when developing health promotion programs for older blacks and other ethnic groups.[31]

Programs enjoy more success when the planners are of the same ethnic group as the participants. Planners must be sensitive to cultural preferences and restrictions related to food, dress, and social behaviors, since all of these will impact the participants' acceptance of any health teaching.

Likewise, successful program outcomes are increased when the health care provider/educator is of the same ethnic group as the participants and is fluent in their language. When it is not possible to achieve the desired cultural match between providers and participants, other strategies must be considered. One might be able to delay initiating the program until the desired providers are available. Another strategy may be to train non-professionals to do the health education. For instance, Haber has demonstrated success with training peer leaders of the target cultural group to conduct some health promotion programs.[26]

More studies are needed in addressing health promotion and disease prevention of the four major minority groups living in the United States: blacks, Native Americans, Asian/Pacific Islanders, and Hispanics. Also, the goal of nursing services is to achieve positive patient outcomes regardless of the patient's race, age, illness, and physical disabilities.

Community-Based Approach

This study has reinforced what other studies have shown: that community-based programs are effective in reaching older blacks. The North Little Rock Community Seniors Health Services project, of which this study was a part, established itself in the community, in the neighborhoods, to deliver health services and health education to the seniors. We presented the health promotion programs in the senior centers, where people were familiar with the surroundings and with each other. Concerns about transportation, safety, membership fees, acceptance within a new social group, and other potential socioeconomic stressors were minimized for the seniors who wished to attend. Outreach such as this has been demonstrated to be important to black seniors and to some other ethnic groups.[31-33] When senior centers are not available, churches may be an acceptable site for health promotion programs.[33] Churches are a culturally significant meeting place, especially for blacks. Such sites could be the key to getting health promotion services to hard to reach groups.

Determination in one's efforts to establish a community-based program is a key ingredient for success. Members of the multidisciplinary health care team in the parent project for this study were all white. Most of the clients were black. Nevertheless, the patients accepted us, attended the health promotion/education programs, and demonstrated positive changes in their health behaviors. The project used strategies for successful community-based efforts. Team members continually reinforced their commitment to working with the patients. They incorporated ideas from the community and supported the participants' efforts to adhere to their care plans. We demonstrated that the project was there for the duration, not just for the limited time of the research project.

Patience, along with determination, is important for obtaining a useful evaluation of a community-based program and its offerings. Researchers as well as program planners are usually eager to know about the effectiveness of their efforts. They often are eager to learn the results and communicate the findings to others. This study has demonstrated the importance of choosing an appropriate time interval for measuring results. No changes were seen in the health behaviors after 6 months; however, significant changes were found after 12 months. Had we not waited an additional 6 months to measure changes in health behaviors, we would have missed those changes and made inaccurate conclusions about the effects of our health promotion/education interventions.

GERONTOLOGICAL NURSING IMPLICATIONS

Older adults have special needs for managing chronic health problems and psychosocial changes related to aging. Nurses must be cognizant of these needs in terms of quality of life issues. They can develop strategies in nursing practice, education, and research to help older adults improve their disease prevention and health promotion behaviors. In clinical nursing practice, nurses can apply the findings of this research study by using the HRA as an assessment tool in managing the care of their older patients. By using the HRA data, nurses can promote continuity of care as they communicate the results to other health care providers and develop multidisciplinary teams. The team can use information obtained from the HRA to develop plans of care with realistic and individualized goals. Using such plans, the team's focus would be on health, rather than just illness. Primary and secondary prevention programs would be geared to an older patient's individual needs, and the outcomes would be evaluated according to health behavior and lifestyle changes. Clinical nurses can use HRA data in discharge planning by obtaining a baseline of measurable health behaviors that health care providers could monitor from setting to setting. Used in this way, the HRA would help to bridge the gap that occurs when a patient moves from one health care environment to another.

As health care delivery continues to move toward community-based care settings and away from institutional settings, nursing education must keep pace. Educators must emphasize the importance of older adults' lifestyle behaviors and their relationship to health promotion and disease prevention. The HRA is a vehicle that could enable nursing students to be prepared to provide individualized care to older adults living in the community. Using the HRA, students could learn nursing care techniques adapted to cultural lifestyles, customs, and individual needs of their older patients. Much greater emphasis is needed in most nursing curricula related to cultural influences on health behaviors. Nursing students need to be taught about the various cultural groups and older people who are individual members of groups. Students need to learn about customs and cultural lifestyles, how those beliefs and behaviors may influence an older patient's health behaviors, and how all of this may affect an older patient's acceptance of health promotion/education.

More clinical nursing research is needed involving community-dwelling older adults and their needs for community-based health care services. Nurse researchers can use the HRA in these endeavors. Researchers could modify the HRA to assess additional risk areas such as falls, cognitive impairment, drug interaction, nutritional deficits, and other domains in which lifestyle behavior changes would reduce risk and promote health.

More studies are needed to identify perceived barriers to health promotion that interfere with older adults undertaking a recommended health promotion program. These studies should include the assessment of the older adult's value system related to health and self-care, self-worth, and self-actualizing traits.[15] These perceived barriers are variables that may affect the motivation of older adults to change life-long negative lifestyle behaviors. Further studies using the HRA with health promotion should include a control group that does not receive the interventions. Such a design could define the effect of directed health promotion interventions on HRA changes. Additionally, there is a great need for research in the area of health behaviors, culturally specific health behaviors, and age specific health behaviors. Attempts have been made to modify Healthier People, the HRA used in this study, to make it more specific to older adults. There is a need to construct an HRA that is specific to older blacks. Data on health behaviors of older blacks and elders of other cultures currently are not sufficient to develop a valid and reliable instrument.[34] Longitudinal studies may be the best method for obtaining such data. Although longitudinal studies are expensive, they may prove to be the most cost effective for developing culture- and elder-sensitive HRAs.

The results of this study indicate that the appropriate time span for administering the HRA to detect health behavior changes is 12 months. The longer testing interval also would avoid the possible effects of test wiseness from more frequent exposure to the HRA.

A longitudinal follow-up to this study is needed with a subject group of patients in a community-based clinic. Nurse researchers could measure the lifestyle and health behavior changes of such subjects by administering the HRA after 5 years and 10 years. The knowledge learned about long-term maintenance of lifestyle changes in older adults could prove invaluable to gerontological nursing and to improving the health care for this country's growing population of older adults.

Based on this study, the HRA appears to be useful not only for assessing the older patient's health risks, but also for measuring changes in their health behaviors. Healthier People HRA was easy to administer, highly comprehensible by the subjects, and significantly demonstrated that older adults change behavior to promote their health.

REFERENCES

1. Kemper D. The healthwise program: Growing younger. In: Dychtwald K., ed *Wellness and health promotion for the elderly.* Rockville, MD: Aspen Publishers; 1986.
2. Lederman M, Farrar M. The wisdom project of the American Red Cross in Greater New York: A blueprint for a community-based health care and health education program. In: Dychtwald K., ed *Wellness and Health Promotion for the Elderly.* Rockville, MD: Aspen Publishers; 1986.
3. Wagner EH, Grothaus LC, Hecht JA, LaCroix AZ. Factors associated with participation in a senior health promotion program. *Gerontologist.* 1991;31(5):598-602.
4. Watkins AJ, Evan W, Kligman EW. Attendance patterns of older adults in a health promotion program. *Public Health Reports.* 1993;108(1):86-90.
5. Mayer JA, Jermanovich A, Wright BL, Elder JP, Drew JA, Williams SJ. Changes in health behaviors of older adults: the San Diego medicare preventive health project. *Preventive Med.* 1994;23:127-133.
6. Schweizer SO, Mayer-Oakes SA. Health promotion and disease prevention for older adults: opportunity for change or preaching to the converted? *Am J Prev Med.* 1994;10(4):223-229.
7. Robbins LC, Hall JC. *How to practice prospective medicine.* Indianapolis: Slaymaker Enterprises; 1960.
8. Pilon BA, Renfrow D. Evaluation of an employee health risk appraisal program. *AAOHN J.* 1990;38(5):230-235.
9. Sherman Z. Health risk appraisal at the worksite. *AAOHN J.* 1990;38(1):18-23.
10. Dychtwald K. *Wellness and Health Promotion for the Elderly.* Rockville, MD: Aspen Publishers; 1986.
11. Bamberg R, Acton R, Goodson L, Go R, Struempler B, Roseman J. The effect of risk assessment in conjunction with health promotion education on compliance with preventive behaviors. *J Allied Health.* 1989;18(2):271-279.
12. Ellis LB, Joo HY, Gross CR. Use of a computer based health risk appraisal by older adults. *J Fam Prac.* 1991;33(4):390-394.
13. Doerr BT, Hutchins EB. Health risk appraisal: Process, problems, and prospects for nursing practice and research. *Nurs Res.* 1981;30(5):299-306.
14. Fultz FG. Effects of an experimental personal health education course and HHA on selected college students in Illinois. In: *Proceedings of the 13th Annual Meeting of the Society of Prospective Medicine.* The Society of Prospective Medicine, Health and Education Resources, Bethesda, MD, 1977.
15. Wheston WR, Reid JC. Health promotion of older adults: perceived barriers. *J Adv Nurs.* 1991;16():1343-1349.
16. Foxman B, Edington D. The accuracy of health risk appraisals in predicting mortality. *Am J Public Health.* 1987;77(8):971-974.
17. Smith KW, Mckinley SM, Mckinley J. The reliability of health risk appraisals: a field trial of four instruments. *Am J Public Health.* 1989;79(12):1603-1607.
18. Thatcher-Winger R, Leath C. *Estimating reliability and validity health risk measures of older adults.* Unpublished raw data, 1990.
19. Smith KW, Mckinley SM, Mckinley J. The validity of health risk appraisals for coronary heart disease: Results from a randomized field trial. *Am J Public Health.* 1991;81(4):466-470.
20. Leath C, Thatcher RM. Team-managed care for older adults. A clinical demonstration of a community model. *J Gerontol Nurs.* 1991;17(7):25-28.
21. American Association of Retired Persons. Making health promotion work for minority elders. *Perspectives In Health Promotion and Aging.* 1990;5(5):1-6.
22. Nickens HW. Health promotion and disease prevention among minorities. *Health Affairs.* 1990;9(2):133-143.
23. Kahn KL, Pearson ML, Harrison ER, Desmond KA, Rogers WH, Rubenstein LV, Brook RH, Keeler EB. Health care for black and poor hospitalized medicare patients. *JAMA.* 1994;271(15):1169-1174.
24. Gibson RC. The age-by gap in health and mortality in the older population: a social science research agenda. *Gerontologist.* 1994;34(4):454-461.
25. Peterson ED, Wright SM, Daley J, Thibault GE. Racial variation in cardiac procedure use and survival following acute myocardial infarction in the Department of Veterans Affairs. *JAMA.* 1994;271(15):1175-1180.
26. Haber D. Health promotion to reduce blood pressure level among older blacks. *Gerontologist.* 1986;26(2):119-21.
27. Surage L, Nichols DC, Brady CA. Use of peer role models to increase Pap smear and mammogram screening in Mexican-American and black women. *Am J Prev Med.* 1993;9(5):290-6.
28. Kane RL, Kane RA, Arnold SB. Prevention and the elderly: risk factors. *Health Services Research.* 1985;19(6):946-995.
29. Lubbin JE, Weiler PG, Chi I. Health practices of the elderly poor. *Am J Public Health.* 1989;79(6):731-733.
30. Kane RL, Ouslander JG, Abass IB. *Essentials of Clinical Geriatrics* (2nd ed.). New York: McGraw-Hill, 1989.
31. Erwin DO, Spatz TS. Development of an African-American Role Model Intervention to Increase Breast Self-Examination and Mammography. *J Cancer Ed.* 1992;7(4):311-318.
32. Tiernan KM. Training volunteers in risk-reduction education: a program in a US-Mexican border community. *Fam Community Health.* 1988;11(1):60-72.
33. Farooqi A. Heath promotion and ethnic patients. *Practitioner.* 1991;235:597-599.
34. DeFriese GH, Crossland CL. Health status and health risk assessment among older adults, current state and future trends in science and practice. *Generations.* Spring, 1994;51-56.

Chapter 30

Tomorrow: Gerontological Nursing in the 21st Century

Virginia Burggraf, RN, C, MSN, and Richard Barry, MDiv, MLS

OVERVIEW

The approaching millennium brings not only a muted but also a challenging vision for the future of gerontological nursing. A vision muted by the rhetoric of the 1990s dictating the elimination of costly programs that have the potential to diminish quality. A vision of challenge to advocate for, protect, demand, and create a new framework that will guarantee our older patients high quality health care.

In an attempt to clarify that vision, this chapter will outline three areas of gerontological nursing: education, practice, and research. The future direction in these areas will dictate how our collective thinking can support health care for older people in the next century and beyond. These components of nursing must be integrated to develop quality care needed by older patients.

INTRODUCTION

"Each passing year confirms one of the great events of modern times: the triumph of survivorship. It is an event so enormous that we have no handy scale to measure it and its consequences."[1] These words, said almost two decades ago, still have relevance as we look at the dramatic gains made in life expectancy. The increased number of people older than age 75 challenges the nursing profession and the health care system to respond to needed services. These services will require a creative integration of many components involving professionals committed to care and a plan that can be consistently implemented in multiple diverse settings. We know from previous chapters that the elderly move in and out of the health care environment, experience multiple chronic illnesses, are in need of preventive/health promoting care, and are cared for, in many instances, by informal caregivers. Their multiple needs are not limited to accurate and timely assessment, immediate treatment of acute and exacerbating problems, an integrated team approach, and participation in the care received. How these needs and services will be linked deserves a look at past history, which can provide some guidance.

The past defines the present, and the present shapes the future. During the past 70 years, we have seen the shaping of many aging policies in the United States. The enactment of

Social Security, in depressed economic times, contributed to the treatment of aging Americans as a separate population in need of services.[2] The elderly were characterized as homogeneous, poor, sick, and possibly feeble. The passage of Medicare and Medicaid led to a major involvement of the government in the development of national policies that would impact on the care of the older adult. The end result of all of this has been a decrease in mortality and morbidity. Older adults are less likely to live in poverty than the rest of the population (12.4% vs. 13.6%), with black elderly experiencing a higher poverty level than whites. Today, most elders are better educated, healthier, have more income, and the freedom to live where they wish, than did their forbears. We now live in the midst of past successes that have been achieved in gerontology.[2]

During the past 30 years, a tremendous growth in the field of gerontology has given rise to increasing academic programs in the health related and social service areas, the numbers of aging organizations, the numbers of professionals and non-professionals working with the elderly, and the involvement of the corporate world in marketing services to the older adult. This has all occurred based on the projected needs of an aging population.[3] Projecting future needs from the present knowledge allows an opportunity to share one's visions while at the same time risking inaccuracy. In order to increase the probability of accuracy about the nursing future in gerontology, many noted gerontological nurses were contacted for their visions of this future. These pages reflect much of their thinking coupled with the vision of the authors.

EDUCATION IN GERONTOLOGICAL NURSING

Faculty, students, and nursing programs are all important spokes in the wheel of education that must first be addressed before curriculum development. All modalities of health care are moving into the community. This shift has an impact on the academic faculty needed to educate/train the numbers of professionals required to care for older adults in the future. The buzz words home care, rehabilitation, senior centers, transitional living, respite care, wellness, health promotion, managed care, collaborative practice, and case management are all incorporated into the aging health care network. Browdie[3] mentions "...the majority of people working in the field of aging will continue to be those who are willing and able to do that kind of work—in other words, true caregivers." It is important to note, that with any specialty, a true commitment to a professional identity is needed. Elder care is not like other service industries. It is labor intensive, requiring more personnel and professionals to not only meet the needs of the older person but also to provide direct services. This is particularly evident when chronicity and disability occur. Specialized therapeutic staff and machine technology are no substitutes for the hands-on care required.[2] Faculty recruitment efforts must focus on personality type and positive attitudes in addition to educational preparation for a hands-on care approach to be a priority. Empathy must be natural and spontaneous in the faculty chosen to teach/mentor others in the field of gerontological nursing. Faculty, frequently with little or no preparation in gerontology, are asked to teach courses in gerontology,[4,5] often passing on inappropriate attitudes and values. The report of the Planning Committee for the White House Conference on Aging[6] revealed that an alarming 40% of the nursing faculty now teaching in graduate level gerontological nursing programs have had no formal preparation in gerontology. Three-fourths (77%) of all clinical preceptors and instructors in all nursing programs have had no formal preparation in working with the elderly.[7] There is also a lack of faculty consensus on the core curriculum in gerontological nursing that has resulted in major gaps, as well as confusion.[8] Faculty of the 20th century who wish to be effective professors for the 21st century will have to be re-educated in the use of technical equipment and new innovative skills as well as computer assisted instruction, and long distance learning. They will have to think primarily of wellness and health promotion, rather than illness. "They will have to accept the fact that the elderly are here in ever increasing numbers, and that people will live their lives as older persons far longer than they did as a child, adolescent, and young adult."[9]

A recent survey of the 15-state Southern Regional Education Board found that only 12% to 13% of nurse educators who responded were prepared in gerontological nursing.[10,11] The Board expressed this view:

> We need to recognize that even if we could provide an ideal grounding in gerontology to every health professions student, the majority of practitioners for years to come would still be graduated with an education that included no course work in aging. In the short term, there may be no area of gerontology education more important than continuing education.[12]

Continuing education programs, specifically for faculty, will continue to provide the opportunity to learn the attitudes, empathy, values, and skills needed to take care of older people. Incentives to attend should be developed in academic institutions, as well as opportunities for research, publication, and tenure options expanded. Research is needed to assess for interest and needs in specific geographical areas. The educational challenges presented to the faculty will impact the student population and also the service providers to make certain that qualified professionals and non-professionals are performing in the manner expected.

To provide adequate health care for older people, it is predicted that at least 36,000 geriatricians and more than 1 million registered nurses will be required. The total need for full-time equivalent (FTE) registered nurses (RNs) by 2020 is forecast to be 1,126,000 (72% of available supply). A multi-cultural nursing staff and unlicensed assistive personnel (UAP) will be needed to optimize the care provided older adults.[13] Professional nursing organizations will be propelled by the managed care settings to better define basic and advanced practice nursing. As nurses assume more autonomy in the community, there will be a shift to enrollments in nursing programs, with larger enrollment in graduate programs vs. basic nursing programs. Managed care is demanding a baccalaureate in nursing as the minimum entry level for practice. This trend demands that schools of nursing provide for bridge courses toward the BSN for associate degree nurses. Social change is forcing the nursing profession to address these challenging issues and see them as positive, not as impediments to practice. Alford[9] predicts that the present baccalaureate programs will be around for the next 30 years, but will look very different from today's formal setting. The electronic classroom, the Internet, and virtual reality laboratories, which are now beginning, will make learning individualized and enjoyable. A Master's in nursing will become the entry level into nursing before the end of the next millennium. A large pool of nurse applicants from diverse professional fields will enter nursing at the graduate level. This will not only provide individuals with second career options but also be an entre for nursing into new fields. Nurse architects, nurse comptrollers, and nurse marketing directors will expand the identity of what nurses can do for their patients.

Community colleges will expand their curriculum base to offer courses leading to an associate degree (AD) in gerontology, gerontological technology, and possibly gerontological nursing. Training will be provided for students to work with the elderly under the supervision and direction of the advanced practice nurse. The LVN/LPN programs will eventually end and mesh into these AD programs. Alford further predicts that a requirement for those who work with older people will be a pre-service certificate of skill and competence in their field of gerontology. A periodic update will be required to maintain this certification.[9]

The present trend toward using unlicensed assistive personnel (UAPs) to care for the older adult will not change. What will change is the consumer demanding that "Every Patient Needs a Nurse," a slogan developed by the American Nurses Association.[14] The demand for UAPs will have to be addressed not only in academic institutions, by service providers, but also by labor and business enterprises. Gerontologists will be forced to develop research that recasts and revalues the low-tech worker in the future. Redesigning their positions, places of employment, and their cultural identity will be very important in the future. The cultural revolution taking place in American will place a large demand on workers from various ethnic and racial backgrounds. The growing ethnic elderly population will want care from those who know and understand their cultures and ways of life. Diversity offers a wild card type of impact upon all elements of the future. With these ideas setting the stage, a brief discussion of curriculum will frame the end of this section on the educational preparation of nurses to care for older people.

Curriculum will be designed around a number of concepts, which will be fashioned from the needs of faculty and students. While "Adult Health" will be retained as the core curriculum, there will be a much greater emphasis on later life issues. Later life issues and health care are currently tacked on to the Adult Health curriculum, which continues to concentrate more on the young and middle-aged adult. The nursing curriculum will become more multidisciplinary in its focus, organization, content, and clinical experiences. Family centered nursing curricula will expand with the demographics of the multi-generational household re-emerging. The pediatric nurse may care for children who are reared by grandparents, and adult children may be caring for aging parents.[10]

Nursing students will study with medical students, which is currently being emphasized in many nurse practitioner programs. This has implications for clinical experiences as a member of a team. Additionally, collaborative practice partnerships will develop.

Case management and managed care concepts will be incorporated into all curriculum structures, however where the older adult is concerned special emphasis on continuity of care from one setting to another will receive greater attention (see Chapter 1, *Health and Long-Term Care: A Perspective on the Older Adult*). Hanchett[15] emphasizes the need to include non-traditional and nonclinical skills in the core curriculum. Additionally, case management strategies, methods of effectiveness/outcome measurement, use of emerging technologies outside of the hospital or community facility, as well as a proficiency (not just a competency) in computer applications will be required.[15] There will be an expanding selection of electives specific to gerontology, such as courses in business applications, consultation, consumer health, political advocacy, and policy development.

The future of gerontological nursing education involves many components: faculty preparation, varied programs, student enrollment, and curriculum development. There is no single answer to the issues presented. A sense of commitment and unity are needed to implement the strategies defined. Once educated, where will the students practice? This becomes another point of interest and vision.

PRACTICE SETTINGS IN GERONTOLOGICAL NURSING

The role of the registered nurse has undergone significant change in the past 5 years. The RN, traditionally seen as the primary caregiver, is shifting to that of primary care coordinator (or care manager) in most practice settings (see Chapter 1, *Health and Long-Term Care: A Perspective on the Older Adult*). Until needs are formally established for more registered nurses to care for older patients, this trend will continue. As stated previously, the consumer will be the driving force behind any changes that occur. Consumers will also demand programs that maintain health and prevent disability. Senior centers will be wellness centers where nurses will staff and direct the operation of nursing clinics. There will be an increased need for RNs to work in occupational health. People are working longer, the retirement age is increasing, and people are taking on second careers after retiring from one work setting perpetuating older workers in business. Health promotion and disease prevention will be emphasized in the work place.

The increasing needs in home care and the number of older adults requiring functional assistance to remain at home will require the RN to play a greater role in the education and training of the UAP. Certification of UAPs will be demanded in all settings. In addition to the home care environment, the gerontological registered nurses will be sought out for their expertise in supervision, administration, consultation, and rehabilitation.

The consulting role of the gerontological nurse will expand with expertise needed by architects designing homes that are adaptable for the older adult and living centers. Increased senior travel will create a role for the nurse to consult with the airlines to make travel for the older person more comfortable. This consultation will provide for appropriate seating, food, and facilities that contribute to seniors traveling to visit family and friends. Nurses have and will continue to provide programs for families caring for elderly relatives. There will be a return to the private duty nurse of years gone by who will be called to work for the more affluent older adult.

Although hospitals will continue to exist, the role of the clinical nurse specialist (CNS) will once again emerge as critical to the team effort to respond to all the needs of the older patients. Gerontological nurses may lease out floors/offices in hospital settings to provide care for their patients (eg, cardiac rehabilitation, diabetes management, stress reduction, and mental health).[9] The concept of the geriatric hospital is very popular in the United Kingdom, and may eventually take hold here in the United States. These settings are all encompassing in the services that are provided to older adults. They offer acute and chronic care, rehabilitation services, and long term-institutional care. A geriatric day care facility is also an integral part of the geriatric hospital.[16]

The idea of the neighborhood nurse has been discussed as a realistic possibility.[17] Urban and rural areas will see the emergence of the community health nurse who will be an adult nurse practitioner (ANP), a family nurse practitioner (FNP), or a gerontological nurse practitioner (GNP) making house calls. They will work independently in a particular region of the community, in emergent care centers, or in collaborative practice with physicians and others. Managed care settings may also sub-contract with them for their services to meet the needs of the population that is difficult to access.

Nurse managed care will become a reality as HMOs expand and include nurse practitioners on their provider panels. In many HMOs, this is fast becoming a reality. Research into outcomes will be very supportive of advanced practice nurses in the future. Lamb relates that primary care and home care will be the two most commonly used nursing services.[18] These will be most evident in community settings, clinics, and nursing HMOs. Nurse-run HMOs will operate as a consortium of entrepreneurial GNPs, GCNSs, colleges of nursing along with home care agencies, and assisted living centers.[9] Faculty will practice in these settings and also provide a clinical laboratory for their students. Collaborative practice models can be developed with medical schools and other allied health providers.

Lastly, the nursing home as it now exists will decline. Many of these institutions were built after the enactment of the Medicare and Medicaid legislation. They are structurally obsolete and in need of renovation. Special care centers are now in existence that are specific to the care of the demented patient, and the sub-acute facility is quickly taking precedence. Sub-acute care needs to be monitored and standards developed to assure that patients receive quality care. Nursing homes will be called care centers and also offer hospice care since many of the elderly may not desire advanced directives. Respite care will be offered as a benefit in most health care plans.

The settings where nurses will care for older patients in the next century are limitless. We need only the ability to imagine, plan for, and get involved in the pursuit of these entities. As nurses committed to the care of the older adult, the time to be idle has passed. In order to make nursing a primary focus in the care of older adults and to implement it as a specialty practice, nurses must act. The need for scientific studies to support these efforts will be necessary and will be discussed next, and provide the final vision into the tomorrow of gerontological nursing.

RESEARCH IN GERONTOLOGICAL NURSING

Advancing the knowledge base for the practice of gerontological nursing is imperative if the rapidly increasing aging society is to have adequate health care.[7] A critical mass of doctorally prepared nurses are needed to conduct this research. Doctoral programs in gerontological nursing must increase as well as the numbers of qualified faculty to mentor these students. Unfortunately, the scarcity of qualified faculty may turn students away from majoring in this specialty. Their lack of expertise in the field of aging may create a negative environment for mentoring, which frustrates students. Students entering doctoral programs are frequently experts in their fields and need to be supported in this environment.

The Southern Council on Collegiate Education for Nursing[7] discussed research needs of the future:

- Effectiveness and efficacy of specific clinical interventions
- Quality of life measures
- Assessment of healthy behaviors and lifestyles
- Development of contemporary theories of aging
- Assessment of the complex phenomena of aging
- Development of culture-sensitive instruments
- Assessment of innovative educational approaches to prepare nurses
- Cost benefit analysis of innovative systems of health care delivery.

These topics should provide some of the priority concerns for gerontological nurse researchers now and in the future.

In relation to the building of a community-based long-term care service system, the Long-Term Task Force of the Gerontological Society of America offered these considerations concerning research on aging.[19]

- Consumer-driven service delivery systems
- Service delivery for the disabled and non-disabled elderly
- Effectiveness of various delivery systems in their provision for recruitment, training, supervision, compensation, and provision of career opportunities for home care
- Effectiveness of various models of service delivery supporting housing allowing the disabled elderly to retain autonomy
- Replication of effective programs and the circumstances surrounding their success.

It would appear that nursing research into these areas in gerontology is vast and challenging, however, there is little mention of the clinical practice of nursing, which has historically framed the profession. Nurses must begin to question the scientific basis and nursing validity of each and every nursing procedure used with older adults. Standards of care for older adults must be tested.[9] Nursing interventions used in all areas need re-evaluation and must be investigated. Nursing research will enter the realm of business where nurses will become members of consortia developing products. They will patent innovations and provide the license for marketing and production. We have been improvising and caring for many a year. In the 21st century, the nurse will become an inventor.

Alford discussed the area of chronotherapeutics, the time when therapy is most effective, as becoming a valid research topic. Nurses have been involved in this modality of knowing what and when is needed for their patients. They will now scientifically test their notions. The potential for the development of a Gerontology Research Institute, in an academic setting, where multidisciplinary research teams work is a vision that holds great promise. Hancett claims that nurses, because of their broad knowledge and skill, will achieve positions of influence and importance in negotiating for key positions in these multidisciplinary teams.[15] Additionally, Jackson claims that research into cultural differences on the aging population will offer significant findings for prevention and quality issues.[20] The framework in which the older adult lives and works on a daily basis will better assist the nurse to understand the patient and how to best treat him or her.

PROJECTIONS FOR GERONTOLOGICAL NURSING

These pages have been replete with numerous nursing implications. It is appropriate to summarize what has been projected for the future. Faculty are needed to teach the diverse numbers of students that will enroll in schools of nursing. More RNs will be needed to work in community settings, workplaces, institutions, and in ambulatory care settings. The role of the UAP will continue to be developed and expanded upon as consumers drive the health care environment and demand nursing care. Nurses in advanced practice will proliferate, deliver primary care and serve as care managers assessing patients for discharge and/or placement for rehabilitative services. There will be more of an emphasis on health promotion and disease prevention to avoid chronic illness in the "well elderly" and to avoid additional exacerbation in the disabled. A changing curriculum structure will meet the increasing need and demand for gerontological technicians as well as specialists. Family care will be a significant entity as more middle aged adults care for aging parents and many aging grandparents care for their grandchildren. The next century will see the development of new gerontological practice models in managed care, neighborhoods, home care, sub-acute care, and in corporations. The nurse will have at his or her disposal the opportunity to practice gerontological nursing in occupational and industrial settings, in collaborative practice models of care, in care centers, and in adult day care. These issues will expand the research opportunities for nurses to impact aging in all areas affecting the older person.

The possibilities for education, practice, and research are as limitless as one's imagination. It is the hope of these authors that this imagination is vivid in all practitioners caring for older people. The excitement of an approaching new century brings with it not only a sense of anxiety but also a sense of promise that we will be the leaders in the tomorrow projected for the older adult.

REFERENCES

1. Butler R. In: Sommers A, Fabian D, eds. *The Geriatric Imperative.* New York: Appleton-Century-Crofts; 1981:xv-xvi.
2. Morris R. Challenges of aging in tomorrow's world: will gerontology grow, stagnate, or change? *Gerontologist.* 1989;29(4):494-500.
3. Browdie R. The best education & training: meeting the needs of the aging network. *Generations.* 1995;19(2):16-18.
4. Bahr RT. Adding years to the educational agenda. *J Gerontol Nurs.* 1987;13(3):6-11.
5. Hartley C. From vision to victory: making significant curriculum revisions. *Newslink, The Community College-Nursing Home Partnership.* Fremont, CA: Ohlone College; 1990.
6. Dye CA. Education and training. *Report on the White House Conference on Aging Planning Committee.* Unpublished; 1992.
7. Gueldner S, Brant B, Joyce-Nagata B, et al. Gerontological nursing issues and demands beyond the year 2000. *J Gerontol Nurs.* 1995;21(6):6-8.
8. Timms J. Needs assessment surveys in gerontological nursing: are we really assessing continuing education needs and priorities? *J Continuing Ed Nurs.* 1995;26(2):84-88.
9. Alford D. *A Twentieth Century Vision of Gerontological Nursing in the Twenty-First Century.* Unpublished; 1995.
10. Morrissey S. In nursing, a study in contradictions. *Generations.* 1995;19(2):6-8.
11. Yurchuck R, Brower T. Faculty preparation for gerontological nursing. *J Gerontol Nurs.* 1994;20(1):17-24.
12. Denton D. Caring for an aging society: issues and strategies for gerontology education. *Southern Regional Education Board.* 1990.
13. Buckwalter K, Mass M. *Gazing Through the Crystal Ball: Gerontological Nursing Issues and Challenges for the 21st Century.* In press.
14. Every patient needs a nurse. *American Nurses Association.* Washington, D.C.: American Nurses Association; 1994.
15. Hanchett M. *Thoughts about the Future of Gerontological Nursing.* unpublished. 1995.
16. Burggraf V. Geriatric nursing: health care reform in Scotland. *J Gerontol Nurs.* 1993:19(8):35-39.
17. Sibbald B. 2020 Vision of nursing. *Canadian Nurse.* 1995;91 (3):33-36.
18. Lamb G. *New Delivery Systems: The Call to Community.* Paper presented at the American Academy of Nursing Scientific Meeting; Phoenix, AZ; 1994.
19. Caro FG, Callahan J. *Toward Improved Federal Support for Research on Delivery of Home and Community Long-Term Care.* Paper presented at the meeting of the Gerontological Society of America; Atlanta, GA; 1994.
20. Jackson M. *Comments on the Future of Gerontological Nursing.* Unpublished paper; 1995.

INDEX